Skill Checklists for

Taylor's Clinical Nursing Skills

A NURSING PROCESS APPROACH

Skill Checklists for

Taylor's Clinical Nursing Skills

A NURSING PROCESS APPROACH

FIFTH EDITION

Pamela Lynn, EdD, MSN, RN
Assistant Professor
Gwynedd Mercy University
Frances M. Maguire School of Nursing and Health Professions
Gwynedd Valley, Pennsylvania

Wolters Kluwer

Philadelphia • Baltimore • New York • London
Buenos Aires • Hong Kong • Sydney • Tokyo

Vice President and Publisher: Julie K. Stegman
Director of Product Development: Jennifer K. Forestieri
Digital Product Manager: Betsy Gentzler
Senior Development Editor: Michael Kerns
Editorial Coordinators: Emily Buccieri and Lindsay Ries
Editorial Assistant: Leo Gray
Marketing Manager: Brittany Clements
Production Project Manager: Bridgett Dougherty
Design Coordinator: Holly Reid McLaughlin
Manufacturing Coordinator: Karin Duffield
Prepress Vendor: Aptara, Inc.

5th Edition

9 8 7 6 5 4 3 2 1

Printed in the United States

ISBN: 9781496387172

shop.lww.com

Introduction

Developing clinical competency is an important challenge for each fundamentals nursing student. To facilitate the mastery of nursing skills, we are happy to provide skill checklists for each skill included in *Taylor's Clinical Nursing Skills: A Nursing Process Approach,* Fifth Edition. Students can use the checklists to facilitate self-evaluation, and faculty will find them useful in measuring and recording student performance. Three-hole-punched and perforated, these checklists can be easily reproduced and brought to the simulation laboratory or clinical area.

The checklists follow each step of the skill to provide a complete evaluative tool. They are designed to record an evaluation of each step of the procedure.

- Checkmark in the "Excellent" column denotes mastering the procedure.
- Checkmark in the "Satisfactory" column indicates use of the recommended technique.
- Checkmark in the "Needs Practice" column indicates use of some but not all of each recommended technique.

The Comments section allows you to highlight suggestions that will improve skills. Space is available at the top of each checklist to record a final pass/fail evaluation, date, and the signature of the student and evaluating faculty member.

Faculty who adopt this book will also find on thePoint website at http://thepoint.lww.com/LynnCklst5e a *Master Skills Competency Checklist* to aid in record keeping.

List of Skills by Chapter

List of Skills in Alphabetical Order

Skill Checklists for Taylor's Clinical Nursing Skills. A Nursing Process Approach, 5th edition

Name ______________________ Date ______________

Unit ______________________ Position ______________

Instructor/Evaluator: ______________________ Position ______________

Excellent	Satisfactory	Needs Practice	SKILL 1-1 **Performing Hand Hygiene Using an Alcohol-Based Handrub** **Goal:** Transient microorganisms are eliminated from the hands.	Comments
____	____	____	1. Remove jewelry prior to patient contact, if possible, and secure in a safe place. (A plain wedding band may remain in place.)	
____	____	____	2. Check the product labeling for correct amount of product needed.	
____	____	____	3. Apply the product to the palm of one hand. Ensure use of the correct amount of product.	
____	____	____	4. Rub hands together, covering all surfaces of hands and fingers, and between fingers. Also clean the fingertips and the area beneath the fingernails.	
____	____	____	5. Rub hands together until they are dry (at least 15 seconds).	
____	____	____	6. Use oil-free lotion on hands, if use of lotion is desired.	

Skill Checklists for Taylor's Clinical Nursing Skills. A Nursing Process Approach, 5th edition

Name ________________________ Date ________________________

Unit ________________________ Position ________________________

Instructor/Evaluator: ________________________ Position ________________________

SKILL 1-2

Performing Hand Hygiene Using Soap and Water (Handwashing)

Goal: The hands will be free of visible soiling and transient microorganisms will be eliminated.

Excellent	Satisfactory	Needs Practice		Comments
___	___	___	1. Gather the necessary supplies. Stand in front of the sink. Do not allow your clothing to touch the sink during the washing procedure.	
___	___	___	2. Remove jewelry, if possible, and secure in a safe place. A plain wedding band may remain in place.	
___	___	___	3. Turn on water and adjust force. Regulate the temperature until the water is warm.	
___	___	___	4. Wet the hands and wrist area. Keep hands lower than elbows to allow water to flow toward fingertips.	
___	___	___	5. Use about 1 teaspoon liquid soap from dispenser or rinse bar of soap and lather thoroughly. Cover all areas of hands with the soap product. If using bar soap, rinse soap bar again and return to soap rack without touching the rack.	
___	___	___	6. With firm rubbing and circular motions, wash the palms and backs of the hands, each finger, the areas between the fingers, and the knuckles, wrists, and forearms. ***Wash at least 1 in above area of contamination.*** If hands are not visibly soiled, wash to 1 in above the wrists.	
___	___	___	7. Continue this friction motion for at least 20 seconds.	
___	___	___	8. Use fingernails of the opposite hand or a clean orangewood stick to clean under fingernails.	
___	___	___	9. Rinse thoroughly with water flowing toward fingertips.	
___	___	___	10. Pat hands dry with a paper towel, beginning with the fingers and moving upward toward forearms, and discard it immediately. Use another clean towel to turn off the faucet. Discard towel immediately without touching other clean hand.	
___	___	___	11. Use oil-free lotion on hands, if desired.	

Skill Checklists for Taylor's Clinical Nursing Skills. A Nursing Process Approach, 5th edition

Name ______________________ Date ______________________

Unit ______________________ Position ______________________

Instructor/Evaluator: ______________________ Position ______________________

Excellent	Satisfactory	Needs Practice	SKILL 1-3 **Using Personal Protective Equipment** **Goal:** The transmission of microorganisms is prevented.	**Comments**
____	____	____	1. Check medical record and nursing care plan for type of precautions and review precautions in infection control manual.	
____	____	____	2. Plan nursing activities before entering patient's room.	
____	____	____	3. Provide instruction about precautions to patient, family members, and visitors.	
____	____	____	4. Perform hand hygiene.	
____	____	____	5. Put on gown, mask, protective eyewear, and gloves based on the type of exposure anticipated and category of isolation precautions.	
____	____	____	a. Put on the gown, with the opening in the back. Tie gown securely at neck and waist.	
____	____	____	b. Put on the mask or respirator over your nose, mouth, and chin. Secure ties or elastic bands at the middle of the head and neck. If respirator is used, perform a fit check. Inhale; the respirator should collapse. Exhale; air should not leak out.	
____	____	____	c. Put on goggles. Place over eyes and adjust to fit. Alternately, a face shield could be used to take the place of the mask and goggles.	
____	____	____	d. Put on clean disposable gloves. Extend gloves to cover the cuffs of the gown.	
____	____	____	6. Identify the patient. Explain the procedure to the patient. Continue with patient care as appropriate.	

SKILL 1-3

Using Personal Protective Equipment *(Continued)*

Excellent	Satisfactory	Needs Practice		Comments
			Remove PPE	
___	___	___	7. Remove PPE: Except for respirator, remove PPE at the doorway or in an anteroom. ***Remove respirator after leaving the patient's room and closing the door.***	
___	___	___	a. If impervious gown has been tied in front of the body at the waistline, untie waist strings before removing gloves.	
___	___	___	b. Grasp the outside of one glove with the opposite gloved hand and peel off, turning the glove inside out as you pull it off. Hold the removed glove in the remaining gloved hand.	
___	___	___	c. Slide fingers of ungloved hand under the remaining glove at the wrist, ***taking care not to touch the outer surface of the glove.***	
___	___	___	d. Peel off the glove over the first glove, containing the one glove inside the other. Discard in appropriate container.	
___	___	___	e. To remove the goggles or face shield: Handle by the headband or earpieces. Lift away from the face. Place in designated receptacle for reprocessing or in an appropriate waste container.	
___	___	___	f. To remove gown: Unfasten ties, if at the neck and back. Allow the gown to fall away from shoulders. ***Touching only the inside of the gown***, pull away from the torso. Keeping hands on the inner surface of the gown, pull gown from arms. Turn gown inside out. Fold or roll into a bundle and discard.	
___	___	___	g. To remove mask or respirator: Grasp the neck ties or elastic, then top ties or elastic and remove. ***Take care to avoid touching front of mask or respirator***. Discard in waste container. If using a respirator, save for future use in the designated area.	
___	___	___	8. Perform hand hygiene immediately after removing all PPE.	

Skill Checklists for Taylor's Clinical Nursing Skills.
A Nursing Process Approach, 5th edition

Name ______________________ Date ______________

Unit ______________________ Position ______________

Instructor/Evaluator: ______________________ Position ______________

SKILL 1-4

Preparing a Sterile Field Using a Packaged Sterile Drape

Goal: The sterile field is created without contamination and the patient remains free of exposure to pathogens.

Excellent	Satisfactory	Needs Practice		Comments
____	____	____	1. Perform hand hygiene and put on PPE, if indicated.	
____	____	____	2. Identify the patient. Explain the procedure to the patient.	
____	____	____	3. Check that the packaged sterile drape is dry and unopened. Also note expiration date, making sure that the date is still valid.	
____	____	____	4. Select a work area that is waist level or higher.	
____	____	____	5. Open the outer covering of the drape. Remove sterile drape, lifting it carefully by its corners. Hold away from body and above the waist and work surface.	
____	____	____	6. Continue to hold only by the corners. Allow the drape to unfold, away from your body and any other surface.	
____	____	____	7. Position the drape on the work surface with the moisture-proof side down. This would be the shiny or blue side. Avoid touching any other surface or object with the drape. If any portion of the drape hangs off the work surface, that part of the drape is considered contaminated.	
____	____	____	8. Place additional sterile items on field as needed. Refer to Skill 1-6. Continue with the procedure as indicated.	
____	____	____	9. When procedure is completed, remove PPE, if used. Perform hand hygiene.	

Skill Checklists for Taylor's Clinical Nursing Skills. A Nursing Process Approach, 5th edition

Name ________________________ Date ________________

Unit ________________________ Position ________________

Instructor/Evaluator: ________________________ Position ________________

SKILL 1-5

Preparing a Sterile Field Using a Commercially Prepared Sterile Kit or Tray

Goal: A sterile field is created without contamination, the contents of the package remain sterile, and the patient remains free of exposure to pathogens.

Excellent	Satisfactory	Needs Practice		Comments
____	____	____	1. Perform hand hygiene and put on PPE, if indicated.	
____	____	____	2. Identify the patient. Explain the procedure to the patient.	
____	____	____	3. Check that the packaged kit or tray is dry and unopened. Also note expiration date, making sure that the date is still valid.	
____	____	____	4. Select a work area that is waist level or higher.	
____	____	____	5. Open the outside cover of the package and remove the kit or tray. Place in the center of the work surface, with the topmost flap positioned on the far side of the package. Discard outside cover.	
____	____	____	6. Reach around the package and grasp the outer surface of the end of the topmost flap, holding no more than 1 in from the border of the flap. Pull open away from the body, keeping the arm outstretched and away from the inside of the wrapper. Allow the wrapper to lie flat on the work surface.	
____	____	____	7. Reach around the package and grasp the outer surface of the first side flap, holding no more than 1 in from the border of the flap. Pull open to the side of the package, keeping the arm outstretched and away from the inside of the wrapper. Allow the wrapper to lie flat on the work surface.	
____	____	____	8. Reach around the package and grasp the outer surface of the remaining side flap, holding no more than 1 in from the border of the flap. Pull open to the side of the package, keeping the arm outstretched and away from the inside of the wrapper. Allow the wrapper to lie flat on the work surface.	

Excellent	Satisfactory	Needs Practice	SKILL 1-5 **Preparing a Sterile Field Using a Commercially Prepared Sterile Kit or Tray** *(Continued)*	Comments
____	____	____	9. Stand away from the package and work surface. Grasp the outer surface of the remaining flap closest to the body, holding not more than 1 in from the border of the flap. Pull the flap back toward the body, keeping arm outstretched and away from the inside of the wrapper. Keep this hand in place. Use other hand to grasp the wrapper on the underside (the side that is down to the work surface). Position the wrapper so that when flat, edges are on the work surface, and do not hang down over sides of work surface. Allow the wrapper to lie flat on the work surface.	
____	____	____	10. The outer wrapper of the package has become a sterile field with the packaged supplies in the center. Do not touch or reach over the sterile field. Place additional sterile items on field as needed. Refer to Skill 1-6. Continue with the procedure as indicated.	
____	____	____	11. When procedure is completed, remove PPE, if used. Perform hand hygiene.	

Skill Checklists for Taylor's Clinical Nursing Skills. A Nursing Process Approach, 5th edition

Name ______________________ Date ______________________

Unit ______________________ Position ______________________

Instructor/Evaluator: ______________________ Position ______________________

SKILL 1-6

Adding Sterile Items to a Sterile Field

Goal: The sterile field is created without contamination, the sterile supplies are not contaminated, and the patient remains free of exposure to pathogens.

Excellent	Satisfactory	Needs Practice		Comments
___	___	___	1. Perform hand hygiene and put on PPE, if indicated.	
___	___	___	2. Identify the patient. Explain the procedure to the patient.	
___	___	___	3. Check that the sterile, packaged drape and supplies are dry and unopened. Also note expiration date, making sure that the date is still valid.	
___	___	___	4. Select a work area that is waist level or higher.	
___	___	___	5. Prepare sterile field as described in Skill 1-4 or Skill 1-5.	
___	___	___	6. Add sterile item:	
			To Add a Facility-Wrapped and Sterilized Item	
___	___	___	a. Hold facility-wrapped item in the dominant hand, with top flap opening away from the body. With other hand, reach around the package and unfold top flap and both sides.	
___	___	___	b. Keep a secure hold on the item through the wrapper with the dominant hand. Grasp the remaining flap of the wrapper closest to the body, taking care not to touch the inner surface of the wrapper or the item. Pull the flap back toward the wrist, so the wrapper covers the hand and wrist.	
___	___	___	c. Grasp all the corners of the wrapper together with the nondominant hand and pull back toward wrist, covering hand and wrist. Hold in place.	
___	___	___	d. Hold the item 6 in above the surface of the sterile field and drop onto the field. Be careful to avoid touching the surface or other items or dropping any item onto the 1-in border.	
			To Add a Commercially Wrapped and Sterilized Item	
___	___	___	a. Hold package in one hand. Pull back top cover with other hand. Alternately, carefully peel the edges apart using both hands.	
___	___	___	b. After top cover or edges are partially separated, hold the item 6 in above the surface of the sterile field. Continue opening the package and drop the item onto the field. ***Be careful to avoid touching the surface or other items or dropping an item onto the 1-in border.***	
___	___	___	c. Discard wrapper.	

SKILL 1-6

Adding Sterile Items to a Sterile Field *(Continued)*

Excellent	Satisfactory	Needs Practice		Comments
			To Add a Sterile Solution	
___	___	___	a. Obtain appropriate solution and check expiration date.	
___	___	___	b. Open solution container according to directions and ***place cap on table away from the field with edges up.***	
___	___	___	c. Hold bottle outside the edge of the sterile field with the label side facing the palm of your hand and prepare to pour from a height of 4 to 6 in (10 to 15 cm). ***Never touch the tip of the bottle to the sterile container or field.***	
___	___	___	d. Pour required amount of solution steadily into sterile container previously added to the sterile field and positioned at side of sterile field or onto dressings. ***Avoid splashing any liquid.***	
___	___	___	e. Touch only the outside of the lid when recapping. Label solution with date and time of opening.	
___	___	___	7. Continue with procedure as indicated.	
___	___	___	8. When procedure is completed, remove PPE, if used. Perform hand hygiene.	

Skill Checklists for Taylor's Clinical Nursing Skills. A Nursing Process Approach, 5th edition

Name ______________________ Date ______________________

Unit ______________________ Position ______________________

Instructor/Evaluator: ______________________ Position ______________________

SKILL 1-7

Putting on Sterile Gloves and Removing Soiled Gloves

Goal: The gloves are applied and removed without contamination.

Excellent	Satisfactory	Needs Practice		Comments
____	____	____	1. Perform hand hygiene and put on PPE, if indicated.	
____	____	____	2. Identify the patient. Explain the procedure to the patient.	
____	____	____	3. Check that the sterile glove package is dry and unopened. Also note expiration date, making sure that the date is still valid.	
____	____	____	4. Place sterile glove package on clean, dry surface at or above your waist.	
____	____	____	5. Open the outside wrapper by carefully peeling the top layer back. Remove inner package, handling only the outside of it.	
____	____	____	6. Place the inner package on the work surface with the side labeled "cuff end" closest to the body.	
____	____	____	7. Carefully open the inner package. Fold open the top flap, then the bottom and sides. *Do not touch the inner surface of the package or the gloves.*	
____	____	____	8. With the thumb and forefinger of the nondominant hand, grasp the folded cuff of the glove for the dominant hand, touching only the exposed inside of the glove.	
____	____	____	9. Keeping the hands above the waistline, lift and hold the glove up and off the inner package with fingers down. *Do not let it touch any unsterile object.*	
____	____	____	10. Carefully insert dominant hand palm up into glove and pull glove on. Leave the cuff folded until the opposite hand is gloved.	
____	____	____	11. Hold the thumb of the gloved hand outward. Place the fingers of the gloved hand inside the cuff of the remaining glove. Lift it from the wrapper, taking care not to touch anything with the gloves or hands.	
____	____	____	12. Carefully insert nondominant hand into glove. Pull the glove on, taking care that the skin does not touch any of the outer surfaces of the gloves.	
____	____	____	13. *Slide the fingers of one hand under the cuff of the other and fully extend the cuff down the arm, touching only the sterile outside of the glove. Repeat for the remaining hand.*	

Excellent	Satisfactory	Needs Practice	SKILL 1-7 **Putting on Sterile Gloves and Removing Soiled Gloves** *(Continued)*	Comments
___	___	___	14. Adjust gloves on both hands, if necessary, ***touching only sterile areas with other sterile areas.***	
___	___	___	15. Continue with procedure as indicated.	
			Removing Soiled Gloves	
___	___	___	16. Use dominant hand to grasp the opposite glove ***near cuff end on the outside exposed area.*** Remove it by pulling it off, inverting it as it is pulled, keeping the contaminated area on the inside. Hold the removed glove in the remaining gloved hand.	
___	___	___	17. Slide fingers of ungloved hand between the remaining glove and the wrist. ***Take care to avoid touching the outside surface of the glove.*** Remove it by pulling it off, inverting it as it is pulled, keeping the contaminated area on the inside, and securing the first glove inside the second.	
___	___	___	18. Discard gloves in appropriate container. Remove additional PPE, if used. Perform hand hygiene.	

Skill Checklists for Taylor's Clinical Nursing Skills. A Nursing Process Approach, 5th edition

Name ______________________ Date ______________________

Unit ______________________ Position ______________________

Instructor/Evaluator: ______________________ Position ______________________

Excellent	Satisfactory	Needs Practice	SKILL 2-1 **Assessing Body Temperature** **Goal:** The patient's temperature is assessed accurately without injury and the patient experiences only minimal discomfort.	**Comments**
___	___	___	1. Check the medical order or nursing care plan for frequency of measurement and route. More frequent temperature measurement may be appropriate based on nursing judgment.	
___	___	___	2. Perform hand hygiene and put on PPE, if indicated.	
___	___	___	3. Identify the patient.	
___	___	___	4. Close the curtains around the bed and close the door to the room, if possible. Discuss the procedure with the patient and assess the patient's ability to assist with the procedure.	
___	___	___	5. Assemble equipment on the overbed table within reach.	
___	___	___	6. Ensure that the electronic or digital thermometer is in working condition.	
___	___	___	7. Put on gloves, if indicated.	
___	___	___	8. Select the appropriate site based on assessment data.	
___	___	___	9. Follow the steps as outlined below for the appropriate type of thermometer.	
___	___	___	10. When measurement is completed, remove gloves, if worn. Remove additional PPE, if used. Perform hand hygiene.	
			Measuring an Oral Temperature	
___	___	___	11. Remove the electronic unit from the charging unit, and remove the probe from within the recording unit.	
___	___	___	12. Cover thermometer probe with disposable probe cover and slide it on until it snaps into place.	
___	___	___	13. ***Place the probe beneath the patient's tongue in the posterior sublingual pocket. Ask the patient to close his or her lips around the probe.***	
___	___	___	14. Continue to hold the probe until you hear a beep. Note the temperature reading.	
___	___	___	15. Remove the probe from the patient's mouth. Dispose of the probe cover by holding the probe over an appropriate receptacle and pressing the probe-release button.	

SKILL 2-1

Assessing Body Temperature *(Continued)*

Excellent	Satisfactory	Needs Practice		Comments
___	___	___	16. Return the thermometer probe to the storage place within the unit. Return the electronic unit to the charging unit, if appropriate.	
			Measuring a Tympanic Membrane Temperature	
___	___	___	17. If necessary, push the "ON" button and wait for the "ready" signal on the unit.	
___	___	___	18. Attach the disposable cover onto the tympanic probe.	
___	___	___	19. ***Insert the probe snugly into the external ear using gentle but firm pressure, angling the thermometer toward the patient's jaw line. Pull the pinna up and back to straighten the ear canal in an adult.***	
___	___	___	20. Activate the unit by pushing the trigger button. The reading is immediate (usually within 2 seconds). Note the reading.	
___	___	___	21. Discard the probe cover in an appropriate receptacle by pushing the probe-release button or use the rim of cover to remove it from the probe. Replace the thermometer in its charger, if necessary.	
			Measuring Temporal Artery Temperature	
___	___	___	22. Brush the patient's hair aside if it is covering the temporal artery area.	
___	___	___	23. Apply a probe cover.	
___	___	___	24. Hold the thermometer like a remote control device, with your thumb on the red "ON" button. Place the probe flush on the center of the forehead, with the body of the instrument sideways (not straight up and down) so that it is not in the patient's face.	
___	___	___	25. Depress the "ON" button. Keep the button depressed throughout the measurement.	
___	___	___	26. Slowly slide the probe straight across the forehead, midline, to the hairline. The thermometer will click; fast clicking indicates a rise to a higher temperature, slow clicking indicates that the instrument is still scanning, but not finding any higher temperature.	
___	___	___	27. If required, based on specific thermometer in use, brush hair aside if it is covering the ear, exposing the area of the neck under the ear lobe. Lift the probe from the forehead and touch on the neck just behind the ear lobe, in the depression just below the mastoid.	
___	___	___	28. Release the button and read the thermometer measurement.	

SKILL 2-1

Assessing Body Temperature *(Continued)*

Excellent	Satisfactory	Needs Practice		Comments
____	____	____	29. Hold the thermometer over a waste receptacle. Gently push the probe cover with your thumb against the proximal edge to dispose of the probe cover.	
____	____	____	30. The instrument will automatically turn off in 30 seconds, or press and release the power button.	
			Measuring Axillary Temperature	
____	____	____	31. Move the patient's clothing to expose only the axilla.	
____	____	____	32. Remove the probe from the recording unit of the electronic thermometer. Place a disposable probe cover on by sliding it on and snapping it securely.	
____	____	____	33. ***Place the end of the probe in the center of the axilla. Have the patient bring the arm down and close to the body.***	
____	____	____	34. Hold the probe in place until you hear a beep, and then carefully remove the probe. Note the temperature reading.	
____	____	____	35. Cover the patient and help him or her to a position of comfort.	
____	____	____	36. Dispose of the probe cover by holding the probe over an appropriate waste receptacle and pushing the release button.	
____	____	____	37. Place the bed in the lowest position and elevate rails, as needed. Leave the patient clean and comfortable.	
____	____	____	38. Return the electronic thermometer to the charging unit.	
			Measuring Rectal Temperature	
____	____	____	39. Adjust the bed to a comfortable working height, usually elbow height of the caregiver (VHACEOSH, 2016). Put on nonsterile gloves.	
____	____	____	40. Assist the patient to a side-lying position. Pull back the covers sufficiently to expose only the buttocks.	
____	____	____	41. Remove the rectal probe from within the recording unit of the electronic thermometer. Cover the probe with a disposable probe cover and slide it until it snaps in place.	
____	____	____	42. ***Lubricate about 1 in of the probe with a water-soluble lubricant.***	
____	____	____	43. Reassure the patient. Separate the buttocks until the anal sphincter is clearly visible.	
____	____	____	44. ***Insert the thermometer probe into the anus about 1.5 in in an adult or no more than 1 in in a child.***	

Excellent	Satisfactory	Needs Practice	SKILL 2-1 **Assessing Body Temperature** *(Continued)*	Comments
___	___	___	45. Hold the probe in place until you hear a beep, then carefully remove the probe. Note the temperature reading on the display.	
___	___	___	46. Dispose of the probe cover by holding the probe over an appropriate waste receptacle and pressing the release button.	
___	___	___	47. Using toilet tissue, wipe the anus of any feces or excess lubricant. Dispose of the toilet tissue. Remove gloves and discard them.	
___	___	___	48. Cover the patient and help him or her to a position of comfort.	
___	___	___	49. Place the bed in the lowest position; elevate rails as needed.	
___	___	___	50. Perform hand hygiene.	
___	___	___	51. Return the thermometer to the charging unit.	

Skill Checklists for Taylor's Clinical Nursing Skills.
A Nursing Process Approach, 5th edition

Name ____________________ Date ____________________

Unit ____________________ Position ____________________

Instructor/Evaluator: ____________________ Position ____________________

SKILL 2-2

Regulating Temperature Using an Overhead Radiant Warmer

Excellent	Satisfactory	Needs Practice	**Goal:** The infant's temperature is maintained within normal limits without injury.	Comments
____	____	____	1. Check the medical order or nursing care plan for the use of a radiant warmer.	
____	____	____	2. Perform hand hygiene and put on PPE, if indicated.	
____	____	____	3. Identify the patient.	
____	____	____	4. Close curtains around the bed and close the door to the room, if possible. Discuss the procedure with the patient's family.	
____	____	____	5. Plug in the warmer. Turn the warmer to the manual setting. Allow the blankets to warm before placing the infant under the warmer.	
____	____	____	6. ***Switch the warmer setting to automatic. Set the warmer to the desired abdominal skin temperature, usually 36.5°C (97.7°F).***	
____	____	____	7. Place the infant under the warmer. Attach the probe to the infant's abdominal skin at mid-epigastrium, halfway between the xiphoid and the umbilicus. Cover with a foil-backed shield. If the infant is prone, attach the probe to the skin over either flank (not between the scapulae) (Bell, 2015).	
____	____	____	8. When the abdominal skin temperature reaches the desired set point, check the patient's temperature using the route specified in facility policy to be sure it is within the normal range.	
____	____	____	9. Adjust the warmer's set point slightly, as needed, if the patient's temperature is abnormal. Do not change the set point if the temperature is normal.	
____	____	____	10. Remove additional PPE, if used. Perform hand hygiene.	
____	____	____	11. Check the position of the probe frequently to ensure the probe maintains contact with the patient's skin. Continue to monitor temperature measurement and other vital signs.	

Skill Checklists for Taylor's Clinical Nursing Skills. A Nursing Process Approach, 5th edition

Name ______________________ Date ______________________

Unit ______________________ Position ______________________

Instructor/Evaluator: ______________________ Position ______________________

SKILL 2-3

Regulating Temperature Using a Hypothermia Blanket

Excellent	Satisfactory	Needs Practice	**Goal**: The patient maintains the desired body temperature.	**Comments**
___	___	___	1. Review the medical order for the application of the hypothermia blanket. Obtain consent for the therapy per facility policy.	
___	___	___	2. Perform hand hygiene and put on PPE, if indicated.	
___	___	___	3. Identify the patient. Determine if the patient has had any previous adverse reaction to hypothermia therapy.	
___	___	___	4. Assemble equipment on the overbed table within reach.	
___	___	___	5. Close curtains around the bed and close the door to the room, if possible. Explain what you are going to do and why you are going to do it to the patient.	
___	___	___	6. Check that the water in the electronic unit is at the appropriate level. Fill the unit two thirds full with distilled water, or to the fill mark, if necessary. Check the temperature setting on the unit to ensure it is within the safe range.	
___	___	___	7. Assess the patient's vital signs, neurologic status, peripheral circulation, and skin integrity.	
___	___	___	8. Adjust bed to comfortable working height, usually elbow height of the caregiver (VHACEOSH, 2016).	
___	___	___	9. Make sure the patient's gown has cloth ties, not snaps or pins.	
___	___	___	10. Apply lanolin or a mixture of lanolin and cold cream to the patient's skin where it will be in contact with the blanket.	
___	___	___	11. Turn on the blanket and make sure the cooling light is on. ***Verify that the temperature limits are set within the desired safety range.***	
___	___	___	12. Cover the hypothermia blanket with a thin sheet or bath blanket.	
___	___	___	13. Position the blanket under the patient so that the top edge of the pad is aligned with the patient's neck.	

Excellent	Satisfactory	Needs Practice	SKILL 2-3 **Regulating Temperature Using a Hypothermia Blanket** *(Continued)*	Comments
___	___	___	14. Put on gloves. Lubricate the rectal probe and insert it into the patient's rectum unless contraindicated. Or tuck the skin probe deep into the patient's axilla and tape it in place. For patients who are comatose or anesthetized, use an esophageal probe. Remove gloves. Perform hand hygiene. Attach the probe to the control panel for the blanket.	
___	___	___	15. Wrap the patient's hands and feet in gauze if ordered, or if the patient desires. For male patients, elevate the scrotum off the hypothermia blanket with towels.	
___	___	___	16. Place the patient in a comfortable position. Lower the bed. Dispose of any other supplies appropriately.	
___	___	___	17. Recheck the thermometer and settings on the control panel.	
___	___	___	18. Remove any additional PPE, if used. Perform hand hygiene.	
___	___	___	19. ***Turn and position the patient regularly (every 30 minutes to 1 hour).*** Keep linens free from condensation. Reapply cream, as needed. Observe the patient's skin for change in color, changes in lips and nail beds, edema, pain, and sensory impairment.	
___	___	___	20. ***Monitor vital signs and perform a neurologic assessment, per facility policy, usually every 15 minutes, until the body temperature is stable.*** In addition, monitor the patient's skin integrity, peripheral circulation and fluid and electrolyte status, as per facility policy.	
___	___	___	21. Avoid cooling to the point of shivering (Morton & Fontaine, 2018). Observe for signs of shivering, including verbalized sensations, facial muscle twitching, hyperventilation, or twitching of extremities.	
___	___	___	22. Assess the patient's level of comfort.	
___	___	___	23. Turn off the blanket according to facility policy, usually when the patient's body temperature reaches 1 degree above the desired temperature. ***Continue to monitor the patient's temperature until it stabilizes.***	

Skill Checklists for Taylor's Clinical Nursing Skills. A Nursing Process Approach, 5th edition

Name ______________________ Date ______________________

Unit ______________________ Position ______________________

Instructor/Evaluator: ______________________ Position ______________________

SKILL 2-4
Assessing a Peripheral Pulse by Palpation

Goal: The patient's pulse is assessed accurately without injury and the patient experiences only minimal discomfort.

Excellent	Satisfactory	Needs Practice	Step	Comments
___	___	___	1. Check medical order or nursing care plan for frequency of pulse assessment. More frequent pulse measurement may be appropriate based on nursing judgment.	
___	___	___	2. Perform hand hygiene and put on PPE, if indicated.	
___	___	___	3. Identify the patient.	
___	___	___	4. Close the curtains around the bed and close the door to the room, if possible. Discuss the procedure with the patient and assess the patient's ability to assist with the procedure.	
___	___	___	5. Put on gloves, if indicated.	
___	___	___	6. Select the appropriate peripheral site based on assessment data.	
___	___	___	7. Move the patient's clothing to expose only the site chosen.	
___	___	___	8. Place your first, second, and third fingers over the artery. Place your fingers over the artery so that the ends of your fingers are flat against the patient's skin when palpating peripheral pulses. Do not press with the tip of the fingers only. ***Lightly compress the artery so pulsations can be felt and counted.***	
___	___	___	9. Using a watch with a second hand, count the number of pulsations felt for 30 seconds. Multiply this number by 2 to calculate the rate for 1 minute. ***If the rate, rhythm, or amplitude of the pulse is abnormal in any way, palpate and count the pulse for 1 minute.***	
___	___	___	10. Note the rhythm and amplitude of the pulse.	
___	___	___	11. When measurement is completed, remove gloves, if worn. Cover the patient and help him or her to a position of comfort.	
___	___	___	12. Remove additional PPE, if used. Perform hand hygiene.	

Skill Checklists for Taylor's Clinical Nursing Skills. A Nursing Process Approach, 5th edition

Name ______________________ Date ______________________

Unit ______________________ Position ______________________

Instructor/Evaluator: ______________________ Position ______________________

SKILL 2-5

Assessing the Apical Pulse by Auscultation

Excellent	Satisfactory	Needs Practice	**Goal:** The patient's pulse is assessed accurately without injury and the patient experiences minimal discomfort.	Comments
___	___	___	1. Check medical order or nursing care plan for frequency of pulse assessment. More frequent pulse measurement may be appropriate based on nursing judgment. Identify the need to obtain an apical pulse measurement.	
___	___	___	2. Perform hand hygiene and put on PPE, if indicated.	
___	___	___	3. Identify the patient.	
___	___	___	4. Close curtains around the bed and close the door to the room, if possible. Discuss the procedure with the patient and assess the patient's ability to assist with the procedure.	
___	___	___	5. Put on gloves, if indicated.	
___	___	___	6. Use an alcohol swab to clean the diaphragm of the stethoscope. Use another swab to clean the earpieces, if necessary.	
___	___	___	7. Assist the patient to a sitting or reclining position and expose the chest area.	
___	___	___	8. Move the patient's clothing to expose only the apical site.	
___	___	___	9. Hold the stethoscope diaphragm against the palm of your hand for a few seconds.	
___	___	___	10. ***Palpate the space between the fifth and sixth ribs (fifth intercostal space), and move to the left midclavicular line.*** Place the stethoscope diaphragm over the apex of the heart.	
___	___	___	11. Listen for heart sounds ("lub-dub"). Each "lub-dub" counts as one beat.	
___	___	___	12. Using a watch with a second hand, count the heartbeat for 1 minute.	
___	___	___	13. Note the rhythm of the beats.	
___	___	___	14. When measurement is completed, cover the patient and help him or her to a position of comfort.	
___	___	___	15. Clean the diaphragm of the stethoscope with an alcohol swab.	
___	___	___	16. Remove gloves and additional PPE, if used. Perform hand hygiene.	

Skill Checklists for Taylor's Clinical Nursing Skills.
A Nursing Process Approach, 5th edition

Name ____________________ Date ____________________

Unit ____________________ Position ____________________

Instructor/Evaluator: ____________________ Position ____________________

SKILL 2-6

Assessing Respiration

Excellent	Satisfactory	Needs Practice	**Goal:** The patient's respirations are assessed accurately without injury and the patient experiences only minimal discomfort.	Comments
____	____	____	1. ***While your fingers are still in place for the pulse measurement, after counting the pulse rate, observe the patient's respirations.***	
____	____	____	2. Note the rise and fall of the patient's chest.	
____	____	____	3. Using a watch with a second hand, count the number of respirations for 30 seconds. Multiply this number by 2 to calculate the respiratory rate per minute.	
____	____	____	4. ***If respirations are abnormal in any way, count the respirations for at least 1 full minute.***	
____	____	____	5. Note the depth and rhythm of the respirations.	
____	____	____	6. When measurement is completed, remove gloves, if worn. Cover the patient and help him or her to a position of comfort.	
____	____	____	7. Remove additional PPE, if used. Perform hand hygiene.	

Skill Checklists for Taylor's Clinical Nursing Skills. A Nursing Process Approach, 5th edition

Name ______________________ Date ______________________

Unit ______________________ Position ______________________

Instructor/Evaluator: ______________________ Position ______________________

SKILL 2-7

Assessing Blood Pressure by Auscultation

Excellent	Satisfactory	Needs Practice	**Goal:** The patient's blood pressure is measured accurately without injury.	**Comments**
___	___	___	1. Check the medical order or nursing care plan for frequency of blood pressure measurement. More frequent measurement may be appropriate based on nursing judgment.	
___	___	___	2. Perform hand hygiene and put on PPE, if indicated.	
___	___	___	3. Identify the patient.	
___	___	___	4. Close the curtains around the bed and close the door to the room, if possible. Discuss the procedure with the patient and assess patient's ability to assist with the procedure. Validate that the patient has relaxed for several minutes.	
___	___	___	5. Put on gloves, if indicated.	
___	___	___	6. Select the appropriate arm for application of the cuff.	
___	___	___	7. Have the patient assume a comfortable lying or sitting position with the forearm supported at the level of the heart and the palm of the hand upward. If the measurement is taken in the supine position, support the arm with a pillow. In the sitting position, support the arm yourself or by using the bedside table. If the patient is sitting, have the patient sit back in the chair so that the chair supports his or her back. In addition, make sure the patient keeps the legs uncrossed.	
___	___	___	8. Expose the brachial artery by removing garments or move a sleeve if it is not too tight, above the area where the cuff will be placed.	
___	___	___	9. Palpate the location of the brachial artery. ***Center the bladder of the cuff over the brachial artery, about midway on the arm, so that the lower edge of the cuff is about 2.5 to 5 cm (1 to 2 in) above the inner aspect of the elbow. Line up the artery marking on the cuff with the patient's brachial artery.*** The tubing should extend from the edge of the cuff nearer the patient's elbow.	
___	___	___	10. Wrap the cuff around the arm smoothly and snugly, and fasten it. Do not allow any clothing to interfere with the proper placement of the cuff.	

Excellent	Satisfactory	Needs Practice	SKILL 2-7 **Assessing Blood Pressure by Auscultation** *(Continued)*	Comments
___	___	___	11. Check that the needle on the aneroid gauge is within the zero mark. If using a mercury manometer, check to see that the manometer is in the vertical position and that the mercury is within the zero level with the gauge at eye level.	
			Estimating Systolic Pressure	
___	___	___	12. Palpate the pulse at the brachial or radial artery by pressing gently with the fingertips.	
___	___	___	13. Tighten the screw valve on the air pump.	
___	___	___	14. ***Inflate the cuff while continuing to palpate the artery. Note the point on the gauge where the pulse disappears.***	
___	___	___	15. Deflate the cuff and wait 1 minute.	
			Obtaining Blood Pressure Measurement	
___	___	___	16. Assume a position that is no more than 3 ft away from the gauge.	
___	___	___	17. Place the stethoscope earpieces in your ears. Direct the earpieces forward into the canal and not against the ear itself.	
___	___	___	18. Place the bell or diaphragm of the stethoscope firmly but with as little pressure as possible over the brachial artery. Do not allow the stethoscope to touch clothing or the cuff.	
___	___	___	19. Pump the pressure 30 mm Hg above the point at which the systolic pressure was palpated and estimated. Open the valve on the manometer and allow air to escape slowly (allowing the gauge to drop 2 to 3 mm per second).	
___	___	___	20. ***Note the point on the gauge at which the first faint, but clear, sound appears that slowly increases in intensity. Note this number as the systolic pressure. Read the pressure to the closest 2 mm Hg.***	
___	___	___	21. Do not reinflate the cuff once the air is being released to recheck the systolic pressure reading.	
___	___	___	22. ***Note the point at which the sound completely disappears. Note this number as the diastolic pressure. Read the pressure to the closest 2 mm Hg.***	
___	___	___	23. Allow the remaining air to escape quickly. Repeat any suspicious reading, but wait at least 1 minute. Deflate the cuff completely between attempts to check the blood pressure.	

Excellent	Satisfactory	Needs Practice	SKILL 2-7 **Assessing Blood Pressure by Auscultation** *(Continued)*	**Comments**
____	____	____	24. When measurement is completed, remove the cuff. Remove gloves, if worn. Cover the patient and help him or her to a position of comfort.	
____	____	____	25. Clean the bell or diaphragm of the stethoscope with the alcohol wipe. Clean and store the sphygmomanometer, according to facility policy.	
____	____	____	26. Remove additional PPE, if used. Perform hand hygiene.	

Skill Checklists for Taylor's Clinical Nursing Skills.
A Nursing Process Approach, 5th edition

Name ______________________ Date ______________________

Unit ______________________ Position ______________________

Instructor/Evaluator: ______________________ Position ______________________

SKILL 3-1

Performing a General Survey

Excellent	Satisfactory	Needs Practice	**Goal:** The assessment is completed without the patient experiencing anxiety or discomfort, an overall impression of the patient is formulated, the findings are documented, and the appropriate referral is made to other healthcare professionals, as needed for further evaluation.	**Comments**
___	___	___	1. Perform hand hygiene and put on PPE, if indicated.	
___	___	___	2. Identify the patient.	
___	___	___	3. Close curtains around the bed and the door to the room, if possible. Explain the purpose of the health examination and what you are going to do. Answer any questions.	
___	___	___	4. Assess the patient's overall appearance and behavior. Observe if the patient appears to be his or her stated age. Note the patient's mental status. Is the person alert and oriented, responsive to questions, and responding appropriately? Are the facial features symmetric? Note any signs of acute distress, such as shortness of breath, pain, or anxiousness.	
___	___	___	5. Assess the patient's body structure. Does the person's height appear within normal range for stated age and genetic heritage? Does the person's weight appear within normal range for height and body build? Note if body fat is evenly distributed. Do body parts appear equal bilaterally and relatively proportionate? Is the patient's posture erect and appropriate for age?	
___	___	___	6. Assess the patient's mobility. Is the patient's gait smooth, even, well balanced, and coordinated? Is joint mobility smooth and coordinated with a general full range of motion (ROM)? Are involuntary movements evident?	
___	___	___	7. Assess the patient's behavior. Are facial expressions appropriate for the situation? Does the patient maintain eye contact, based on cultural norms? Does the person appear comfortable and relaxed with you? Is the patient's speech clear and understandable? Observe the person's hygiene and grooming. Is the clothing appropriate for climate, fit well, appear clean, and appropriate for the person's culture and age group? Does the person appear clean and well groomed, appropriate for age and culture?	

Excellent	Satisfactory	Needs Practice	SKILL 3-1 **Performing a General Survey** *(Continued)*	Comments
____	____	____	8. Assess for pain.	
____	____	____	9. Have the patient remove shoes and heavy outer clothing. Weigh the patient using a scale. Compare the measurement with previous weight measurements and recommended range for height.	
____	____	____	10. With shoes off, and standing erect, measure the patient's height using a wall-mounted measuring device or measuring pole.	
____	____	____	11. Use the patient's weight and height measurements to calculate the patient's BMI. $$\text{Body mass index} = \frac{\text{weight in kilograms}}{\text{height in meters}^2}$$	
____	____	____	12. Using the tape measure, measure the patient's waist circumference. Place the tape measure snugly around the patient's waist at the level of the umbilicus.	
____	____	____	13. Measure the patient's temperature, pulse, respirations, blood pressure, and oxygen saturation.	
____	____	____	14. Remove PPE, if used. Clean equipment, based on facility policy. Perform hand hygiene. Continue with assessments of specific body systems as appropriate or indicated. Initiate appropriate referral to other health care providers for further evaluation as indicated.	

Skill Checklists for Taylor's Clinical Nursing Skills. A Nursing Process Approach, 5th edition

Name ______________________ Date ______________________

Unit ______________________ Position ______________________

Instructor/Evaluator: ______________________ Position ______________________

SKILL 3-2
Using a Portable Bed Scale

Excellent	Satisfactory	Needs Practice	**Goal:** The patient's weight is measured accurately without injury, and the patient experiences minimal discomfort.	Comments
___	___	___	1. Check the medical order or nursing care plan for frequency of weight measurement. More frequent measurement of the patient's weight may be appropriate based on nursing judgment. Obtain the assistance of a second caregiver, based on the patient's mobility and ability to cooperate with the procedure.	
___	___	___	2. Perform hand hygiene and put on PPE, if indicated.	
___	___	___	3. Identify the patient.	
___	___	___	4. Close the curtains around the bed and close the door to the room if possible. Discuss the procedure with the patient and assess the patient's ability to assist with the procedure.	
___	___	___	5. Place a cover over the sling of the bed scale.	
___	___	___	6. Attach the sling to the bed scale. Lay the sheet or bath blanket in the sling. Turn on the scale. ***Balance the scale so that weight reads 0.0.***	
___	___	___	7. Adjust the bed to a comfortable working position, usually elbow height of the caregiver (VHACEOSH, 2016). Position one caregiver on each side of the bed, if two caregivers are present. Raise side rail on the opposite side of the bed from where the scale is located, if not already in place. Cover the patient with the sheet or bath blanket. Remove other covers and any pillows.	
___	___	___	8. Turn the patient onto his or her side facing the side rail, keeping his or her body covered with the sheet or blanket. Remove the sling from the scale. Place the cover on the sling. Roll cover and sling lengthwise. Place rolled sling under the patient, making sure the patient is centered in the sling.	
___	___	___	9. Roll the patient back over the sling and onto the other side. Pull the sling through, as if placing sheet under patient, unrolling the sling as it is pulled through.	
___	___	___	10. Roll the scale over the bed so that the arms of the scale are directly over the patient. ***Spread the base of the scale.*** Lower the arms of the scale and place the arm hooks into the holes on the sling.	

SKILL 3-2

Using a Portable Bed Scale *(Continued)*

Excellent	Satisfactory	Needs Practice		Comments
___	___	___	11. Once the scale arms are hooked onto the sling, gradually elevate the sling so that the patient is lifted up off the bed. ***Assess all tubes and drains, making sure that none have tension placed on them as the scale is lifted. Once the sling is no longer touching the bed, ensure that nothing else is hanging onto the sling (e.g., ventilator or IV tubing). If any tubing is connected to the patient, raise it up so that it is not adding any weight to the patient.***	
___	___	___	12. Note the weight reading on the scale. Slowly and gently, lower the patient back onto the bed. Disconnect the scale arms from the sling. Close the base of the scale and pull it away from the bed.	
___	___	___	13. Raise the side rail. Turn the patient to the side rail. Roll the sling up against the patient's backside.	
___	___	___	14. Raise the other side rail. Roll the patient back over the sling and up facing the other side rail. Remove the sling from the bed. Remove gloves, if used. Raise the remaining side rail.	
___	___	___	15. Cover the patient and help him or her to a position of comfort. Place the bed in the lowest position.	
___	___	___	16. Remove the disposable cover from the sling and discard in the appropriate receptacle.	
___	___	___	17. Remove additional PPE, if used. Clean equipment based on facility policy. Perform hand hygiene.	
___	___	___	18. Replace the scale and sling in the appropriate spot. Plug the scale into the electrical outlet.	

Skill Checklists for Taylor's Clinical Nursing Skills.
A Nursing Process Approach, 5th edition

Name ______________________ Date ______________________

Unit ______________________ Position ______________________

Instructor/Evaluator: ______________________ Position ______________________

SKILL 3-3

Assessing the Skin, Hair, and Nails

Goal: The assessment is completed without the patient experiencing anxiety or discomfort, the findings are documented, and the appropriate referral is made to the other healthcare professionals, as needed, for further evaluation.

Excellent	Satisfactory	Needs Practice	Step	Comments
___	___	___	1. Perform hand hygiene and put on PPE, if indicated.	
___	___	___	2. Identify the patient.	
___	___	___	3. Close curtains around the bed and the door to room, if possible. Explain the purpose of the integumentary examination and what you are going to do. Answer any questions.	
___	___	___	4. Ask the patient to remove all clothing and put on an examination gown (if appropriate). The patient remains in the sitting position for most of the examination, but will need to stand or lie on the side when the posterior part of the body is examined, exposing only the body part being examined.	
___	___	___	5. Use the bath blanket or drape to cover any exposed area other than the one being assessed. Inspect the overall skin coloration.	
___	___	___	6. Inspect skin for vascularity, bleeding, or ecchymosis.	
___	___	___	7. Inspect the skin for lesions. Note bruises, scratches, cuts, insect bites, and wounds. If present, note size, shape, color, exudates, and distribution/pattern, and presence of drainage or odor. Assess the location and condition of body piercings and/or tattoos.	
___	___	___	8. Palpate skin using the backs of your hands to assess temperature. Wear gloves when palpating any potentially open area of the skin.	
___	___	___	9. Palpate for texture and moisture.	
___	___	___	10. Assess skin turgor by gently pinching the skin under the clavicle.	
___	___	___	11. Palpate for edema, which is characterized by swelling, with taut and shiny skin over the edematous area.	
___	___	___	12. If lesions are present, put on gloves and palpate the lesion.	
___	___	___	13. Inspect the nail condition, including the shape, texture, and color as well as the nail angle; note if any clubbing is present.	

Excellent	Satisfactory	Needs Practice	SKILL 3-3 **Assessing the Skin, Hair, and Nails** *(Continued)*	Comments
____	____	____	14. Palpate nails for texture and capillary refill.	
____	____	____	15. Inspect the hair and scalp for color, texture, and distribution. Wear gloves for palpation if lesions or infestation is suspected or if hygiene is poor.	
____	____	____	16. Remove gloves and any additional PPE, if used. Perform hand hygiene. Continue with assessments of specific body systems, as appropriate or indicated. Initiate appropriate referral to other health care providers for further evaluation, as indicated.	

Skill Checklists for Taylor's Clinical Nursing Skills. A Nursing Process Approach, 5th edition

Name ______________________ Date ______________________

Unit ______________________ Position ______________________

Instructor/Evaluator: ______________________ Position ______________________

Excellent	Satisfactory	Needs Practice	SKILL 3-4 **Assessing the Head and Neck** **Goal**: The assessment is completed without the patient experiencing anxiety or discomfort, the findings are documented, and the appropriate referral is made to the other healthcare professionals, as needed, for further evaluation.	**Comments**
____	____	____	1. Perform hand hygiene and put on PPE, if indicated.	
____	____	____	2. Identify the patient.	
____	____	____	3. Close the curtains around the bed and close the door to the room, if possible. Explain the purpose of the head and neck examination and what you are going to do. Answer any questions.	
____	____	____	4. Inspect the head for size and shape. Inspect the face for color, symmetry, lesions, and distribution of facial hair. Note facial expression. Palpate the skull.	
____	____	____	5. Inspect the external eye structures (eyelids, eyelashes, eyeball, and eyebrows), cornea, conjunctiva, and sclera. Note color, edema, symmetry, and alignment.	
____	____	____	6. Examine the pupils for equality of size and shape. Examine the pupillary reaction to light:	
____	____	____	a. Darken the room.	
____	____	____	b. Ask the patient to look straight ahead.	
____	____	____	c. Bring the penlight from the side of the patient's face and briefly shine the light on the pupil.	
____	____	____	d. Observe the pupil's reaction; it normally constricts rapidly (direct response). Note pupil size.	
____	____	____	e. Repeat the procedure and observe the other eye; it too normally will constrict (consensual reflex).	
____	____	____	f. Repeat the procedure with the other eye.	
____	____	____	7. Test for pupillary accommodation:	
____	____	____	a. Hold the forefinger, a pencil, or other straight object about 10 to 15 cm (4 to 6 in) from the bridge of the patient's nose.	
____	____	____	b. Ask the patient to first look at the object, then at a distant object, and then back to the object being held. The pupil normally constricts when looking at a near object and dilates when looking at a distant object.	

Excellent	Satisfactory	Needs Practice	SKILL 3-4 **Assessing the Head and Neck** *(Continued)*	Comments
____	____	____	8. Assess extraocular movements.	
____	____	____	a. Ask the patient to hold the head still and follow the movement of your forefinger or a penlight with the eyes as you move the patient's eyes through the six cardinal positions of gaze.	
____	____	____	b. Keeping your finger or penlight about 1 ft from the patient's face, move it slowly through the cardinal positions: up and down, right and left, diagonally up and down to the left, diagonally up and down to the right.	
____	____	____	9. Test convergence:	
____	____	____	a. Hold your finger about 6 to 8 in from the bridge of the patient's nose.	
____	____	____	b. Move your finger toward the patient's nose. The patient's eyes should normally converge (assume a cross-eyed appearance).	
____	____	____	10. Test the patient's visual acuity with a Snellen chart. Have the patient stand 20 ft from the chart and ask the patient to read the smallest line of letters possible, first with both eyes and then with one eye at a time (with the opposite eye covered). Note whether the patient's vision is being tested with or without corrective lenses.	
____	____	____	11. Inspect the external ear bilaterally for shape, size, and lesions. Palpate the ear and mastoid process. Inspect the visible portion of the ear canal. Note cerumen (wax), edema, discharge, or foreign bodies.	
____	____	____	12. Use a whispered voice to test hearing. Stand about 1 to 2 ft away from the patient out of the patient's line of vision. Ask the patient to cover the ear not being tested. Determine whether the patient can hear a whispered sentence or group of numbers from a distance of 1 to 2 ft. Perform test on each ear.	
____	____	____	13. Put on gloves. Inspect and palpate the external nose.	
____	____	____	14. Palpate over the frontal and maxillary sinuses.	
____	____	____	15. Occlude one nostril externally with a finger while patient breathes through the other; repeat for the other side.	
____	____	____	16. Inspect each anterior nares and turbinates by tipping the patient's head back slightly and shining a light into the nares. Examine the mucous membranes for color and the presence of lesions, exudate, or growths.	

SKILL 3-4

Assessing the Head and Neck *(Continued)*

Excellent	Satisfactory	Needs Practice		Comments
___	___	___	17. Inspect the lips, oral mucosa, hard and soft palates, gingivae, teeth, and salivary gland openings. Ask the patient to open the mouth wide and use a tongue blade and penlight to visualize structures.	
___	___	___	18. Inspect the tongue. Ask the patient to stick out the tongue. Place a tongue blade at the side of the tongue while patient pushes it to the left and right with the tongue. Inspect the uvula by asking the patient to say "ahh" while sticking out the tongue. Palpate the tongue for muscle tone and tenderness. Remove gloves.	
___	___	___	19. Inspect and palpate the lymph nodes for enlargement, tenderness, and mobility, using the fingerpads in a slow, circular motion.	
___	___	___	20. Inspect and palpate the left and then the right carotid arteries. ***Palpate only one carotid artery at a time.*** Note the strength of the pulse and grade it as with peripheral pulses. Use the bell of the stethoscope to auscultate the carotid arteries.	
___	___	___	21. Inspect and palpate the trachea.	
___	___	___	22. Assess the thyroid gland with the patient's neck slightly hyperextended. Observe the lower portion of the neck overlying the thyroid gland. Assess for symmetry and visible masses. Ask the patient to swallow. Observe the area while the patient swallows. Offer a glass of water, if necessary, to make it easier for the patient to swallow.	
___	___	___	23. Inspect the ability of the patient to move the neck. Ask the patient to touch chin to chest and to each shoulder, each ear to the corresponding shoulder, and then tip the head back as far as possible.	
___	___	___	24. Remove any additional PPE, if used. Perform hand hygiene. Continue with assessments of specific body systems, as appropriate or indicated. Initiate appropriate referral to other health care providers for further evaluation, as indicated.	

Skill Checklists for Taylor's Clinical Nursing Skills. A Nursing Process Approach, 5th edition

Name ______________________ Date ______________

Unit ______________________ Position ______________

Instructor/Evaluator: ______________________ Position ______________

SKILL 3-5

Assessing the Thorax, Lungs, and Breasts

Goal: The assessment is completed without causing the patient to experience anxiety or discomfort, the findings are documented, and the appropriate referral is made to other healthcare professionals, as needed, for further evaluation.

Excellent	Satisfactory	Needs Practice		Comments
___	___	___	1. Perform hand hygiene and put on PPE, if indicated.	
___	___	___	2. Identify the patient.	
___	___	___	3. Close the curtains around the bed and close the door to the room, if possible. Explain the purpose of the thorax, lung, breast, and axillae examination and what you are going to do. Answer any questions.	
___	___	___	4. Help the patient undress, if needed, and provide a patient gown. Assist the patient to a sitting position and expose the posterior thorax.	
___	___	___	5. Use the bath blanket to cover any exposed area other than the one being assessed.	
___	___	___	6. Inspect the posterior thorax. Examine the skin, bones, and muscles of the spine, shoulder blades, and back as well as symmetry of expansion and accessory muscle use during respirations.	
___	___	___	7. Assess the anteroposterior (AP) and lateral diameters of the thorax.	
___	___	___	8. Palpate over the spine and posterior thorax. Use the dorsal surface of the hand to palpate for temperature. Use the palmar surface of the hand to palpate in a sequential pattern for tenderness, muscle development, and masses.	
___	___	___	9. Assess thoracic expansion by standing behind the patient and placing both thumbs on either side of the patient's spine at the level of T9 or T10. Ask the patient to take a deep breath and note movement of your hands.	
___	___	___	10. As the patient breathes slowly and deeply through the mouth, auscultate the lungs across and down the posterior thorax to the bases of lungs in a sequential pattern, comparing sides.	
___	___	___	11. Inspect the anterior thorax. With the patient sitting, rearrange the gown so the anterior chest is exposed. Inspect the skin, bones, and muscles, as well as symmetry of lung expansion and accessory muscle use.	

SKILL 3-5

Assessing the Thorax, Lungs, and Breasts *(Continued)*

Excellent	Satisfactory	Needs Practice		Comments
___	___	___	12. Palpate the anterior thorax across and down the anterior thorax to the bases of lungs in a sequential pattern. Use the palmar surface of the hand to palpate for temperature, tenderness, muscle development, and masses.	
___	___	___	13. As the patient breathes slowly and deeply through the mouth, auscultate the lungs across and down the anterior thorax to the bases of lungs in a sequential pattern, comparing sides.	
___	___	___	14. If assessment of the breasts is required, inspect the breasts. Ask the patient to rest hands on both sides of the body, then on the hips and finally above the head. With the patient holding each position, inspect the breasts for size, shape, symmetry, color, texture, and skin lesions. Inspect the areola and nipples for size and shape and the nipples for discharge, crusting, and inversion.	
___	___	___	15. Palpate the axillae with the patient's arms resting against the side of the body. If any nodes are palpable, assess their location, size, shape, consistency, tenderness, and mobility.	
___	___	___	16. Assist the patient into a supine position. Place a small pillow or towel under the patient's back and ask the patient to place a hand on the side being examined under the head, if possible.	
___	___	___	17. Wear gloves if there is any discharge from the nipples or if a lesion is present. Palpate each quadrant of each breast in a systematic method, using either the circular, wedge, or vertical strip technique. Palpate the nipple and areola and gently compress the nipple between the thumb and forefinger to assess for discharge.	
___	___	___	18. Assist the patient into a comfortable position and in replacing the gown. Remove gloves and any additional PPE, if used. Perform hand hygiene. Continue with assessments of specific body systems, as appropriate or indicated. Initiate appropriate referral to other health care providers for further evaluation, as indicated.	

Skill Checklists for Taylor's Clinical Nursing Skills. A Nursing Process Approach, 5th edition

Name ______________________ Date ______________________

Unit ______________________ Position ______________________

Instructor/Evaluator: ______________________ Position ______________________

SKILL 3-6

Assessing the Cardiovascular System

Goal: The assessment is completed without causing the patient to experience anxiety or discomfort, the findings are documented, and the appropriate referral is made to other healthcare professionals, as needed, for further evaluation.

Excellent	Satisfactory	Needs Practice		Comments
___	___	___	1. Perform hand hygiene and put on PPE, if indicated.	
___	___	___	2. Identify the patient.	
___	___	___	3. Close the curtains around the bed and close the door to the room, if possible. Explain the purpose of the cardiovascular examination and what you are going to do. Answer any questions.	
___	___	___	4. Help the patient undress, if needed, and provide a patient gown. Assist the patient to a supine position with the head elevated about 30 to 45 degrees, if possible, and expose the anterior chest. Use the bath blanket to cover any exposed area other than the one being assessed.	
___	___	___	5. If not performed previously with the assessment of the head and neck, inspect and palpate the left and then the right carotid arteries. ***Palpate only one carotid artery at a time.*** Note the strength of the pulse and grade it as with peripheral pulses.	
___	___	___	6. Inspect the neck for distention of the jugular veins.	
___	___	___	7. Inspect the precordium for contour, pulsations, and heaves. Observe for the apical impulse at the fourth to fifth intercostal space (ICS) at the left midclavicular line.	
___	___	___	8. Using the palmar surface, with the four fingers held together, gently palpate the precordium for pulsations. Remember that hands should be warm. Palpation proceeds in a systematic manner, with assessment of specific cardiac landmarks—the aortic, pulmonic, tricuspid, and mitral areas and Erb's point. Palpate the apical impulse in the mitral area. Note size, duration, force, and location in relationship to the midclavicular line.	

Excellent	Satisfactory	Needs Practice	SKILL 3-6 **Assessing the Cardiovascular System** *(Continued)*	Comments
___	___	___	9. Auscultate heart sounds. Ask the patient to breathe normally. Use the diaphragm of the stethoscope first to listen to high-pitched sounds. Then use the bell to listen to low-pitched sounds. Focus on the overall rate and rhythm of the heart and the normal heart sounds. Begin at the aortic area, move to the pulmonic area, then to Erb's point, then the tricuspid area, and finally listen at the mitral area.	
___	___	___	10. Assist the patient in replacing the gown. Remove PPE, if used. Perform hand hygiene. Continue with assessments of specific body systems as appropriate or indicated. Initiate appropriate referral to other health care providers for further evaluation, as indicated.	

Skill Checklists for Taylor's Clinical Nursing Skills.
A Nursing Process Approach, 5th edition

Name ______________________ Date ______________________

Unit ______________________ Position ______________________

Instructor/Evaluator: ______________________ Position ______________________

SKILL 3-7

Assessing the Abdomen

Excellent	Satisfactory	Needs Practice	**Goal:** The assessments are completed without causing the patient to experience anxiety or discomfort, the findings are documented, and the appropriate referral is made to other healthcare professionals, as needed, for further evaluation.	Comments
___	___	___	1. Perform hand hygiene and put on PPE, if indicated.	
___	___	___	2. Identify the patient.	
___	___	___	3. Close the curtains around bed and close the door to the room, if possible. Explain the purpose of the abdominal examination and what you are going to do. Answer any questions.	
___	___	___	4. Help the patient undress, if needed, and provide a patient gown. Assist the patient to a supine position, if possible, and expose the abdomen. Use the bath blanket to cover any exposed area other than the one being assessed.	
___	___	___	5. Inspect the abdomen for skin color, contour, pulsations, the umbilicus, and other surface characteristics (rashes, lesions, masses, scars).	
___	___	___	6. Auscultate all four quadrants of the abdomen for bowel sounds. Warm the stethoscope and, using light pressure, place the flat diaphragm on the right lower quadrant of the abdomen, then move to the right upper quadrant, left upper quadrant, and finally left lower quadrant. Listen carefully for bowel sounds (gurgles and clicks), and note their frequency and character.	
___	___	___	7. Auscultate the abdomen for vascular sounds. Using the bell of the stethoscope, auscultate over the abdominal aorta, femoral arteries, and iliac arteries for bruits.	
___	___	___	8. Palpate the abdomen lightly in all four quadrants. The pads of the fingers are used to palpate with a light, gentle, dipping motion approximately 1 cm (approx. 0.5 in) (Jensen, 2015). Watch the patient's face for nonverbal signs of pain during palpation. Palpate each quadrant in a systematic manner, noting muscular resistance, tenderness, enlargement of the organs, or masses. ***If the patient complains of pain or discomfort in a particular area of the abdomen, palpate that area last.***	

Excellent	Satisfactory	Needs Practice	SKILL 3-7 **Assessing the Abdomen** *(Continued)*	Comments
___	___	___	9. Palpate and then auscultate the femoral pulses in the groin. Note the strength of the pulse and grade it as with peripheral pulses. Use the bell of the stethoscope to auscultate the arteries.	
___	___	___	10. Assist the patient into a comfortable position and in replacing the gown. Remove PPE, if used. Perform hand hygiene. Continue with assessments of specific body systems, as appropriate, or indicated. Initiate appropriate referral to other health care providers for further evaluation, as indicated.	

Skill Checklists for Taylor's Clinical Nursing Skills. A Nursing Process Approach, 5th edition

Name ______________________ Date ______________________

Unit ______________________ Position ______________________

Instructor/Evaluator: ______________________ Position ______________________

SKILL 3-8

Assessing the Female Genitalia

Goal: The assessments are completed without causing the patient to experience anxiety or discomfort, the findings are documented, and the appropriate referral is made to other health care professionals, as needed, for further evaluation.

Excellent	Satisfactory	Needs Practice		Comments
___	___	___	1. Perform hand hygiene and put on PPE, if indicated.	
___	___	___	2. Identify the patient.	
___	___	___	3. Close the curtains around bed and close the door to the room, if possible. Explain the purpose of the examination of genitalia and what you are going to do. Answer any questions.	
___	___	___	4. Help the patient undress, if needed, and provide a patient gown. Assist the patient to a supine position, or lying on her side, if possible. Use the bath blanket to cover any exposed area other than the one being assessed.	
___	___	___	5. Inspect the external genitalia for color, size of the labia majora and vaginal opening, lesions, and discharge.	
___	___	___	6. Palpate the labia for masses.	
___	___	___	7. Assist the patient to a comfortable position.	
___	___	___	8. Remove PPE, if used. Perform hand hygiene. Continue with assessments of specific body systems, as appropriate, or indicated. Initiate appropriate referral to other health care providers for further evaluation, as indicated.	

Skill Checklists for Taylor's Clinical Nursing Skills.
A Nursing Process Approach, 5th edition

Name ______________________ Date ______________________

Unit ______________________ Position ______________________

Instructor/Evaluator: ______________________ Position ______________________

SKILL 3-9

Assessing the Male Genitalia

Goal: Assessments are completed without causing the patient to experience anxiety or discomfort, the findings are documented, and the appropriate referral is made to other health care professionals, as needed, for further evaluation.

Excellent	Satisfactory	Needs Practice		Comments
___	___	___	1. Perform hand hygiene and put on PPE, if indicated.	
___	___	___	2. Identify the patient.	
___	___	___	3. Close the curtains around the bed and close the door to the room, if possible. Explain the purpose of the examination of genitalia and what you are going to do. Answer any questions.	
___	___	___	4. Help the patient undress, if needed, and provide a patient gown. Assist the patient to a supine or sitting position, if possible. Use a bath blanket to cover any exposed area other than the one being assessed.	
___	___	___	5. Put on gloves. Inspect the external genitalia for size, placement, contour, appearance of the skin, redness, edema, and discharge. If the patient is uncircumcised, retract the foreskin for inspection of the glans penis. Assess the location of the urinary meatus. Inspect the scrotum for symmetry.	
___	___	___	6. Palpate the scrotum for consistency, nodules, masses, and tenderness.	
___	___	___	7. Inspect the inguinal area. Ask the patient to bear down and look for bulging of the area.	
___	___	___	8. Assist the patient to a comfortable position.	
___	___	___	9. Remove PPE, if used. Perform hand hygiene. Continue with assessments of specific body systems, as appropriate, or indicated. Initiate appropriate referral to other health care providers for further evaluation, as indicated.	

Skill Checklists for Taylor's Clinical Nursing Skills. A Nursing Process Approach, 5th edition

Name ______________________ Date ______________________

Unit ______________________ Position ______________________

Instructor/Evaluator: ______________________ Position ______________________

SKILL 3-10

Assessing the Neurologic, Musculoskeletal, and Peripheral Vascular Systems

Goal: The assessments are completed without causing the patient to experience anxiety or discomfort, the findings are documented, and the appropriate referral is made to other healthcare professionals, as needed, for further evaluation.

Excellent	Satisfactory	Needs Practice		Comments
___	___	___	1. Perform hand hygiene and put on PPE, if indicated.	
___	___	___	2. Identify the patient.	
___	___	___	3. Close the curtains around the bed and close the door to the room, if possible. Explain the purpose of the neurologic, musculoskeletal, and peripheral vascular examinations and what you are going to do. Answer any questions.	
___	___	___	4. Help the patient undress, if needed, and provide a patient gown. Assist the patient to a supine position, if possible. Use the bath blanket to cover any exposed area other than the one being assessed.	
___	___	___	5. Begin with a survey of the patient's overall hygiene and physical appearance.	
___	___	___	6. Assess the patient's mental status.	
___	___	___	a. Evaluate level of consciousness. Refer to Chapter 17 for standardized assessment tools to assess level of consciousness.	
___	___	___	b. Evaluate the patient's orientation to person, place, and time.	
___	___	___	c. Assess memory (immediate recall and past memory).	
___	___	___	d. Evaluate the patient's ability to understand spoken and written word.	
___	___	___	7. Test cranial nerve (CN) function, as indicated.	
___	___	___	a. Ask the patient to close the eyes, occlude one nostril, and then identify the smell of different substances, such as coffee, chocolate, or alcohol. Repeat with other nostril.	
___	___	___	b. Test visual acuity and pupillary constriction. Refer to previous discussion in the assessment of the head and neck.	
___	___	___	c. Move the patient's eyes through the six cardinal positions of gaze. Refer to previous discussion in the assessment of the head and neck.	

Excellent	Satisfactory	Needs Practice	SKILL 3-10 **Assessing the Neurologic, Musculoskeletal, and Peripheral Vascular Systems** *(Continued)*	Comments
___	___	___	d. Ask the patient to smile, frown, wrinkle the forehead, and puff out cheeks.	
___	___	___	e. Ask the patient to protrude tongue and push against the cheek with the tongue.	
___	___	___	f. Palpate the jaw muscles. Ask the patient to open and clench jaws. Stroke the patient's face with a cotton ball.	
___	___	___	g. Test hearing with the whispered voice test. Refer to previous discussion in the assessment of the head and neck.	
___	___	___	h. Put on gloves. Ask patient to open mouth. While observing soft palate, ask patient to say "ah"; observe upward movement of the soft palate. Test the gag reflex by touching the posterior pharynx with the tongue depressor. Explain to patient that this may be uncomfortable. Ask the patient to swallow. Remove gloves.	
___	___	___	i. Place your hands on the patient's shoulders while he or she shrugs against resistance. Then place your hand on the patient's left cheek, then the right cheek, and have the patient push against it.	
___	___	___	8. Check the patient's ability to move his or her neck. Ask the patient to touch his or her chin to the chest and to each shoulder, then move each ear to the corresponding shoulder, and then tip the head back as far as possible.	
___	___	___	9. Inspect the upper extremities. Observe for skin color, presence of lesions, rashes, and muscle mass. Palpate for skin temperature, texture, and presence of masses.	
___	___	___	10. Ask the patient to extend arms forward and then rapidly turn palms up and down.	
___	___	___	11. Ask the patient to flex upper arm and to resist examiner's opposing force.	
___	___	___	12. Inspect and palpate the hands, fingers, wrists, and elbow joints.	
___	___	___	13. Ask the patient to bend and straighten the elbow, and flex and extend the wrists and hands.	
___	___	___	14. Palpate the skin and the radial and brachial pulses. Assess the pulse rate, quality or amplitude, and rhythm. Test capillary refill.	
___	___	___	15. Have the patient squeeze your index and middle fingers.	

Excellent	Satisfactory	Needs Practice	SKILL 3-10 **Assessing the Neurologic, Musculoskeletal, and Peripheral Vascular Systems** *(Continued)*	Comments
___	___	___	16. Assist the patient to a supine position. Palpate and then use the bell of the stethoscope to auscultate the femoral pulses in the groin, if not done during assessment of the abdomen. Note the strength of the pulse and grade it as with peripheral pulses.	
___	___	___	17. Examine the lower extremities. Inspect the legs and feet for color, lesions, varicosities, hair growth, nail growth, edema, and muscle mass.	
___	___	___	18. Assess for pitting edema in the lower extremities by pressing fingers into the skin at the pretibial area and dorsum of the foot. If an indentation remains in the skin after the fingers have been lifted, pitting edema is present.	
___	___	___	19. Palpate for pulses and skin temperature at the posterior tibial, dorsalis pedis, and popliteal areas. Assess the pulse rate, quality or amplitude, and rhythm. Test capillary refill.	
___	___	___	20. Ask the patient to move one leg laterally with the knee straight to test abduction of the hip. Keeping knee straight, move leg medially to test adduction of the hip. Repeat with other leg.	
___	___	___	21. Ask the patient to raise the thigh against the resistance of your hand; next have the patient push outward against the resistance of your hand; then have the patient pull backward against the resistance of your hand. Repeat on the opposite side.	
___	___	___	22. Ask the patient to dorsiflex and then plantarflex both feet against opposing resistance.	
___	___	___	23. As needed, assist the patient to a standing position. Observe the patient as he or she walks with a regular gait, on the toes, on the heels, and then heel to toe.	
___	___	___	24. Perform the Romberg's test; ask the patient to stand straight with feet together, both eyes closed with arms at side. Wait 20 seconds and observe for patient swaying and ability to maintain balance. Be alert to prevent patient fall or injury related to losing balance during this assessment.	
___	___	___	25. Assist the patient to a comfortable position.	
___	___	___	26. Remove PPE, if used. Perform hand hygiene. Continue with assessments of specific body systems, as appropriate, or indicated. Initiate appropriate referral to other health care providers for further evaluation, as indicated.	

Skill Checklists for Taylor's Clinical Nursing Skills.
A Nursing Process Approach, 5th edition

Name ______________________ Date ______________________

Unit ______________________ Position ______________________

Instructor/Evaluator: ______________________ Position ______________________

SKILL 4-1

Performing a Situational Assessment

Goal: A situational assessment is completed; the patient's needs are met; and the patient remains free from injury.

Excellent	Satisfactory	Needs Practice		Comments
___	___	___	1. Perform hand hygiene and put on PPE, if indicated.	
___	___	___	2. Identify the patient. Explain the purpose of the assessment to the patient.	
___	___	___	3. Assess for data that suggest a problem with the patient's airway, breathing, or circulation. If a problem is present, identify if it is urgent or nonurgent in nature. Refer to Chapter 3 for specific related assessments.	
___	___	___	4. Assess the patient's level of consciousness, orientation, and speech. Observe the patient's behavior and affect. Refer to Chapter 3 for specific related assessments.	
___	___	___	5. Assess the patency of an oxygen delivery device, if in use. Refer to Chapter 14 for specific related assessments.	
___	___	___	6. Survey the patient's environment. Assess the bed position and call bell location. Bed should be in the lowest positon and the call bell (based on specific patient care setting) should be within the patient's reach.	
___	___	___	7. Assess for clutter and hazards. Remove excess equipment, supplies, furniture, and other objects from rooms and walkways. Pay particular attention to high traffic areas and the route to the bathroom.	
___	___	___	8. Note the presence and location of appropriate emergency equipment, based on individual patient situation.	
___	___	___	9. Note the presence and location of appropriate assistive devices and mobility aids, based on individual patient situation. Ensure any devices are within the patient's reach.	
___	___	___	10. Assess for the presence of an intravenous access and/or infusion. Assess patency of the device and the insertion site. If an infusion is present, assess the solution and rate. Refer to Chapter 15 for specific related assessments.	
___	___	___	11. Assess for the presence of any tubes, such as gastric tubes, chest tubes, surgical drains, or urinary catheters. Assess patency of device and insertion site. Refer to Chapters 8 and 11 to 14 for specific related assessments.	
___	___	___	12. Provide a bedside commode and/or urinal/bedpan, if appropriate. Ensure that it is near the bed at all times.	

Excellent	Satisfactory	Needs Practice	SKILL 4-1 **Performing a Situational Assessment** *(Continued)*	Comments
____	____	____	13. Ensure that the bedside table, telephone, and other personal items are within the patient's reach at all times.	
____	____	____	14. Consider what further assessments should be completed and additional interventions that may be indicated. Identify problems that need to be reported and whom to contact.	
____	____	____	15. Remove PPE, if used. Perform hand hygiene.	

Skill Checklists for Taylor's Clinical Nursing Skills.
A Nursing Process Approach, 5th edition

Name ______________________________ Date ______________

Unit ______________________________ Position ______________

Instructor/Evaluator: ______________________________ Position ______________

SKILL 4-2

Fall Prevention

Excellent	Satisfactory	Needs Practice	**Goal:** The patient does not experience a fall and remains free of injury.	Comments
___	___	___	1. Perform hand hygiene and put on PPE, if indicated.	
___	___	___	2. Identify the patient. Assess fall risk as outlined above.	
___	___	___	3. Review the results of the fall risk assessment and fall risk factors with the patient and family.	
___	___	___	4. Explain the rationale for fall prevention interventions to the patient and family/significant others.	
___	___	___	5. Include the patient's family and/or significant others in the plan of care.	
___	___	___	6. Provide time for the patient and family to discuss concerns about falling, identify fall risk factors not identified by the risk assessment, confirm their understanding of risk factors and interventions, and to verbalize concerns or questions (Quigley, 2015).	
___	___	___	7. Provide adequate lighting. Use a night light during sleeping hours.	
___	___	___	8. Remove excess equipment, supplies, furniture, and other objects from rooms and walkways. Pay particular attention to high traffic areas and the route to the bathroom.	
___	___	___	9. Orient patient and significant others to new surroundings, including use of the telephone, call bell, patient bed, and room illumination. Indicate the location of the patient's bathroom.	
___	___	___	10. Provide a "low bed" to replace regular hospital bed.	
___	___	___	11. Use floor mats if patient is at risk for serious injury.	
___	___	___	12. Provide nonskid footwear and/or walking shoes.	
___	___	___	13. Institute a toileting regimen and/or continence program, if appropriate.	
___	___	___	14. Provide a bedside commode and/or urinal/bedpan, if appropriate. Ensure that it is near the bed at all times, if appropriate for individual patient.	
___	___	___	15. Ensure that the call bell, bedside table, telephone, and other personal items are within the patient's reach at all times.	
___	___	___	16. Confer with primary care provider regarding and encourage appropriate exercise and physical therapy.	

SKILL 4-2

Fall Prevention *(Continued)*

Excellent	Satisfactory	Needs Practice		Comments
___	___	___	17. Confer with primary care provider regarding appropriate mobility aids, such as a cane or walker.	
___	___	___	18. Confer with primary care provider regarding the use of bone-strengthening medications, such as calcium, vitamin D, and drugs to prevent/treat osteoporosis.	
___	___	___	19. Encourage the patient to rise or change position slowly and sit for several minutes before standing.	
___	___	___	20. Evaluate the appropriateness of elastic stockings for lower extremities.	
___	___	___	21. Review medications for potential hazards.	
___	___	___	22. Keep the bed in the lowest position. If elevated to provide care (to reduce caregiver strain), ensure that it is lowered when care is completed.	
___	___	___	23. Make sure locks on the bed or wheelchair are secured at all times.	
___	___	___	24. Use bed rails according to facility policy, when appropriate, based on individual patient assessment.	
___	___	___	25. Anticipate patient needs and provide assistance with activities instead of waiting for the patient to ask.	
___	___	___	26. Consider the use of an electronic personal alarm or pressure sensor alarm for the bed or chair.	
___	___	___	27. Discuss the possibility of appropriate family member(s) staying with patient.	
___	___	___	28. Consider the use of patient attendant or sitter.	
___	___	___	29. Increase the frequency of patient observation and surveillance. Utilize 1- or 2-hour nursing rounds, including pain assessment, toileting assistance, patient comfort, making sure personal items are in reach, and meeting patient needs.	
___	___	___	30. Remove PPE, if used. Perform hand hygiene.	

Skill Checklists for Taylor's Clinical Nursing Skills. A Nursing Process Approach, 5th edition

Name ______________________ Date ______________________

Unit ______________________ Position ______________________

Instructor/Evaluator: ______________________ Position ______________________

SKILL 4-3

Implementing Alternatives to the Use of Restraints

Goal: The use of restraints is avoided and the patient and others remain free from harm.

Excellent	Satisfactory	Needs Practice		Comments
___	___	___	1. Perform hand hygiene and put on PPE, if indicated.	
___	___	___	2. Identify the patient.	
___	___	___	3. Explain the rationale for interventions to the patient and family/significant others.	
___	___	___	4. Include the patient's family and/or significant others in the plan of care.	
___	___	___	5. Identify behavior(s) that place the patient at risk for restraint use. Assess the patient's status and environment, as outlined above.	
___	___	___	6. Identify triggers or contributing factors to patient behaviors. Evaluate medication usage for medications that can contribute to cognitive and movement dysfunction and to increased risk for falls.	
___	___	___	7. Assess the patient's functional, mental, and psychological status and the environment, as outlined above.	
___	___	___	8. Provide adequate lighting. Use a night light during sleeping hours.	
___	___	___	9. Consult with primary care provider and other appropriate health care providers regarding the continued need for treatments/therapies and the use of the least invasive method to deliver care.	
___	___	___	10. Assess the patient for pain and discomfort. Provide appropriate pharmacologic and nonpharmacologic interventions.	
___	___	___	11. Ask a family member or significant other to stay with the patient.	
___	___	___	12. Reduce unnecessary environmental stimulation and noise.	
___	___	___	13. Provide simple, clear, and direct explanations for treatments and care. Repeat to reinforce, as needed.	
___	___	___	14. Distract and redirect using a calm voice.	
___	___	___	15. Increase the frequency of patient observation and surveillance; 1- or 2-hour nursing rounds, including pain assessment, toileting assistance, patient comfort, keeping personal items in reach, and meeting patient needs.	

Excellent	Satisfactory	Needs Practice	SKILL 4-3 **Implementing Alternatives to the Use of Restraints** *(Continued)*	Comments
___	___	___	16. Implement fall precaution interventions.	
___	___	___	17. Camouflage tube and other treatment sites with clothing, elastic sleeves, or bandaging.	
___	___	___	18. Ensure the use of glasses and hearing aids, if necessary.	
___	___	___	19. Consider relocation to a room close to the nursing station.	
___	___	___	20. Encourage daily exercise/provide exercise and activities or relaxation techniques.	
___	___	___	21. Make the environment as homelike as possible; provide familiar objects.	
___	___	___	22. Allow restless patients to walk after ensuring that the environment is safe. Use a large plant or a piece of furniture as a barrier to limit wandering from the designated area.	
___	___	___	23. Consider the use of a patient attendant or sitter.	
___	___	___	24. Remove PPE, if used. Perform hand hygiene.	

Skill Checklists for Taylor's Clinical Nursing Skills. A Nursing Process Approach, 5th edition

Name ____________________ Date ____________

Unit ____________________ Position ____________

Instructor/Evaluator: ____________________ Position ____________

SKILL 4-4

Applying an Extremity Restraint

Goal: The patient is constrained by the restraint, remains free from injury, and the restraint does not interfere with therapeutic devices.

Excellent	Satisfactory	Needs Practice		Comments
___	___	___	1. Determine the need for restraints. Assess the patient's physical condition, behavior, and mental status.	
___	___	___	2. Confirm facility policy for the application of restraints. ***Secure an order from the primary care provider, or validate that the order has been obtained within the required time frame.***	
___	___	___	3. Perform hand hygiene and put on PPE, if indicated.	
___	___	___	4. Identify the patient.	
___	___	___	5. Explain the reason for restraint use to patient and family. Clarify how care will be given and how needs will be met. Explain that restraint is a temporary measure.	
___	___	___	6. Include the patient's family and/or significant others in the plan of care.	
___	___	___	7. Apply restraint according to the manufacturer's directions:	
___	___	___	a. Choose the least restrictive type of device that allows the greatest possible degree of mobility.	
___	___	___	b. Pad bony prominences.	
___	___	___	c. Wrap the restraint around the extremity with the soft part in contact with the skin. If a hand mitt is being used, pull over the hand with cushion to the palmar aspect of the hand.	
___	___	___	8. Secure in place with the Velcro straps or other mechanism, depending on specific restraint device. Depending on the characteristics of the specific restraint, it may be necessary to tie a knot in the restraint ties, to ensure the restraint remains secure on the extremity.	
___	___	___	9. ***Ensure that two fingers can be inserted between the restraint and patient's extremity.***	
___	___	___	10. Maintain restrained extremity in normal anatomic position. ***Use a quick-release knot to tie the restraint to the bed frame, not side rail.*** The restraint may also be attached to a chair frame. The site should not be readily accessible to the patient.	
___	___	___	11. Remove PPE, if used. Perform hand hygiene.	

SKILL 4-4

Applying an Extremity Restraint *(Continued)*

Excellent	Satisfactory	Needs Practice		Comments
___	___	___	12. Assess the patient at least every hour or according to facility policy. Assessment should include the placement of the restraint, neurovascular assessment of the affected extremity, and skin integrity. In addition, assess for signs of sensory deprivation, such as increased sleeping, daydreaming, anxiety, panic, and hallucinations. Monitor the patient's vital signs.	
___	___	___	13. ***Remove the restraint at least every 2 hours, or according to facility policy and patient need.*** Perform range-of-motion (ROM) exercises.	
___	___	___	14. Evaluate the patient for continued need of restraint. Reapply restraint only if continued need is evident and order is still valid.	
___	___	___	15. Reassure the patient at regular intervals. Provide continued explanation of rationale for interventions, reorientation if necessary, and plan of care. ***Keep the call bell within the patient's easy reach.***	

Skill Checklists for Taylor's Clinical Nursing Skills. A Nursing Process Approach, 5th edition

Name ______________________ Date ______________________

Unit ______________________ Position ______________________

Instructor/Evaluator: ______________________ Position ______________________

SKILL 4-5
Applying a Waist Restraint

Goal: The patient is constrained by the restraint, remains free from injury, and the restraint does not interfere with therapeutic devices.

Excellent	Satisfactory	Needs Practice		Comments
___	___	___	1. Determine the need for restraints. Assess the patient's physical condition, behavior, and mental status.	
___	___	___	2. Confirm facility policy for application of restraints. ***Secure an order from the primary care provider, or validate that the order has been obtained within the required time frame.***	
___	___	___	3. Perform hand hygiene and put on PPE, if indicated.	
___	___	___	4. Identify the patient.	
___	___	___	5. Explain reason for the use of restraint to patient and family. Clarify how care will be given and how needs will be met. Explain that restraint is a temporary measure.	
___	___	___	6. Include the patient's family and/or significant others in the plan of care.	
___	___	___	7. Apply restraint according to the manufacturer's directions.	
___	___	___	a. Choose the correct size of the least restrictive type of device that allows the greatest possible degree of mobility.	
___	___	___	b. Pad bony prominences that may be affected by the waist restraint.	
___	___	___	c. Assist patient to a sitting position, if not contraindicated.	
___	___	___	d. Place waist restraint on patient over gown. Bring ties through slots in restraint. Position slots at patient's back.	
___	___	___	e. Pull the ties secure. ***Ensure that the restraint is not too tight and has no wrinkles.***	
___	___	___	f. ***Insert fist between restraint and patient to ensure that breathing is not constricted. Assess respirations after restraint is applied.***	
___	___	___	8. ***Use a quick-release knot to tie the restraint to the bed frame, not side rail.*** If patient is in a wheelchair, lock the wheels and place the ties under the arm rests and tie behind the chair. Site should not be readily accessible to the patient.	
___	___	___	9. Remove PPE, if used. Perform hand hygiene.	

SKILL 4-5

Applying a Waist Restraint *(Continued)*

Excellent	Satisfactory	Needs Practice		Comments
___	___	___	10. Assess the patient at least every hour or according to facility policy. An assessment should include the placement of the restraint, respirations, and skin integrity. Assess for signs of sensory deprivation, such as increased sleeping, daydreaming, anxiety, panic, and hallucinations. Monitor the patient's vital signs.	
___	___	___	11. ***Remove restraint at least every 2 hours or according to facility policy and patient need.*** Perform ROM exercises.	
___	___	___	12. Evaluate patient for continued need of restraint. Reapply restraint only if continued need is evident and order is still valid.	
___	___	___	13. Reassure patient at regular intervals. Provide continued explanation of rationale for interventions, reorientation if necessary, and plan of care. ***Keep call bell within easy reach of patient.***	

Skill Checklists for Taylor's Clinical Nursing Skills.
A Nursing Process Approach, 5th edition

Name ______________________________ Date ______________________

Unit ______________________________ Position ______________________

Instructor/Evaluator: ______________________ Position ______________________

SKILL 4-6
Applying an Elbow Restraint

Goal: The patient is constrained by the restraint, remains free from injury, and the restraint does not interfere with therapeutic devices.

Excellent	Satisfactory	Needs Practice		Comments
___	___	___	1. Determine the need for restraints. Assess the patient's physical condition, behavior, and mental status.	
___	___	___	2. Confirm facility policy for application of restraints. ***Secure an order from the primary care provider, or validate that the order has been obtained within the required time frame.***	
___	___	___	3. Perform hand hygiene and put on PPE, if indicated.	
___	___	___	4. Identify the patient.	
___	___	___	5. Explain the reason for use to the patient and family. Clarify how care will be given and how needs will be met. Explain that the restraint is a temporary measure.	
___	___	___	6. Apply the restraint according to manufacturer's directions:	
___	___	___	a. Choose the correct size of the least restrictive type of device that allows the greatest possible degree of mobility.	
___	___	___	b. Pad bony prominences that may be affected by the restraint.	
___	___	___	c. Spread elbow restraint out flat. Place the middle of the elbow restraint behind the patient's elbow. ***The restraint should not extend below the wrist or place pressure on the axilla.***	
___	___	___	d. ***Wrap the restraint snugly around the patient's arm, but make sure that two fingers can easily fit under the restraint.***	
___	___	___	e. Secure Velcro straps around the restraint.	
___	___	___	f. Apply the restraint to the opposite arm if the patient can move the arm.	
___	___	___	g. Thread Velcro strap from one elbow restraint across the back and into the loop on the opposite elbow restraint.	
___	___	___	7. ***Assess circulation to fingers and hand.***	
___	___	___	8. Remove PPE, if used. Perform hand hygiene.	

Excellent	Satisfactory	Needs Practice	SKILL 4-6 **Applying an Elbow Restraint** *(Continued)*	Comments
___	___	___	9. Assess the patient at least every hour or according to facility policy. An assessment should include the placement of the restraint, neurovascular assessment, and skin integrity. Assess for signs of sensory deprivation, such as increased sleeping, daydreaming, anxiety, inconsolable crying, and panic. Monitor the patient's vital signs.	
___	___	___	10. ***Remove the restraint at least every 2 hours or according to facility policy and patient need. Remove the restraint at least every 2 hours for children ages 9 to 17 years and at least every 1 hour for children under age 9, or according to facility policy and patient need.*** Perform ROM exercises.	
___	___	___	11. Evaluate the patient for continued need of restraint. Reapply the restraint only if continued need is evident.	
___	___	___	12. Reassure the patient at regular intervals. ***Keep call bell within easy reach of the patient.***	

Skill Checklists for Taylor's Clinical Nursing Skills.
A Nursing Process Approach, 5th edition

Name ______________________ Date ______________________

Unit ______________________ Position ______________________

Instructor/Evaluator: ______________________ Position ______________________

SKILL 4-7

Applying a Mummy Restraint

Goal: The patient is constrained by the restraint, remains free from injury, and the restraint does not interfere with therapeutic devices.

Excellent	Satisfactory	Needs Practice		Comments
___	___	___	1. Determine the need for restraints. Assess the patient's physical condition, behavior, and mental status.	
___	___	___	2. Confirm facility policy for application of restraints. ***Secure an order from the primary care provider, or validate that the order has been obtained within the required time frame.***	
___	___	___	3. Perform hand hygiene and put on PPE, if indicated.	
___	___	___	4. Identify the patient.	
___	___	___	5. Explain the reason for use to the patient and family. Clarify how care will be given and how needs will be met. Explain that restraint is a temporary measure.	
___	___	___	6. Open the blanket or sheet. Place the child on the blanket, with the edge of the blanket at or above neck level.	
___	___	___	7. Position the child's right arm alongside the child's body. Left arm should not be constrained at this time. Pull the right side of the blanket tightly over the child's right shoulder and chest. Secure under the left side of the child's body.	
___	___	___	8. Position the left arm alongside the child's body. Pull the left side of the blanket tightly over the child's left shoulder and chest. Secure under the right side of the child's body.	
___	___	___	9. Fold the lower part of the blanket up and pull over the child's body. Secure under the child's body on each side or with safety pins.	
___	___	___	10. Stay with the child while the mummy wrap is in place. Reassure the child and parents at regular intervals. Once examination or treatment is completed, unwrap the child.	
___	___	___	11. Remove PPE, if used. Perform hand hygiene.	

Skill Checklists for Taylor's Clinical Nursing Skills. A Nursing Process Approach, 5th edition

Name ______________________ Date ______________________

Unit ______________________ Position ______________________

Instructor/Evaluator: ______________________ Position ______________________

SKILL 5-1

Administering Oral Medications

Excellent	Satisfactory	Needs Practice	**Goal:** The medication is successfully administered via the oral route; the patient experiences the desired effect from the medication; the patient does not aspirate; the patient experiences decreased anxiety; the patient does not experience adverse effects; and the patient complies with the medication regime.	**Comments**
___	___	___	1. Gather equipment. Check each medication order against the original in the medical record, according to facility policy. Clarify any inconsistencies. Check the patient's medical record for allergies.	
___	___	___	2. Know the actions, special nursing considerations, safe dose ranges, purpose of administration, and potential adverse effects of the medications to be administered. Consider the appropriateness of the medication for this patient.	
___	___	___	3. Perform hand hygiene.	
___	___	___	4. Move the medication supply system to the outside of the patient's room or prepare for administration at the medication supply system in the medication area. Alternatively, access the medication administration supply system at or inside the patient's room.	
___	___	___	5. Unlock the medication supply system or drawer. Enter pass code into the computer and scan employee identification, if required.	
___	___	___	6. ***Prepare medications for one patient at a time.***	
___	___	___	7. Read the eMAR/MAR and select the proper medication from the medication supply system or patient's medication drawer.	
___	___	___	8. Compare the medication label with the eMAR/MAR. Check expiration dates and perform calculations, if necessary. Scan the bar code on the package, if required.	
___	___	___	9. Prepare the required medications:	
___	___	___	a. *Unit dose packages:* ***Do not open the wrapper until at the bedside.*** Keep opioids and medications that require special nursing assessments separate from other medication packages.	
___	___	___	b. *Multidose containers:* When removing tablets or capsules from a multidose bottle, pour the necessary number into the bottle cap and then place the tablets or capsules in a medication cup. Break only scored tablets, if necessary, to obtain the proper dosage. Do not touch tablets or capsules with hands.	

Excellent	Satisfactory	Needs Practice	SKILL 5-1 **Administering Oral Medications** *(Continued)*	Comments
___	___	___	c. *Liquid medication in multidose bottle:* When pouring liquid medications out of a multidose bottle, hold the bottle so the label is against the palm. Use the appropriate measuring device when pouring liquids, and read the amount of medication at the bottom of the meniscus at eye level. Wipe the lip of the bottle with a paper towel.	
___	___	___	10. ***Depending on facility policy, the third check of the label may occur at this point. If so, when all medications for one patient have been prepared, recheck the labels with the eMAR/MAR before taking the medications to the patient. However, many facilities require the third check to occur at the bedside, after identifying the patient.***	
___	___	___	11. Replace any multidose containers in the patient's drawer or medication supply system. ***Lock the medication supply system before leaving it.***	
___	___	___	12. Transport medications to the patient's bedside carefully, and keep the medications in sight at all times.	
___	___	___	13. ***Ensure that the patient receives the medications at the correct time.***	
___	___	___	14. Perform hand hygiene and put on PPE, if indicated.	
___	___	___	15. ***Identify the patient. Compare the information with the eMAR/MAR. The patient should be identified using at least two of the following methods*** (The Joint Commission, 2018):	
___	___	___	a. Check the name on the patient's identification band.	
___	___	___	b. Check the identification number on the patient's identification band.	
___	___	___	c. Check the birth date on the patient's identification band.	
___	___	___	d. Ask the patient to state his or her name and birth date, based on facility policy.	
___	___	___	16. ***Complete necessary assessments before administering medications. Check the patient's allergy bracelet or ask the patient about allergies. Explain the purpose and action of each medication to the patient.***	
___	___	___	17. Scan the patient's bar code on the identification band, if required.	
___	___	___	18. ***Based on facility policy, the third check of the medication label may occur at this point. If so, recheck the label with the eMAR/MAR before administering the medications to the patient.***	

Excellent	Satisfactory	Needs Practice	SKILL 5-1 **Administering Oral Medications** *(Continued)*	Comments
___	___	___	19. Assist the patient to an upright or lateral (side-lying) position.	
___	___	___	20. Administer medications:	
___	___	___	a. Offer water or other permitted fluids with pills, capsules, tablets, and some liquid medications.	
___	___	___	b. Ask whether the patient prefers to take the medications by hand or in a cup.	
___	___	___	21. ***Remain with the patient until each medication is swallowed. Never leave medication at the patient's bedside.***	
___	___	___	22. Assist the patient to a comfortable position. Remove PPE, if used. Perform hand hygiene.	
___	___	___	23. Document the administration of the medication immediately after administration.	
___	___	___	24. Evaluate the patient's response to the medication within the appropriate time frame.	

Skill Checklists for Taylor's Clinical Nursing Skills. A Nursing Process Approach, 5th edition

Name ________________ Date ________________

Unit ________________ Position ________________

Instructor/Evaluator: ________________ Position ________________

SKILL 5-2

Administering Medications via a Gastric Tube

Excellent	Satisfactory	Needs Practice	**Goal:** The patient receives the medication via the tube and experiences the intended effect of the medication.	Comments
___	___	___	1. Gather equipment. Check each medication order against the original in the medical record, according to facility policy. Clarify any inconsistencies. Check the patient's health record for allergies.	
___	___	___	2. Know the actions, special nursing considerations, safe dose ranges, purpose of administration, and adverse effects of the medications to be administered. Consider the appropriateness of the medication for this patient.	
___	___	___	3. Perform hand hygiene.	
___	___	___	4. Move the medication supply system to the outside of the patient's room or prepare for administration at the medication supply system in the medication area. Alternatively, access the medication administration supply system at or inside the patient's room.	
___	___	___	5. Unlock the medication supply system or drawer. Enter pass code into the computer and scan employee identification, if required.	
___	___	___	6. ***Prepare medications for one patient at a time.***	
___	___	___	7. Read the eMAR/MAR and select the proper medication from the medication supply system or patient's medication drawer.	
___	___	___	8. Compare the label with the eMAR/MAR. Check expiration dates and perform calculations, if necessary. Scan the bar code on the package, if required.	
___	___	___	9. Check to see if medications to be administered come in a liquid form. ***If pills or capsules are to be given, check with pharmacy or drug reference to verify the ability to crush tablets or open capsules.***	
___	___	___	10. Prepare medication. *Pills:* Using a pill crusher, crush each pill one at a time. Dissolve the powder with water or other recommended liquid in a liquid medication cup, keeping each medication separate from the others. Keep the package label with the medication cup, for future comparison of information.	

Excellent	Satisfactory	Needs Practice	SKILL 5-2 **Administering Medications via a Gastric Tube** *(Continued)*	Comments
			Liquid: When pouring liquid medications from a multidose bottle, hold the bottle with the label against the palm. Use the appropriate measuring device when pouring liquids, and read the amount of medication at the bottom of the meniscus at eye level. Wipe the lip of the bottle with a paper towel.	
___	___	___	11. ***Depending on facility policy, the third check of the label may occur at this point. If so, when all medications for one patient have been prepared, recheck the labels with the eMAR/MAR before taking the medications to the patient. However, many facilities require the third check to occur at the bedside, after identifying the patient.***	
___	___	___	12. Replace any multidose containers in the patient's drawer or medication supply system.	
___	___	___	13. ***Lock the medication supply system before leaving it.***	
___	___	___	14. Transport medications to the patient's bedside carefully, and keep the medications in sight at all times.	
___	___	___	15. ***Ensure that the patient receives the medications at the correct time.***	
___	___	___	16. Perform hand hygiene and put on PPE, if indicated.	
___	___	___	17. ***Identify the patient. Compare the information with the eMAR/MAR. The patient should be identified using at least two of the following methods*** (The Joint Commission, 2018):	
___	___	___	a. Check the name on the patient's identification band.	
___	___	___	b. Check the identification number on the patient's identification band.	
___	___	___	c. Check the birth date on the patient's identification band.	
___	___	___	d. Ask the patient to state his or her name and birth date, based on facility policy.	
___	___	___	18. ***Complete necessary assessments before administering medications. Check the patient's allergy bracelet or ask the patient about allergies. Explain what you are going to do, and the reason for doing it, to the patient.***	
___	___	___	19. Scan the patient's bar code on the identification band, if required.	
___	___	___	20. ***Based on facility policy, the third check of the label may occur at this point. If so, recheck the labels with the eMAR/MAR before administering the medications to the patient.***	

SKILL 5-2

Administering Medications via a Gastric Tube *(Continued)*

Excellent	Satisfactory	Needs Practice		Comments
			21. Assist the patient to the high-Fowler's position, unless contraindicated.	
			22. Put on gloves.	
			23. If patient is receiving continuous tube feedings, pause the tube-feeding pump.	
			24. Pour the water into the irrigation container. Measure 30 mL of water. Apply clamp on feeding tube, if present. Alternatively, pinch gastric tube below port with fingers, or position stopcock to correct direction. Open port on gastric tube delegated to medication administration or disconnect tubing for feeding from gastric tube and place cap on end of feeding tubing.	
			25. ***Check tube placement, depending on type of tube and facility policy.***	
			26. Note the amount of any residual. Replace residual back into stomach, based on facility policy.	
			27. Apply clamp on feeding tube, if present. Alternatively, pinch the gastric tube below port with fingers, or position stop-cock to correct direction. Remove 60-mL syringe from gastric tube. Remove the plunger of the syringe. Reinsert the syringe in the gastric tube without the plunger. Pour 30 mL of water into the syringe. ***Unclamp the tube and allow the water to enter the stomach via gravity infusion.***	
			28. Administer the first dose of medication by pouring it into the syringe. Follow with a 5- to 10-mL water flush between medication doses. Follow the last dose of medication with 30 to 60 mL of water flush.	
			29. Clamp the tube, remove the syringe, and replace the feeding tubing. If a stopcock is used, position it to correct direction. If a tube medication port was used, cap the port. Unclamp the gastric tube and restart tube feeding, if appropriate for medications administered.	
			30. Remove gloves. Assist the patient to a comfortable position. If receiving a tube feeding, the head of the bed must remain elevated at least 30 degrees.	
			31. Remove additional PPE, if used. Perform hand hygiene.	
			32. Document the administration of the medication immediately after administration.	
			33. Evaluate the patient's response to the medication within the appropriate time frame.	

Skill Checklists for Taylor's Clinical Nursing Skills.
A Nursing Process Approach, 5th edition

Name ______________________ Date ______________________

Unit ______________________ Position ______________________

Instructor/Evaluator: ______________________ Position ______________________

SKILL 5-3

Removing Medication From an Ampule

Goal: The medication is removed in a sterile manner; the medication is free from glass shards and contamination; and the proper dose is prepared.

Excellent	Satisfactory	Needs Practice		Comments
___	___	___	1. Gather equipment. Check the medication order against the original order in the medical record, according to facility policy. Clarify any inconsistencies. Check the patient's health record for allergies.	
___	___	___	2. Know the actions, special nursing considerations, safe dose ranges, purpose of administration, and adverse effects of the medications to be administered. Consider the appropriateness of the medication for this patient.	
___	___	___	3. Perform hand hygiene.	
___	___	___	4. Move the medication supply system to the outside of the patient's room or prepare for administration at the medication supply system in the medication area. Alternatively, access the medication administration supply system at or inside the patient's room.	
___	___	___	5. Unlock the medication supply system or drawer. Enter pass code and scan employee identification, if required.	
___	___	___	6. ***Prepare medications for one patient at a time.***	
___	___	___	7. Read the eMAR/MAR and select the proper medication from the medication supply system or the patient's medication drawer.	
___	___	___	8. Compare the label with the eMAR/MAR. Check expiration dates and perform calculations, if necessary. Scan the bar code on the package, if required.	
___	___	___	9. Tap the stem of the ampule or twist your wrist quickly while holding the ampule vertically.	
___	___	___	10. Using the antimicrobial swab, scrub the neck of the ampule (Dolan et al, 2016). Wrap a small sterile gauze pad around the neck of the ampule.	
___	___	___	11. Breaking away from your body, use a snapping motion to break off the top of the ampule along the scored line at its neck. ***Always break away from your body.***	
___	___	___	12. Attach filter needle to syringe. Remove the cap from the filter needle by pulling it straight off.	

Excellent	Satisfactory	Needs Practice	SKILL 5-3 **Removing Medication From an Ampule** *(Continued)*	Comments
___	___	___	13. Withdraw medication in the amount ordered plus a small amount more (approximately 30% more). ***Do not inject air into the solution. While inserting the filter needle into the ampule, be careful not to touch the rim.*** Use either of the following methods to withdraw the medication:	
___	___	___	a. Insert the tip of the needle into the ampule, which is upright on a flat surface, and withdraw fluid into the syringe. ***Touch the plunger only at the knob.***	
___	___	___	b. Insert the tip of the needle into the ampule and invert the ampule. Keep the needle centered and not touching the sides of the ampule. Withdraw fluid into syringe. ***Touch the plunger only at the knob.***	
___	___	___	14. Wait until the needle has been withdrawn to tap the syringe and expel the air carefully by pushing on the plunger. ***Check the amount of medication in the syringe with the medication dose and discard any surplus, according to facility policy.***	
___	___	___	15. ***Depending on facility policy, the third check of the label may occur at this point. If so, when all medications for one patient have been prepared, recheck the labels with the eMAR/MAR before taking the medications to the patient. However, many facilities require the third check to occur at the bedside, after identifying the patient.***	
___	___	___	16. ***Engage safety guard on filter needle and remove the needle. Discard the filter needle in a suitable container. Attach appropriate administration device to syringe.***	
___	___	___	17. Discard the ampule in a suitable container.	
___	___	___	18. ***Lock the medication supply system before leaving it.***	
___	___	___	19. Perform hand hygiene.	
___	___	___	20. Proceed with administration, based on prescribed route.	

Skill Checklists for Taylor's Clinical Nursing Skills.
A Nursing Process Approach, 5th edition

Name ______________________ Date ______________________

Unit ______________________ Position ______________________

Instructor/Evaluator: ______________________ Position ______________________

SKILL 5-4

Removing Medication From a Vial

Goal: The medication is withdrawn into a syringe in a sterile manner; the medication is free from contamination; and the proper dose is prepared.

Excellent	Satisfactory	Needs Practice		Comments
___	___	___	1. Gather equipment. Check the medication order against the original order in the medical record, according to facility policy. Clarify any inconsistencies. Check the patient's health record for allergies.	
___	___	___	2. Know the actions, special nursing considerations, safe dose ranges, purpose of administration, and adverse effects of the medications to be administered. Consider the appropriateness of the medication for this patient.	
___	___	___	3. Perform hand hygiene.	
___	___	___	4. Move the medication supply system to the outside of the patient's room or prepare for administration at the medication supply system in the medication area. Alternatively, access the medication administration supply system at or inside the patient's room.	
___	___	___	5. Unlock the medication supply system or drawer. Enter pass code and scan employee identification, if required.	
___	___	___	6. ***Prepare medications for one patient at a time.***	
___	___	___	7. Read the eMAR/MAR and select the proper medication from the medication supply system or the patient's medication drawer.	
___	___	___	8. Compare the label with the eMAR/MAR. Check expiration dates and perform calculations, if necessary. Scan the bar code on the package, if required.	
___	___	___	9. Remove the metal or plastic cap on the vial that protects the self-sealing stopper.	
___	___	___	10. ***Scrub the self-sealing stopper top with the antimicrobial swab and allow to dry.***	
___	___	___	11. Remove the cap from the needle or blunt cannula by pulling it straight off. ***If the vial in use is a multidose vial,*** touch the plunger only at the knob and draw back an amount of air into the syringe that is equal to the specific dose of medication to be withdrawn. If the vial in use is a single-use vial, there is no need to draw air into the syringe.	

Excellent	Satisfactory	Needs Practice	SKILL 5-4 **Removing Medication From a Vial** *(Continued)*	Comments
___	___	___	12. Hold the vial on a flat surface. Pierce the self-sealing stopper in the center with the needle tip and inject the measured air into the space above the solution. ***Do not inject air into the solution.*** If the vial in use is a single-use vial, there is no need to inject air into the vial.	
___	___	___	13. Invert the vial. ***Keep the tip of the needle or blunt cannula below the fluid level.***	
___	___	___	14. Hold the vial in one hand and use the other to withdraw the medication. ***Touch the plunger only at the knob. Draw up the prescribed amount of medication while holding the syringe vertically and at eye level.***	
___	___	___	15. If any air bubbles accumulate in the syringe, tap the barrel of the syringe sharply and move the needle past the fluid into the air space to re-inject the air bubble into the vial. Return the needle tip to the solution and continue withdrawal of the medication.	
___	___	___	16. After the correct dose is withdrawn, remove the needle from the vial and carefully replace the cap over the needle. Some facilities require changing the needle, if one was used to withdraw the medication, before administering the medication.	
___	___	___	17. ***Check the amount of medication in the syringe with the medication dose and discard any surplus.***	
___	___	___	18. ***Depending on facility policy, the third check of the label may occur at this point. If so, when all medications for one patient have been prepared, recheck the labels with the eMAR/MAR before taking the medications to the patient. However, many facilities require the third check to occur at the bedside, after identifying the patient.***	
___	___	___	19. ***If a multidose vial is being used, label the vial with the date and time opened and the beyond-use date, and store the vial containing the remaining medication according to facility policy.*** Limit the use of multiple-dose vials and dedicate them to a single patient whenever possible (CDC, n.d.b).	
___	___	___	20. ***Lock the medication supply system before leaving it.***	
___	___	___	21. Perform hand hygiene.	
___	___	___	22. Proceed with administration, based on prescribed route.	

Skill Checklists for Taylor's Clinical Nursing Skills. A Nursing Process Approach, 5th edition

Name ______________________ Date ______________________

Unit ______________________ Position ______________________

Instructor/Evaluator: ______________________ Position ______________________

SKILL 5-5

Mixing Medications From Two Vials in One Syringe

Excellent	Satisfactory	Needs Practice	**Goal:** The accurate withdrawal of the medication into a syringe in a sterile manner; the medication is free from contamination; and the proper dose is prepared.	**Comments**
___	___	___	1. Gather equipment. Check medication order against the original order in the medical record, according to facility policy.	
___	___	___	2. Know the actions, special nursing considerations, safe dose ranges, purpose of administration, and adverse effects of the medications to be administered. Consider the appropriateness of the medication for this patient.	
___	___	___	3. Perform hand hygiene.	
___	___	___	4. Move the medication supply system to the outside of the patient's room or prepare for administration at the medication supply system in the medication area. Alternatively, access the medication administration supply system at or inside the patient's room.	
___	___	___	5. Unlock the medication supply system or drawer. Enter pass code and scan employee identification, if required.	
___	___	___	6. ***Prepare medications for one patient at a time.***	
___	___	___	7. Read the eMAR/MAR and select the proper medications from the medication supply system or the patient's medication drawer.	
___	___	___	8. Compare the labels with the eMAR/MAR. Check expiration dates and perform dosage calculations, if necessary. Scan the bar code on the package, if required.	
___	___	___	9. If necessary, remove the cap that protects the self-sealing stopper on each vial.	
___	___	___	10. ***If medication is a suspension (e.g., a modified insulin, such as NPH insulin), roll and agitate the vial to mix it well.***	
___	___	___	11. ***Scrub the self-sealing stopper top with the antimicrobial swab and allow to dry.***	
___	___	___	12. Remove cap from needle by pulling it straight off. Touch the plunger only at the knob. Draw back an amount of air into the syringe that is equal to the dose of modified insulin to be withdrawn.	
___	___	___	13. Hold the modified vial on a flat surface. Pierce the self-sealing stopper in the center with the needle tip and inject the measured air into the space above the solution. Do not inject air into the solution. Withdraw the needle.	

SKILL 5-5
Mixing Medications From Two Vials in One Syringe *(Continued)*

Excellent	Satisfactory	Needs Practice		Comments
___	___	___	14. Draw back an amount of air into the syringe that is equal to the dose of unmodified insulin to be withdrawn.	
___	___	___	15. Hold the unmodified vial on a flat surface. Pierce the self-sealing stopper in the center with the needle tip and inject the measured air into the space above the solution. Do not inject air into the solution. Keep the needle in the vial.	
___	___	___	16. Invert the vial of unmodified insulin. Hold the vial in one hand and use the other to withdraw the medication. ***Touch the plunger only at the knob. Draw up the prescribed amount of medication while holding the syringe at eye level and vertically.*** Turn the vial over and then remove the needle from the vial.	
___	___	___	17. Check that there are no air bubbles in the syringe.	
___	___	___	18. ***Check the amount of medication in the syringe with the medication dose and discard any surplus.***	
___	___	___	19. ***Recheck the vial label with the eMAR/MAR.***	
___	___	___	20. Calculate the endpoint on the syringe for the combined insulin amount by adding the number of units for each dose together.	
___	___	___	21. Insert the needle into the modified vial and invert it, taking care not to push the plunger and inject medication from the syringe into the vial. Invert vial of modified insulin. Hold the vial in one hand and use the other to withdraw the medication. ***Touch the plunger only at the knob. Draw up the prescribed amount of medication while holding the syringe at eye level and vertically. Take care to withdraw only the prescribed amount.*** Turn the vial over and then remove the needle from the vial. Carefully recap the needle. Carefully replace the cap over the needle.	
___	___	___	22. ***Check the amount of medication in the syringe with the medication dose.***	
___	___	___	23. ***Depending on facility policy, the third check of the label may occur at this point. If so, recheck the label with the MAR before taking the medications to the patient. However, many facilities require the third check to occur at the bedside, after identifying the patient.***	
___	___	___	24. ***Label the vials with the date and time opened and beyond-use date, and store the vials containing the remaining medication, according to facility policy.***	
___	___	___	25. ***Lock the medication supply system before leaving it.***	
___	___	___	26. Perform hand hygiene.	
___	___	___	27. Proceed with administration, based on prescribed route.	

Skill Checklists for Taylor's Clinical Nursing Skills. A Nursing Process Approach, 5th edition

Name ______________________ Date ______________________

Unit ______________________ Position ______________________

Instructor/Evaluator: ______________________ Position ______________________

SKILL 5-6

Administering an Intradermal Injection

Excellent	Satisfactory	Needs Practice	**Goal:** The medication is injected and a wheal appears at the site of injection.	**Comments**
___	___	___	1. Gather equipment. Check each medication order against the original order in the medical record according to facility policy. Clarify any inconsistencies. Check the patient's health record for allergies.	
___	___	___	2. Know the actions, special nursing considerations, safe dose ranges, purpose of administration, and adverse effects of the medications to be administered. Consider the appropriateness of the medication for this patient.	
___	___	___	3. Perform hand hygiene.	
___	___	___	4. Move the medication supply system to the outside of the patient's room or prepare for administration at the medication supply system in the medication area. Alternatively, access the medication administration supply system at or inside the patient's room.	
___	___	___	5. Unlock the medication supply system or drawer. Enter pass code and scan employee identification, if required.	
___	___	___	6. *Prepare medications for one patient at a time.*	
___	___	___	7. Read the eMAR/MAR and select the proper medication from the medication supply system or the patient's medication drawer.	
___	___	___	8. Compare the label with the eMAR/MAR. Check expiration dates and perform calculations, if necessary. Scan the bar code on the package, if required.	
___	___	___	9. If necessary, withdraw the medication from an ampule or vial.	
___	___	___	10. *Depending on facility policy, the third check of the label may occur at this point. If so, when all medications for one patient have been prepared, recheck the labels with the eMAR/MAR before taking the medications to the patient. However, many facilities require the third check to occur at the bedside, after identifying the patient.*	
___	___	___	11. *Lock the medication supply system before leaving it.*	
___	___	___	12. Transport medications to the patient's bedside carefully, and keep the medications in sight at all times.	

Excellent	Satisfactory	Needs Practice	SKILL 5-6 **Administering an Intradermal Injection** *(Continued)*	**Comments**
___	___	___	13. ***Ensure that the patient receives the medications at the correct time.***	
___	___	___	14. Perform hand hygiene and put on PPE, if indicated.	
___	___	___	15. ***Identify the patient. Compare the information with the eMAR/MAR. The patient should be identified using at least two of the following methods*** (The Joint Commission, 2018):	
___	___	___	a. Check the name on the patient's identification band.	
___	___	___	b. Check the identification number on the patient's identification band.	
___	___	___	c. Check the birth date on the patient's identification band.	
___	___	___	d. Ask the patient to state his or her name and birth date, based on facility policy.	
___	___	___	16. Close the door to the room or pull the bedside curtain.	
___	___	___	17. ***Complete necessary assessments before administering medications. Check allergy bracelet or ask the patient about allergies. Explain the purpose and action of the medication to the patient.***	
___	___	___	18. Scan the patient's bar code on the identification band, if required.	
___	___	___	19. ***Based on facility policy, the third check of the label may occur at this point. If so, recheck the labels with the eMAR/MAR before administering the medications to the patient.***	
___	___	___	20. Put on clean gloves.	
___	___	___	21. Select an appropriate administration site. Assist the patient to the appropriate position for the site chosen. Drape, as needed, to expose only site area to be used.	
___	___	___	22. Cleanse the site with an antimicrobial swab while wiping with a firm, circular motion and moving outward from the injection site. Allow the skin to dry.	
___	___	___	23. Remove the needle cap with the nondominant hand by pulling it straight off.	
___	___	___	24. Use the nondominant hand to spread the skin taut over the injection site.	
___	___	___	25. Hold the syringe in the dominant hand, between the thumb and forefinger with the bevel of the needle up.	
___	___	___	26. Hold the syringe at a 5- to 15-degree angle from the site. Place the needle almost flat against the patient's skin, bevel side up, and insert the needle into the skin. Insert the needle only about 1/8 in with entire bevel under the skin.	

SKILL 5-6

Administering an Intradermal Injection *(Continued)*

Excellent	Satisfactory	Needs Practice		Comments
___	___	___	27. Once the needle is in place, steady the lower end of the syringe. Slide your dominant hand to the end of the plunger.	
___	___	___	28. Slowly inject the agent while watching for a small wheal to appear.	
___	___	___	29. Withdraw the needle quickly at the same angle that it was inserted. Do not recap the used needle. Engage the safety shield or needle guard.	
___	___	___	30. ***Do not massage the area after removing needle. Tell the patient not to rub or scratch the site. If necessary, gently blot the site with a dry gauze square. Do not apply pressure or rub the site.***	
___	___	___	31. Assist the patient to a position of comfort.	
___	___	___	32. Discard the needle and syringe in the appropriate receptacle.	
___	___	___	33. Remove gloves and additional PPE, if used. Perform hand hygiene.	
___	___	___	34. Document the administration of the medication immediately after administration.	
___	___	___	35. Evaluate the patient's response to the medication within the appropriate time frame.	
___	___	___	36. Observe the area for signs of a reaction at determined intervals after administration. Inform the patient of the need for inspection.	

Skill Checklists for Taylor's Clinical Nursing Skills.
A Nursing Process Approach, 5th edition

Name ________________________ Date ____________

Unit ________________________ Position ____________

Instructor/Evaluator: ________________________ Position ____________

SKILL 5-7

Administering a Subcutaneous Injection

Goal: The patient receives medication via the subcutaneous route and experiences the intended effect of the medication.

Excellent	Satisfactory	Needs Practice		Comments
___	___	___	1. Gather equipment. Check each medication order against the original order in the medical record, according to facility policy. Clarify any inconsistencies. Check the patient's health record for allergies.	
___	___	___	2. Know the actions, special nursing considerations, safe dose ranges, purpose of administration, and adverse effects of the medications to be administered. Consider the appropriateness of the medication for this patient.	
___	___	___	3. Perform hand hygiene.	
___	___	___	4. Move the medication supply system to the outside of the patient's room or prepare for administration at the medication supply system in the medication area. Alternatively, access the medication administration supply system at or inside the patient's room.	
___	___	___	5. Unlock the medication supply system or drawer. Enter pass code and scan employee identification, if required.	
___	___	___	6. ***Prepare medications for one patient at a time.***	
___	___	___	7. Read the eMAR/MAR and select the proper medication from the medication supply system or the patient's medication drawer.	
___	___	___	8. Compare the medication label with the eMAR/MAR. Check expiration dates and perform calculations, if necessary. Scan the bar code on the package, if required.	
___	___	___	9. If necessary, withdraw medication from an ampule or vial.	
___	___	___	10. ***Depending on facility policy, the third check of the label may occur at this point. If so, when all medications for one patient have been prepared, recheck the labels with the eMAR/MAR before taking the medications to the patient. However, many facilities require the third check to occur at the bedside, after identifying the patient.***	
___	___	___	11. ***Lock the medication supply system before leaving it.***	
___	___	___	12. Transport medications to the patient's bedside carefully, and keep the medications in sight at all times.	

SKILL 5-7

Administering a Subcutaneous Injection *(Continued)*

Excellent	Satisfactory	Needs Practice		Comments
___	___	___	13. ***Ensure that the patient receives the medications at the correct time.***	
___	___	___	14. Perform hand hygiene and put on PPE, if indicated.	
___	___	___	15. ***Identify the patient. Compare the information with the eMAR/MAR. The patient should be identified using at least two of the following methods*** (The Joint Commission, 2018):	
___	___	___	a. Check the name on the patient's identification band.	
___	___	___	b. Check the identification number on the patient's identification band.	
___	___	___	c. Check the birth date on the patient's identification band.	
___	___	___	d. Ask the patient to state his or her name and birth date, based on facility policy.	
___	___	___	16. Close the door to the room or pull the bedside curtain.	
___	___	___	17. ***Complete necessary assessments before administering medications. Check the patient's allergy bracelet or ask the patient about allergies.*** Explain the purpose and action of the medication to the patient.	
___	___	___	18. Scan the patient's bar code on the identification band, if required.	
___	___	___	19. ***Based on facility policy, the third check of the label may occur at this point. If so, recheck the labels with the eMAR/MAR before administering the medications to the patient.***	
___	___	___	20. Put on clean gloves.	
___	___	___	21. Select an appropriate administration site.	
___	___	___	22. Assist the patient to the appropriate position for the site chosen. Drape, as needed, to expose only site area to be used.	
___	___	___	23. Identify the appropriate landmarks for the site chosen.	
___	___	___	24. Cleanse the area around the injection site with an antimicrobial swab. Use a firm, circular motion while moving outward from the injection site. Allow the area to dry.	
___	___	___	25. Remove the needle cap with the nondominant hand, pulling it straight off.	
___	___	___	26. Create a skin fold, if necessary, by pinching the area surrounding the injection site. Alternatively, spread the skin taut at the site, based on assessment of the patient and needle length used for the injection.	

SKILL 5-7

Administering a Subcutaneous Injection *(Continued)*

Excellent	Satisfactory	Needs Practice		Comments
___	___	___	27. Hold the syringe in the dominant hand between the thumb and forefinger. Inject the needle quickly at a 45- or 90-degree angle, depending on the amount of underlying subcutaneous tissue.	
___	___	___	28. If pinching is used, once the needle is inserted, release the skin and stabilize the base of the needle to avoid injecting into the compressed tissue. Slide your dominant hand to the end of the plunger. Avoid moving the syringe.	
___	___	___	29. Inject the medication slowly (at a rate of 10 sec/mL).	
___	___	___	30. Withdraw the needle quickly at the same angle at which it was inserted, while supporting the surrounding tissue with your nondominant hand.	
___	___	___	31. Do not recap the used needle. Engage the safety shield or needle guard.	
___	___	___	32. If blood or clear fluid appears at the site after withdrawing the needle, use a gauze square to apply gentle pressure to the site. ***Do not massage the site.***	
___	___	___	33. Assist the patient to a position of comfort.	
___	___	___	34. Discard the needle and syringe in the appropriate receptacle.	
___	___	___	35. Remove gloves and additional PPE, if used. Perform hand hygiene.	
___	___	___	36. Document the administration of the medication immediately after administration.	
___	___	___	37. Evaluate the patient's response to the medication within the appropriate time frame for the particular medication.	

Skill Checklists for Taylor's Clinical Nursing Skills. A Nursing Process Approach, 5th edition

Name ______________________ Date ______________________

Unit ______________________ Position ______________________

Instructor/Evaluator: ______________________ Position ______________________

SKILL 5-8

Administering an Intramuscular Injection

Excellent	Satisfactory	Needs Practice	**Goal:** The patient receives the medication via the intramuscular route and experiences the intended effect of the medication.	**Comments**
___	___	___	1. Gather equipment. Check each medication order against the original order in the health record according to facility policy. Clarify any inconsistencies. Check the patient's health record for allergies.	
___	___	___	2. Know the actions, special nursing considerations, safe dose ranges, purpose of administration, and adverse effects of the medications to be administered. Consider the appropriateness of the medication for this patient.	
___	___	___	3. Perform hand hygiene.	
___	___	___	4. Move the medication supply system to the outside of the patient's room or prepare for administration at the medication supply system in the medication area. Alternatively, access the medication administration supply system at or inside the patient's room.	
___	___	___	5. Unlock the medication supply system or drawer. Enter pass code and scan employee identification, if required.	
___	___	___	6. *Prepare medications for one patient at a time.*	
___	___	___	7. Read the eMAR/MAR and select the proper medication from medication supply system or the patient's medication drawer.	
___	___	___	8. Compare the label with the eMAR/MAR. Check expiration dates and perform calculations, if necessary. Scan the bar code on the package, if required.	
___	___	___	9. If necessary, withdraw medication from an ampule or vial.	
___	___	___	10. *Depending on facility policy, the third check of the label may occur at this point. If so, when all medications for one patient have been prepared, recheck the labels with the eMAR/MAR before taking the medications to the patient. However, many facilities require the third check to occur at the bedside, after identifying the patient.*	
___	___	___	11. *Lock the medication supply system before leaving it.*	
___	___	___	12. Transport medications to the patient's bedside carefully, and keep the medications in sight at all times.	
___	___	___	13. *Ensure that the patient receives the medications at the correct time.*	

SKILL 5-8

Administering an Intramuscular Injection *(Continued)*

Excellent	Satisfactory	Needs Practice		Comments
___	___	___	14. Perform hand hygiene and put on PPE, if indicated.	
___	___	___	15. ***Identify the patient. Compare the information with the eMAR/MAR. The patient should be identified using at least two of the following methods*** (The Joint Commission, 2018):	
___	___	___	a. Check the name on the patient's identification band.	
___	___	___	b. Check the identification number on the patient's identification band.	
___	___	___	c. Check the birth date on the patient's identification band.	
___	___	___	d. Ask the patient to state his or her name and birth date, based on facility policy.	
___	___	___	16. Close the door to the room or pull the bedside curtain.	
___	___	___	17. ***Complete necessary assessments before administering medications. Check the patient's allergy bracelet or ask the patient about allergies. Explain the purpose and action of the medication to the patient.***	
___	___	___	18. Scan the patient's bar code on the identification band, if required.	
___	___	___	19. ***Based on facility policy, the third check of the label may occur at this point. If so, recheck the labels with the eMAR/MAR before administering the medications to the patient.***	
___	___	___	20. Put on clean gloves.	
___	___	___	21. Select an appropriate administration site.	
___	___	___	22. Assist the patient to the appropriate position for the site chosen. Drape, as needed, to expose only the site area being used.	
___	___	___	23. ***Identify the appropriate landmarks for the site chosen.***	
___	___	___	24. Cleanse the area around the injection site with an antimicrobial swab. Use a firm, circular motion while moving outward from the injection site. Allow the area to dry.	
___	___	___	25. Remove the needle cap by pulling it straight off. Hold the syringe in your dominant hand between the thumb and forefinger.	

SKILL 5-8

Administering an Intramuscular Injection *(Continued)*

Excellent	Satisfactory	Needs Practice		Comments
___	___	___	26. Displace the skin in a Z-track manner. Pull the skin and underlying tissue down or to one side about 1 in (2.5 cm) with your nondominant hand and hold the skin and tissue in this position. Hand and fingers should remain in the appropriate position for the site chosen to continue accurate identification of landmarks and ensure safe injection technique. Alternatively, if, based on assessment of the particular circumstances for an individual patient, the nurse decides not to use the Z-Track technique, the skin should be stretched flat between two fingers and held taut for needle insertion.	
___	___	___	27. Quickly dart the needle into the tissue so that the needle is perpendicular to the patient's body, with the goal of an angle of 90 degrees.	
___	___	___	28. As soon as the needle is in place, use the thumb and forefinger of your nondominant hand to hold the lower end of the syringe, taking care to maintain the displacement of the skin and tissue. Slide your dominant hand to the end of the plunger. Inject the solution slowly (10 sec/mL of medication).	
___	___	___	29. Once the medication has been instilled, wait 10 seconds before withdrawing the needle.	
___	___	___	30. Withdraw the needle smoothly and steadily at the same angle at which it was inserted, supporting tissue around the injection site with your nondominant hand. ***Remove the hand holding the displaced skin and tissue only after removal of the needle.***	
___	___	___	31. Do not recap the used needle. Engage the safety shield or needle guard, if present.	
___	___	___	32. Apply gentle pressure at the site with a dry gauze. ***Do not massage the site.***	
___	___	___	33. Assist the patient to a position of comfort.	
___	___	___	34. Discard the needle and syringe in the appropriate receptacle.	
___	___	___	35. Remove gloves and additional PPE, if used. Perform hand hygiene.	
___	___	___	36. Document the administration of the medication immediately after administration.	
___	___	___	37. Evaluate the patient's response to the medication within the appropriate time frame. Assess site, if possible, within 2 to 4 hours after administration.	

Skill Checklists for Taylor's Clinical Nursing Skills. A Nursing Process Approach, 5th edition

Name ______________________ Date ______________________

Unit ______________________ Position ______________________

Instructor/Evaluator: ______________________ Position ______________________

SKILL 5-9

Administering a Continuous Subcutaneous Infusion: Applying an Insulin Pump

Goal: The device is applied successfully; the medication is administered correctly; and the patient experiences the intended effect of the medication.

Excellent	Satisfactory	Needs Practice		Comments
___	___	___	1. Gather equipment. Check each medication order against the original order in the health record, according to facility policy. Clarify any inconsistencies. Check the patient's health record for allergies.	
___	___	___	2. Know the actions, special nursing considerations, safe dose ranges, purpose of administration, and adverse effects of the medications to be administered. Consider the appropriateness of the medication for this patient.	
___	___	___	3. Perform hand hygiene.	
___	___	___	4. Move the medication supply system to the outside of the patient's room or prepare for administration at the medication supply system in the medication area. Alternatively, access the medication administration supply system at or inside the patient's room.	
___	___	___	5. Unlock the medication supply system or drawer. Enter pass code and scan employee identification, if required.	
___	___	___	6. *Prepare medications for one patient at a time.*	
___	___	___	7. Read the eMAR/MAR and select the proper medication from medication supply system or the patient's medication drawer.	
___	___	___	8. Compare the label with the eMAR/MAR. Check expiration dates and perform calculations, if necessary. Scan the bar code on the package, if required.	
___	___	___	9. Attach a blunt-ended needle or a small-gauge needle to a syringe. Follow Skill 5-4 to prepare insulin from a vial, if necessary. Prepare enough insulin to last the patient 2 to 3 days, plus 30 units for priming tubing. If using a prepackaged insulin syringe or cartridge, remove from packaging.	
___	___	___	10. *Depending on facility policy, the third check of the label may occur at this point. If so, when all medications for one patient have been prepared, recheck the labels with the eMAR/MAR before taking the medications to the patient. However, many facilities require the third check to occur at the bedside, after identifying the patient.*	

Excellent	Satisfactory	Needs Practice	SKILL 5-9 **Administering a Continuous Subcutaneous Infusion: Applying an Insulin Pump** *(Continued)*	**Comments**
___	___	___	11. ***Lock the medication supply system before leaving it.***	
___	___	___	12. Transport medications to the patient's bedside carefully, and keep the medications in sight at all times.	
___	___	___	13. ***Ensure that the patient receives the medications at the correct time.***	
___	___	___	14. Perform hand hygiene and put on PPE, if indicated.	
___	___	___	15. ***Identify the patient. Compare the information with the eMAR/MAR. The patient should be identified using at least two of the following methods*** (The Joint Commission, 2018):	
___	___	___	a. Check the name on the patient's identification band.	
___	___	___	b. Check the identification number on the patient's identification band.	
___	___	___	c. Check the birth date on the patient's identification band.	
___	___	___	d. Ask the patient to state his or her name and birth date, based on facility policy.	
___	___	___	16. Close the door to the room or pull the bedside curtain.	
___	___	___	17. ***Complete necessary assessments before administering medications. Check the patient's allergy bracelet or ask the patient about allergies. Explain the purpose and action of the medication to the patient.***	
___	___	___	18. Scan the patient's bar code on the identification band, if required.	
___	___	___	19. ***Based on facility policy, the third check of the label may occur at this point. If so, recheck the labels with the eMAR/MAR before administering the medications to the patient.***	
___	___	___	20. Perform hand hygiene. Put on gloves.	
___	___	___	21. Remove the cap from the syringe or insulin cartridge. Attach sterile tubing to the syringe or insulin cartridge. Open the pump and place the syringe or cartridge in compartment according to manufacturer's directions. Close the pump.	
___	___	___	22. Initiate priming of the tubing, according to manufacturer's directions. Program the pump according to manufacturer's recommendations following primary care provider's orders. ***Check for any bubbles in the tubing.***	
___	___	___	23. Activate the delivery device. Place the needle between prongs of the insertion device with the sharp edge facing out. Push insertion set down until a click is heard.	

Excellent	Satisfactory	Needs Practice	SKILL 5-9 **Administering a Continuous Subcutaneous Infusion: Applying an Insulin Pump** *(Continued)*	Comments
___	___	___	24. Select an appropriate administration site.	
___	___	___	25. Assist the patient to the appropriate position for the site chosen. Drape, as needed, to expose only site area to be used.	
___	___	___	26. ***Identify the appropriate landmarks for the site chosen.***	
___	___	___	27. Cleanse area around injection site with antimicrobial swab. Use a firm, circular motion while moving outward from insertion site. Allow antiseptic to dry.	
___	___	___	28. Remove paper from adhesive backing. Remove the needle guard. Pinch skin at insertion site, press insertion device on site, and press release button to insert needle. Remove triggering device. Alternatively, if a needle was used to introduce a subcutaneous catheter and then withdrawn, engage the safety shield or needle guard.	
___	___	___	29. Apply sterile occlusive dressing over the insertion site, if not part of the insertion device. Attach the pump to patient's clothing, as desired.	
___	___	___	30. Assist the patient to a position of comfort.	
___	___	___	31. If a needle was used to introduce a subcutaneous catheter and then withdrawn, discard the needle and syringe in the appropriate receptacle.	
___	___	___	32. Remove gloves and additional PPE, if used. Perform hand hygiene.	
___	___	___	33. Document the administration of the medication immediately after administration.	
___	___	___	34. Evaluate the patient's response to the medication within the appropriate time frame. Monitor the patient's blood glucose levels, as appropriate, or as ordered.	

Skill Checklists for Taylor's Clinical Nursing Skills. A Nursing Process Approach, 5th edition

Name ______________________ Date ______________________

Unit ______________________ Position ______________________

Instructor/Evaluator: ______________________ Position ______________________

SKILL 5-10

Administering Medications by Intravenous Bolus or Push Through an Intravenous Infusion

Goal: The medication is given safely via the IV route and the patient experiences the intended effect of the medication.

Excellent	Satisfactory	Needs Practice		Comments
___	___	___	1. Gather equipment. Check medication order against the original order in the medical record, according to facility policy. Clarify any inconsistencies. Check the patient's health record for allergies. Check a drug resource to clarify whether the medication needs to be diluted before administration. Check the administration rate.	
___	___	___	2. Know the actions, special nursing considerations, safe dose ranges, purpose of administration, and adverse effects of the medications to be administered. Consider the appropriateness of the medication for this patient.	
___	___	___	3. Perform hand hygiene.	
___	___	___	4. Move the medication supply system to the outside of the patient's room or prepare for administration at the medication supply system in the medication area. Alternatively, access the medication administration supply system at or inside the patient's room.	
___	___	___	5. Unlock the medication supply system or drawer. Enter pass code and scan employee identification, if required.	
___	___	___	6. *Prepare medication for one patient at a time.*	
___	___	___	7. Read the eMAR/MAR and select the proper medication from the medication supply system or the patient's medication drawer.	
___	___	___	8. Compare the label with the eMAR/MAR. Check expiration dates and perform calculations, if necessary. Scan the bar code on the package, if required.	
___	___	___	9. If necessary, withdraw medication from an ampule or vial.	
___	___	___	10. *Depending on facility policy, the third check of the label may occur at this point. If so, when all medications for one patient have been prepared, recheck the labels with the eMAR/MAR before taking the medications to the patient. However, many facilities require the third check to occur at the bedside, after identifying the patient.*	
___	___	___	11. *Lock the medication supply system before leaving it.*	

Excellent	Satisfactory	Needs Practice	SKILL 5-10 **Administering Medications by Intravenous Bolus or Push Through an Intravenous Infusion** *(Continued)*	Comments
___	___	___	12. Transport medications and equipment to the patient's bedside carefully, and keep the medications in sight at all times.	
___	___	___	13. ***Ensure that the patient receives the medications at the correct time.***	
___	___	___	14. Perform hand hygiene and put on PPE, if indicated.	
___	___	___	15. ***Identify the patient. Compare the information with the eMAR/MAR. The patient should be identified using at least two of the following methods*** (The Joint Commission, 2018):	
___	___	___	a. Check the name on the patient's identification band.	
___	___	___	b. Check the identification number on the patient's identification band.	
___	___	___	c. Check the birth date on the patient's identification band.	
___	___	___	d. Ask the patient to state his or her name and birth date, based on facility policy.	
___	___	___	16. Close the door to the room or pull the bedside curtain.	
___	___	___	17. ***Complete necessary assessments before administering medications. Check the patient's allergy bracelet or ask the patient about allergies. Explain the purpose and action of the medication to the patient.***	
___	___	___	18. Scan the patient's bar code on the identification band, if required.	
___	___	___	19. ***Based on facility policy, the third check of the label may occur at this point. If so, recheck the label with the eMAR/MAR before administering the medications to the patient.***	
___	___	___	20. Assess IV site for presence of inflammation or infiltration or other signs of complications.	
___	___	___	21. If IV infusion is being administered via an infusion pump, pause the pump.	
___	___	___	22. Put on clean gloves.	
___	___	___	23. Select injection port on the administration set that is closest to the patient. Close the clamp on the administration set immediately above the injection port. Do not disconnect the administration set from the venous access device hub (INS, 2016a).	
___	___	___	24. Remove the passive disinfection cap from the needleless connector or end cap on the infusion set injection port. Alternatively, if a passive disinfection cap is not in place, use an antimicrobial swab to vigorously scrub the needleless connector or end cap on the injection port and allow to dry.	

Excellent	Satisfactory	Needs Practice	SKILL 5-10 **Administering Medications by Intravenous Bolus or Push Through an Intravenous Infusion** *(Continued)*	Comments
___	___	___	25. Uncap saline flush syringe. Insert the saline flush syringe into the needleless connector or end cap on the injection port on the administration tubing.	
___	___	___	26. Pull back on the syringe plunger to aspirate the catheter for positive blood return. If positive, instill the solution over 1 minute or flush the line according to facility policy. Remove syringe.	
___	___	___	27. Use an antimicrobial swab to vigorously scrub the needleless connector or end cap on the injection port and allow to dry.	
___	___	___	28. Uncap the medication syringe. Insert the medication syringe into the needleless connector or end cap on the injection port. Using a watch or clock with a second-hand to time the rate, ***inject the medication at the recommended rate.***	
___	___	___	29. While administering the medication, observe the infusion site and assess patient for any adverse reaction. If signs of adverse reaction occur, stop infusion immediately and notify the primary health provider.	
___	___	___	30. Detach the medication syringe. Use a new antimicrobial swab to vigorously scrub the needleless connector or end cap on the injection port, and allow to dry. Uncap the second saline flush syringe. Insert the saline flush syringe into the needleless connector or end cap on injection port. Instill the flush solution at the same rate as the administered medication (INS, 2016a).	
___	___	___	31. Remove the flush syringe. Unclamp the administration set above the injection port.	
___	___	___	32. Using an antimicrobial swab, vigorously scrub the needleless connector or end cap on the extension tubing and allow to dry. Attach a passive disinfection cap to the needleless connector or end cap on the extension tubing or the injection port on the administration set.	
___	___	___	33. Restart the infusion pump and check IV fluid infusion rate.	
___	___	___	34. Discard the syringe in the appropriate receptacle.	
___	___	___	35. Remove gloves and additional PPE, if used. Perform hand hygiene.	
___	___	___	36. Document the administration of the medication immediately after administration.	
___	___	___	37. Evaluate the patient's response to the medication within the appropriate time frame.	

Skill Checklists for Taylor's Clinical Nursing Skills. A Nursing Process Approach, 5th edition

Name ______________________ Date ______________________

Unit ______________________ Position ______________________

Instructor/Evaluator: ______________________ Position ______________________

SKILL 5-11

Administering Medications by Intravenous Bolus or Push Through a Medication or Drug-Infusion Lock

Goal: The medication is delivered via the IV route and the patient experiences the intended effect of the medication.

Excellent	Satisfactory	Needs Practice		Comments
___	___	___	1. Gather equipment. Check the medication order against the original order in the health record, according to facility policy. Clarify any inconsistencies. Check the patient's health record for allergies. Check a drug resource to clarify whether medication needs to be diluted before bolus administration. Verify the recommended administration rate.	
___	___	___	2. Know the actions, special nursing considerations, safe dose ranges, purpose of administration, and adverse effects of the medications to be administered. Consider the appropriateness of the medication for this patient.	
___	___	___	3. Perform hand hygiene.	
___	___	___	4. Move the medication supply system to the outside of the patient's room or prepare for administration at the medication supply system in the medication area. Alternatively, access the medication administration supply system at or inside the patient's room.	
___	___	___	5. Unlock the medication supply system or drawer. Enter pass code and scan employee identification, if required.	
___	___	___	6. ***Prepare medication for one patient at a time.***	
___	___	___	7. Read the eMAR/MAR and select the proper medication from medication supply system or the patient's medication drawer.	
___	___	___	8. Compare the label with the eMAR/MAR. Check expiration dates and perform calculations, if necessary. Scan the bar code on the package, if required.	
___	___	___	9. If necessary, withdraw medication from an ampule or vial.	
___	___	___	10. ***Depending on facility policy, the third check of the label may occur at this point. If so, when all medications for one patient have been prepared, recheck the labels with the eMAR/MAR before taking the medications to the patient. However, many facilities require the third check to occur at the bedside, after identifying the patient.***	
___	___	___	11. ***Lock the medication supply system before leaving it.***	
___	___	___	12. Transport medications and equipment to the patient's bedside carefully, and keep the medications in sight at all times.	

Excellent	Satisfactory	Needs Practice	SKILL 5-11 **Administering Medications by Intravenous Bolus or Push Through a Medication or Drug-Infusion Lock** *(Continued)*	Comments
___	___	___	13. *Ensure that the patient receives the medications at the correct time.*	
___	___	___	14. Perform hand hygiene and put on PPE, if indicated.	
___	___	___	15. ***Identify the patient. Compare the information with the eMAR/ MAR. The patient should be identified using at least two of the following methods*** (The Joint Commission, 2018):	
___	___	___	a. Check the name on the patient's identification band.	
___	___	___	b. Check the identification number on the patient's identification band.	
___	___	___	c. Check the birth date on the patient's identification band.	
___	___	___	d. Ask the patient to state his or her name and birth date, based on facility policy.	
___	___	___	16. Close the door to the room or pull the bedside curtain.	
___	___	___	17. ***Complete necessary assessments before administering medications. Check the patient's allergy bracelet or ask the patient about allergies. Explain the purpose and action of the medication to the patient.***	
___	___	___	18. Scan the patient's bar code on the identification band, if required.	
___	___	___	19. ***Based on facility policy, the third check of the label may occur at this point. If so, recheck the labels with the eMAR/ MAR before administering the medications to the patient.***	
___	___	___	20. Assess IV site for presence of inflammation or infiltration.	
___	___	___	21. Put on clean gloves.	
___	___	___	22. Remove the passive disinfection cap from the needleless connector or access port of the medication lock. Alternatively, if a passive disinfection cap is not in place, use an antimicrobial swab to vigorously scrub the needleless connector or access port of the medication lock and allow to dry.	
___	___	___	23. Uncap saline flush syringe. Stabilize the port with your nondominant hand and insert the saline flush syringe into the needleless connector or end cap on the access port of the medication lock.	
___	___	___	24. Release the clamp on the extension tubing of the medication lock. Pull back on the syringe plunger to aspirate the catheter for positive blood return. If positive, instill the solution over 1 minute or flush the line according to facility policy. Observe the insertion site while inserting the saline. Remove syringe.	

Excellent	Satisfactory	Needs Practice	SKILL 5-11 **Administering Medications by Intravenous Bolus or Push Through a Medication or Drug-Infusion Lock** *(Continued)*	Comments
___	___	___	25. Use an antimicrobial swab to vigorously scrub the needleless connector or end cap on the access port of the medication lock and allow to dry.	
___	___	___	26. Uncap the medication syringe. Insert the medication syringe into the needleless connector or end cap on the access port of the medication lock. Using a watch or clock with a second-hand to time the rate, ***inject the medication at the recommended rate. Do not force the injection if resistance is felt.***	
___	___	___	27. While administering the medication, observe the infusion site and assess patient for any adverse reaction. If signs of adverse reaction occur, stop infusion immediately and notify the primary health provider.	
___	___	___	28. Remove the medication syringe from the access port. Use a new antimicrobial swab to vigorously scrub the needleless connector or end cap on the access port and allow to dry. Stabilize the port with your nondominant hand. Uncap the second saline flush syringe. Insert the saline flush syringe into the needleless connector or end cap on the access port. Instill the flush solution at the same rate as the administered medication (INS, 2016a).	
___	___	___	29. If the medication lock is capped with positive pressure valve/device, remove syringe, and then clamp the extension tubing. Alternatively, to gain positive pressure if positive pressure valve/device is not present, clamp the extension tubing as you are still flushing the last of the saline into the medication lock. Remove syringe.	
___	___	___	30. Using an antimicrobial swab, vigorously scrub the needleless connector or end cap on the access port of the medication lock and allow to dry. Attach a passive disinfection cap to the needleless connector or end cap on the access port of the medication lock.	
___	___	___	31. Discard the syringe in the appropriate receptacle.	
___	___	___	32. Remove gloves and additional PPE, if used. Perform hand hygiene.	
___	___	___	33. Document the administration of the medication immediately after administration.	
___	___	___	34. Evaluate the patient's response to the medication within an appropriate time frame.	

Skill Checklists for Taylor's Clinical Nursing Skills. A Nursing Process Approach, 5th edition

Name ______________________ Date ______________________

Unit ______________________ Position ______________________

Instructor/Evaluator: ______________________ Position ______________________

SKILL 5-12

Administering a Piggyback Intermittent Intravenous Infusion of Medication

Excellent	Satisfactory	Needs Practice	**Goal:** The medication is delivered via the intravenous route and the patient experiences the intended effect of the medication.	Comments
___	___	___	1. Gather equipment. Check each medication order against the original order in the health record, according to facility policy. Clarify any inconsistencies. Check the patient's health record for allergies.	
___	___	___	2. Know the actions, special nursing considerations, safe dose ranges, purpose of administration, and adverse effects of the medications to be administered. Consider the appropriateness of the medication for this patient. ***Assess the compatibility of the ordered medication, diluent, and the infusing IV fluid.***	
___	___	___	3. Perform hand hygiene.	
___	___	___	4. Move the medication supply system to the outside of the patient's room or prepare for administration at the medication supply system in the medication area. Alternatively, access the medication administration supply system at or inside the patient's room.	
___	___	___	5. Unlock the medication supply system or drawer. Enter pass code and scan employee identification, if required.	
___	___	___	6. ***Prepare medications for one patient at a time.***	
___	___	___	7. Read the eMAR/MAR and select the proper medication from the medication supply system or the patient's medication drawer.	
___	___	___	8. Compare the label with the eMAR/MAR. Check expiration dates. Confirm the prescribed or appropriate infusion rate. Calculate the drip rate if using a gravity system. Scan the bar code on the package, if required.	
___	___	___	9. ***Depending on facility policy, the third check of the label may occur at this point. If so, when all medications for one patient have been prepared, recheck the labels with the eMAR/MAR before taking the medications to the patient. However, many facilities require the third check to occur at the bedside, after identifying the patient.***	
___	___	___	10. ***Lock the medication supply system before leaving it.***	
___	___	___	11. Transport medications to the patient's bedside carefully, and keep the medications in sight at all times.	

Excellent	Satisfactory	Needs Practice	SKILL 5-12 **Administering a Piggyback Intermittent Intravenous Infusion of Medication** *(Continued)*	Comments
___	___	___	12. ***Ensure that the patient receives the medications at the correct time.***	
___	___	___	13. Perform hand hygiene and put on PPE, if indicated.	
___	___	___	14. ***Identify the patient. Compare the information with the eMAR/MAR. The patient should be identified using at least two of the following methods*** (The Joint Commission, 2018):	
___	___	___	a. Check the name on the patient's identification band.	
___	___	___	b. Check the identification number on the patient's identification band.	
___	___	___	c. Check the birth date on the patient's identification band.	
___	___	___	d. Ask the patient to state his or her name and birth date, based on facility policy.	
___	___	___	15. Close the door to the room or pull the bedside curtain.	
___	___	___	16. ***Complete necessary assessments before administering medications. Check the patient's allergy bracelet or ask the patient about allergies. Explain the purpose and action of the medication to the patient.***	
___	___	___	17. Scan the patient's bar code on the identification band, if required.	
___	___	___	18. ***Based on facility policy, the third check of the label may occur at this point. If so, recheck the labels with the eMAR/MAR before administering the medications to the patient.***	
___	___	___	19. Assess the IV site for the presence of complications.	
___	___	___	20. Close the clamp on the short secondary infusion tubing. Using aseptic technique, remove the cap on the tubing spike and the cap on the port of the medication container, taking care to avoid contaminating either end.	
___	___	___	21. Attach infusion tubing to the medication container by inserting the tubing spike into the port with a firm push and twisting motion, taking care to avoid contaminating either end.	
___	___	___	22. Hang piggyback container on IV pole, positioning it higher than primary IV according to manufacturer's recommendations. If necessary for the particular infusion pump in use, use the metal or plastic hook to lower primary IV fluid container. If using gravity infusion, primary IV fluid container must be lowered.	
___	___	___	23. Place label on administration tubing with the current date.	

Excellent	Satisfactory	Needs Practice	SKILL 5-12 **Administering a Piggyback Intermittent Intravenous Infusion of Medication** *(Continued)*	**Comments**
___	___	___	24. Squeeze drip chamber on administration tubing and release. Fill chamber to the line or about half full. Open clamp on administration tubing and prime tubing. Close clamp. Place needleless connector on the end of the tubing, using sterile technique, if required.	
___	___	___	25. Remove the passive disinfection cap from the needleless connector or end cap on the infusion set injection port. Alternatively, if a passive disinfection cap is not in place, use an antimicrobial swab to vigorously scrub the access port or stopcock on the administration set above where the tubing enters the infusion pump or above the roller clamp on the primary IV infusion tubing (gravity infusion).	
___	___	___	26. Connect piggyback setup to the access port or stopcock. If using, turn the stopcock to the open position.	
___	___	___	27. Open clamp on the secondary infusion tubing. Set rate for secondary infusion on infusion pump and begin infusion. If using gravity infusion, use the roller clamp on the primary infusion tubing to regulate the flow at the prescribed delivery rate. Monitor medication infusion at periodic intervals.	
___	___	___	28. Clamp tubing on piggyback set when solution is infused. Follow facility policy regarding disposal of equipment.	
___	___	___	29. Raise primary IV fluid container to original height. ***Check primary infusion rate on infusion pump. If using gravity infusion, readjust flow rate of primary IV.***	
___	___	___	30. Remove PPE, if used. Perform hand hygiene.	
___	___	___	31. Document the administration of the medication immediately after administration. Document the volume of fluid administered on the intake and output record, if necessary.	
___	___	___	32. Evaluate the patient's response to the medication within an appropriate time frame. Monitor IV site at periodic intervals.	

Skill Checklists for Taylor's Clinical Nursing Skills. A Nursing Process Approach, 5th edition

Name ______________________ Date ______________

Unit ______________________ Position ______________

Instructor/Evaluator: ______________________ Position ______________

SKILL 5-13

Administering an Intermittent Intravenous Infusion of Medication via a Mini-Infusion Pump

Excellent	Satisfactory	Needs Practice	**Goal:** The medication is delivered via the intravenous route and the patient experiences the intended effect of the medication.	**Comments**
___	___	___	1. Gather equipment. Check each medication order against the original order in the health record according to facility policy. Clarify any inconsistencies. Check the patient's health record for allergies.	
___	___	___	2. Know the actions, special nursing considerations, safe dose ranges, purpose of administration, and adverse effects of the medications to be administered. Consider the appropriateness of the medication for this patient. ***Assess the compatibility of the ordered medication, diluent, and the infusing IV fluid.***	
___	___	___	3. Perform hand hygiene.	
___	___	___	4. Move the medication supply system to the outside of the patient's room or prepare for administration at the medication supply system in the medication area. Alternatively, access the medication administration supply system at or inside the patient's room.	
___	___	___	5. Unlock the medication supply system or drawer. Enter pass code and scan employee identification, if required.	
___	___	___	6. ***Prepare medications for one patient at a time.***	
___	___	___	7. Read the eMAR/MAR and select the proper medication from the medication supply system or the patient's medication drawer.	
___	___	___	8. Compare the label with the eMAR/MAR. Check expiration dates. Confirm the prescribed or appropriate infusion rate. Scan the bar code on the package, if required.	
___	___	___	9. ***Depending on facility policy, the third check of the label may occur at this point. If so, when all medications for one patient have been prepared, recheck the labels with the eMAR/MAR before taking the medications to the patient. However, many facilities require the third check to occur at the bedside, after identifying the patient.***	
___	___	___	10. ***Lock the medication supply system before leaving it.***	
___	___	___	11. Transport medications to the patient's bedside carefully, and keep the medications in sight at all times.	

Excellent	Satisfactory	Needs Practice	SKILL 5-13 **Administering an Intermittent Intravenous Infusion of Medication via a Mini-Infusion Pump** *(Continued)*	**Comments**
___	___	___	12. ***Ensure that the patient receives the medications at the correct time.***	
___	___	___	13. Perform hand hygiene and put on PPE, if indicated.	
___	___	___	14. ***Identify the patient. Compare the information with the eMAR/MAR. The patient should be identified using at least two of the following methods*** (The Joint Commission, 2018):	
___	___	___	a. Check the name on the patient's identification band.	
___	___	___	b. Check the identification number on the patient's identification band.	
___	___	___	c. Check the birth date on the patient's identification band.	
___	___	___	d. Ask the patient to state his or her name and birth date, based on facility policy.	
___	___	___	15. Close the door to the room or pull the bedside curtain.	
___	___	___	16. ***Complete necessary assessments before administering medications. Check the patient's allergy bracelet or ask the patient about allergies. Explain the purpose and action of the medication to the patient.***	
___	___	___	17. Scan the patient's bar code on the identification band, if required.	
___	___	___	18. ***Based on facility policy, the third check of the label may occur at this point. If so, recheck the labels with the eMAR/MAR before administering the medications to the patient.***	
___	___	___	19. Assess the IV site for the presence of complications.	
___	___	___	20. Using aseptic technique, remove the cap on the administration tubing and the cap on the medication syringe, taking care not to contaminate either end.	
___	___	___	21. Attach administration tubing to the syringe, taking care not to contaminate either end.	
___	___	___	22. Place label on tubing with current date.	
___	___	___	23. Fill administration tubing (prime) with medication by applying gentle pressure to syringe plunger. Place needleless connector on the end of the tubing, if required, using sterile technique.	
___	___	___	24. Insert syringe into mini-infusion pump according to manufacturer's directions.	

Excellent	Satisfactory	Needs Practice	SKILL 5-13 **Administering an Intermittent Intravenous Infusion of Medication via a Mini-Infusion Pump** *(Continued)*	Comments
___	___	___	25. Remove the passive disinfection cap from the needleless connector or end cap on the access port on the primary IV infusion tubing, closest to the IV insertion site. Alternatively, if a passive disinfection cap is not in place, use an antimicrobial swab to vigorously scrub the access port or stopcock above the roller clamp on the primary IV infusion tubing, usually the port closest to the IV insertion site.	
___	___	___	26. Connect the secondary infusion to the primary infusion at the access port.	
___	___	___	27. Program the mini-infusion pump to the appropriate rate and begin infusion. Set the alarm if recommended by the manufacturer.	
___	___	___	28. Clamp tubing on secondary IV infusion administration set when solution is infused. Follow facility policy regarding disposal of equipment.	
___	___	___	29. Check rate of primary infusion.	
___	___	___	30. Remove PPE, if used. Perform hand hygiene.	
___	___	___	31. Document the administration of the medication immediately after administration. Document the volume of fluid administered on the intake and output record, if necessary.	
___	___	___	32. Evaluate the patient's response to the medication within appropriate time frame. Monitor IV site at periodic intervals.	

Skill Checklists for Taylor's Clinical Nursing Skills. A Nursing Process Approach, 5th edition

Name ______________________ Date ______________________

Unit ______________________ Position ______________________

Instructor/Evaluator: ______________________ Position ______________________

SKILL 5-14

Applying a Transdermal Patch

Goal: The medication is delivered via the transdermal route and the patient experiences the intended effect of the medication.

Excellent	Satisfactory	Needs Practice		Comments
___	___	___	1. Gather equipment. Check medication order against the original order in the patient's health record, according to facility policy. Clarify any inconsistencies. Check the patient's health record for allergies.	
___	___	___	2. Know the actions, special nursing considerations, safe dose ranges, purpose of administration, and adverse effects of the medications to be administered. Consider the appropriateness of the medication for this patient.	
___	___	___	3. Perform hand hygiene.	
___	___	___	4. Move the medication supply system to the outside of the patient's room or prepare for administration at the medication supply system in the medication area. Alternatively, access the medication administration supply system at or inside the patient's room.	
___	___	___	5. Unlock the medication supply system or drawer. Enter pass code and scan employee identification, if required.	
___	___	___	6. ***Prepare medications for one patient at a time.***	
___	___	___	7. Read the eMAR/MAR and select the proper medication from medication supply system or the patient's medication drawer.	
___	___	___	8. Compare the label with the eMAR/MAR. Check expiration dates and perform calculations, if necessary. Scan the bar code on the package, if required.	
___	___	___	9. ***Depending on facility policy, the third check of the label may occur at this point. If so, when all medications for one patient have been prepared, recheck the labels with the eMAR/MAR before taking the medications to the patient. However, many facilities require the third check to occur at the bedside, after identifying the patient.***	
___	___	___	10. ***Lock the medication supply system before leaving it.***	
___	___	___	11. Transport medications to the patient's bedside carefully, and keep the medications in sight at all times.	
___	___	___	12. ***Ensure that the patient receives the medications at the correct time.***	
___	___	___	13. Perform hand hygiene and put on PPE, if indicated.	

Excellent	Satisfactory	Needs Practice	SKILL 5-14 **Applying a Transdermal Patch** *(Continued)*	Comments
___	___	___	14. ***Identify the patient. Compare the information with the eMAR/MAR. The patient should be identified using at least two of the following methods*** (The Joint Commission, 2018):	
___	___	___	a. Check the name on the patient's identification band.	
___	___	___	b. Check the identification number on the patient's identification band.	
___	___	___	c. Check the birth date on the patient's identification band.	
___	___	___	d. Ask the patient to state his or her name and birth date, based on facility policy.	
___	___	___	15. ***Complete necessary assessments before administering medications. Check the patient's allergy bracelet or ask the patient about allergies. Explain the purpose and action of each medication to the patient.***	
___	___	___	16. Scan the patient's bar code on the identification band, if required.	
___	___	___	17. ***Based on facility policy, the third check of the label may occur at this point. If so, recheck the labels with the eMAR/MAR before administering the medications to the patient.***	
___	___	___	18. Put on gloves.	
___	___	___	19. Assess the patient's skin where patch is to be placed, looking for any signs of irritation or breakdown. Site should be clean, dry, and free of hair. Rotate application sites.	
___	___	___	20. ***Remove any old transdermal patches of the same kind from the patient's skin.*** Fold the old patch in half with the adhesive sides sticking together and discard according to facility policy. Gently wash the area where the old patch was with a disposable washcloth or soap and water.	
___	___	___	21. Remove the patch from its protective covering. Remove the covering on the patch without touching the medication surface. Apply the patch to the patient's skin. Use the palm of your hand to press firmly for about 10 seconds. Do not massage.	
___	___	___	22. Depending on facility policy, initial and write the date and time of administration on a piece of medical tape. Apply the tape to the patient's skin in close proximity to the patch. ***Do not write directly on the medication patch.***	
___	___	___	23. Remove gloves and additional PPE, if used. Perform hand hygiene.	
___	___	___	24. Document the administration of the medication immediately after administration.	
___	___	___	25. Evaluate the patient's response to the medication within the appropriate time frame.	

Skill Checklists for Taylor's Clinical Nursing Skills.
A Nursing Process Approach, 5th edition

Name ____________________ Date ____________________

Unit ____________________ Position ____________________

Instructor/Evaluator: ____________________ Position ____________________

SKILL 5-15

Administering Eye Drops

Goal: The medication is delivered successfully into the eye and the patient experiences the intended effect of the medication.

Excellent	Satisfactory	Needs Practice		Comments
___	___	___	1. Gather equipment. Check medication order against the original order in the health record, according to facility policy. Clarify any inconsistencies. Check the patient's health record for allergies.	
___	___	___	2. Know the actions, special nursing considerations, safe dose ranges, purpose of administration, and adverse effects of the medications to be administered. Consider the appropriateness of the medication for this patient.	
___	___	___	3. Perform hand hygiene.	
___	___	___	4. Move the medication supply system to the outside of the patient's room or prepare for administration at the medication supply system in the medication area. Alternatively, access the medication administration supply system at or inside the patient's room.	
___	___	___	5. Unlock the medication supply system or drawer. Enter pass code and scan employee identification, if required.	
___	___	___	6. *Prepare medications for one patient at a time.*	
___	___	___	7. Read the eMAR/MAR and select the proper medication from the patient's medication drawer or medication supply system.	
___	___	___	8. Compare the label with the eMAR/MAR. Check expiration dates and perform calculations, if necessary. Scan the bar code on the package, if required.	
___	___	___	9. *Depending on facility policy, the third check of the label may occur at this point. If so, when all medications for one patient have been prepared, recheck the labels with the eMAR/MAR before taking the medications to the patient. However, many facilities require the third check to occur at the bedside, after identifying the patient.*	
___	___	___	10. *Lock the medication supply system before leaving it.*	
___	___	___	11. Transport medications to the patient's bedside carefully, and keep the medications in sight at all times.	
___	___	___	12. *Ensure that the patient receives the medications at the correct time.*	
___	___	___	13. Perform hand hygiene and put on PPE, if indicated.	

Excellent	Satisfactory	Needs Practice	SKILL 5-15 **Administering Eye Drops** *(Continued)*	Comments
___	___	___	14. ***Identify the patient. Compare the information with the eMAR/MAR. The patient should be identified using at least two of the following methods*** (The Joint Commission, 2018):	
___	___	___	a. Check the name on the patient's identification band.	
___	___	___	b. Check the identification number on the patient's identification band.	
___	___	___	c. Check the birth date on the patient's identification band.	
___	___	___	d. Ask the patient to state his or her name and birth date, based on facility policy.	
___	___	___	15. ***Complete necessary assessments before administering medications. Check the patient's allergy bracelet or ask the patient about allergies. Explain the purpose and action of each medication to the patient.***	
___	___	___	16. Scan the patient's bar code on the identification band, if required.	
___	___	___	17. ***Based on facility policy, the third check of the label may occur at this point. If so, recheck the labels with the eMAR/MAR before administering the medications to the patient.***	
___	___	___	18. Put on gloves.	
___	___	___	19. Offer tissue to patient.	
___	___	___	20. Cleanse the eyelids and eyelashes of any drainage with a washcloth, cotton balls, or gauze squares moistened with water or normal saline solution, as indicated by the patient's condition. Use each area of the cleaning surface once, moving from the inner toward the outer canthus.	
___	___	___	21. Tilt the patient's head back slightly if sitting, or place the patient's head over a pillow if lying down. ***Tilting the patient's head should be avoided if the patient has a cervical spine injury or other condition resulting in limited range-of-notion.*** The head may be turned slightly to the affected side to prevent solution or tears from flowing toward the opposite eye.	
___	___	___	22. Remove the cap from the medication bottle, being careful not to touch the inner side of the cap or the tip of the container.	
___	___	___	23. Invert the monodrip plastic container that is commonly used to instill eye drops. Have the patient look up and focus on something on the ceiling.	

SKILL 5-15

Administering Eye Drops *(Continued)*

Excellent	Satisfactory	Needs Practice		Comments
___	___	___	24. Place thumb or two fingers near margin of lower eyelid immediately below eyelashes, and apply pressure downward over bony cheek prominence. The lower conjunctival sac is exposed as the lower lid is pulled down.	
___	___	___	25. Rest the lateral side of your hand on the patient's forehead, just above the eyebrow. ***Hold the dropper close to the eye, but avoid touching eyelids or lashes.*** Squeeze container and allow prescribed number of drops to fall in lower conjunctival sac.	
___	___	___	26. Release lower lid after eye drops are instilled. Ask patient to close eyes gently.	
___	___	___	27. Apply gentle pressure over inner canthus to prevent eye drops from flowing into tear duct.	
___	___	___	28. Instruct patient not to rub affected eye. Replace the cover on the medication bottle.	
___	___	___	29. Remove gloves. Assist the patient to a comfortable position.	
___	___	___	30. Remove additional PPE, if used. Perform hand hygiene.	
___	___	___	31. Document the administration of the medication immediately after administration.	
___	___	___	32. Evaluate the patient's response to the medication within an appropriate time frame.	

Skill Checklists for Taylor's Clinical Nursing Skills. A Nursing Process Approach, 5th edition

Name ______________________ Date ______________________

Unit ______________________ Position ______________________

Instructor/Evaluator: ______________________ Position ______________________

SKILL 5-16
Administering an Eye Irrigation

Excellent	Satisfactory	Needs Practice	**Goal:** The eye is cleansed successfully.	Comments
___	___	___	1. Gather equipment. Check the original order in the patient's health record for the irrigation, according to facility policy. Clarify any inconsistencies. Check the patient's health record for allergies.	
___	___	___	2. Know the actions, special nursing considerations, purpose of administration, and potential adverse effects of the medications to be administered. Consider the appropriateness of the medication for this patient.	
___	___	___	3. Perform hand hygiene and put on PPE, if indicated.	
___	___	___	4. Move the medication supply system to the outside of the patient's room or prepare for administration at the medication supply system in the medication area. Alternatively, access the medication administration supply system at or inside the patient's room.	
___	___	___	5. Unlock the medication supply system or drawer. Enter pass code into the computer and scan employee identification, if required.	
___	___	___	6. ***Prepare medications for one patient at a time.***	
___	___	___	7. Read the eMAR/MAR and select the proper irrigation solution from the medication supply system or patient's medication drawer.	
___	___	___	8. Compare the medication label with the eMAR/MAR. Check expiration dates and perform calculations, if necessary. Scan the bar code on the package, if required.	
___	___	___	9. ***Depending on facility policy, the third check of the label may occur at this point. If so, when all medications for one patient have been prepared, recheck the labels with the eMAR/MAR before taking the medications to the patient. However, many facilities require the third check to occur at the bedside, after identifying the patient.***	
___	___	___	10. ***Lock the medication supply system before leaving it.***	
___	___	___	11. ***Ensure that the patient receives the medications at the correct time.***	
___	___	___	12. Perform hand hygiene and put on PPE, if indicated.	

Excellent	Satisfactory	Needs Practice	SKILL 5-16 **Administering an Eye Irrigation** *(Continued)*	Comments
___	___	___	13. ***Identify the patient. Compare the information with the eMAR/MAR. The patient should be identified using at least two of the following methods*** (The Joint Commission, 2018):	
___	___	___	a. Check the name on the patient's identification band.	
___	___	___	b. Check the identification number on the patient's identification band.	
___	___	___	c. Check the birth date on the patient's identification band.	
___	___	___	d. Ask the patient to state his or her name and birth date, based on facility policy.	
___	___	___	14. ***Complete necessary assessments before administering medications. Check the patient's allergy bracelet or ask the patient about allergies. Explain the purpose and action of each medication to the patient.***	
___	___	___	15. Scan the patient's bar code on the identification band, if required.	
___	___	___	16. Assemble equipment at the patient's bedside.	
___	___	___	17. ***Based on facility policy, the third check of the medication label may occur at this point. If so, recheck the label with the eMAR/MAR before administering the medications to the patient.***	
___	___	___	18. Have the patient sit or lie with head tilted toward side of affected eye. Protect the patient and bed with a waterproof pad.	
___	___	___	19. Put on gloves. Clean lids and lashes with washcloth moistened with water or normal saline or the solution ordered for the irrigation, as indicated by the patient's condition. Wipe from inner canthus toward outer canthus. Use a different corner of washcloth with each wipe.	
___	___	___	20. Put on face shield/splash guard. Place curved basin at cheek on the side of the affected eye to receive irrigating solution. If patient is able, ask him/her to support the basin.	
___	___	___	21. Place thumb near margin of lower eyelid immediately below eyelashes and two fingers above eye. Apply pressure downward over bony cheek prominence to expose the lower conjunctival sac as the lower lid is pulled down. Hold upper lid open with your fingers.	
___	___	___	22. Fill the irrigation syringe with the prescribed fluid. ***Hold irrigation syringe about 2.5 cm (1 in) from eye. Direct flow of solution from inner to outer canthus along the conjunctival sac.***	

Excellent	Satisfactory	Needs Practice	SKILL 5-16 **Administering an Eye Irrigation** *(Continued)*	Comments
___	___	___	23. Irrigate until the solution is clear or all the solution has been used. ***Use only enough force to remove secretions gently from the conjunctiva. Avoid touching any part of the eye with the irrigating tip.***	
___	___	___	24. Pause the irrigation and have the patient close the eye periodically during the procedure.	
___	___	___	25. Dry the periorbital area after irrigation with gauze sponge. Offer a towel to the patient if face and neck are wet.	
___	___	___	26. Remove gloves. Assist the patient to a comfortable position.	
___	___	___	27. Remove face shield and splash guard and additional PPE, if used. Perform hand hygiene.	
___	___	___	28. Evaluate the patient's response to the medication within an appropriate time frame.	

Skill Checklists for Taylor's Clinical Nursing Skills. A Nursing Process Approach, 5th edition

Name ______________________ Date ______________________

Unit ______________________ Position ______________________

Instructor/Evaluator: ______________________ Position ______________________

SKILL 5-17

Administering Ear Drops

Excellent	Satisfactory	Needs Practice	**Goal:** The drops are administered successfully and the patient experiences the intended effect of the medication.	Comments
___	___	___	1. Gather equipment. Check medication order against the original order in the health record, according to facility policy. Clarify any inconsistencies. Check the patient's health record for allergies.	
___	___	___	2. Know the actions, special nursing considerations, safe dose ranges, purpose of administration, and adverse effects of the medication to be administered. Consider the appropriateness of the medication for this patient.	
___	___	___	3. Perform hand hygiene.	
___	___	___	4. Move the medication supply system to the outside of the patient's room or prepare for administration at the medication supply system in the medication area. Alternatively, access the medication administration supply system at or inside the patient's room.	
___	___	___	5. Unlock the medication supply system or drawer. Enter pass code and scan employee identification, if required.	
___	___	___	6. ***Prepare medications for one patient at a time.***	
___	___	___	7. Read the eMAR/MAR and select the proper medication from the patient's medication drawer or medication supply system.	
___	___	___	8. Compare the label with the eMAR/MAR. Check expiration dates and perform calculations, if necessary. Scan the bar code on the package, if required.	
___	___	___	9. ***Depending on facility policy, the third check of the label may occur at this point. If so, when all medications for one patient have been prepared, recheck the labels with the eMAR/MAR before taking the medications to the patient. However, many facilities require the third check to occur at the bedside, after identifying the patient.***	
___	___	___	10. ***Lock the medication supply system before leaving it.***	
___	___	___	11. Transport medications to the patient's bedside carefully, and keep the medications in sight at all times.	
___	___	___	12. ***Ensure that the patient receives the medications at the correct time.***	
___	___	___	13. Perform hand hygiene and put on PPE, if indicated.	

Excellent	Satisfactory	Needs Practice	SKILL 5-17 **Administering Ear Drops** *(Continued)*	Comments
___	___	___	14. ***Identify the patient. Compare the information with the eMAR/MAR. The patient should be identified using at least two of the following methods*** (The Joint Commission, 2018):	
___	___	___	a. Check the name on the patient's identification band.	
___	___	___	b. Check the identification number on the patient's identification band.	
___	___	___	c. Check the birth date on the patient's identification band.	
___	___	___	d. Ask the patient to state his or her name and birth date, based on facility policy.	
___	___	___	15. ***Complete necessary assessments before administering medications. Check the patient's allergy bracelet or ask the patient about allergies. Explain the purpose and action of each medication to the patient.***	
___	___	___	16. Scan the patient's bar code on the identification band, if required.	
___	___	___	17. ***Based on facility policy, the third check of the label may occur at this point. If so, recheck the labels with the eMAR/MAR before administering the medications to the patient.***	
___	___	___	18. Put on gloves.	
___	___	___	19. Cleanse external ear of any drainage with cotton ball or washcloth moistened with normal saline or water.	
___	___	___	20. Place patient on his or her unaffected side in bed, or, if ambulatory, have patient sit with head well tilted to the side so that the affected ear is uppermost.	
___	___	___	21. Remove the cap from the medication bottle, being careful not to touch the inner side of the cap or the tip of the container.	
___	___	___	22. Straighten auditory canal by pulling cartilaginous portion of pinna up and back for an adult.	
___	___	___	23. Invert and hold medication bottle in the ear with its tip above the auditory canal. Do not touch the dropper to the ear.	
___	___	___	24. ***Squeeze container and allow drops to fall on the side of the canal. Avoid instilling in the middle of the canal, to avoid instilling directly onto the tympanic membrane.***	
___	___	___	25. Release pinna after instilling drops, and have patient maintain the head position to prevent escape of medication.	
___	___	___	26. Gently press on the tragus a few times.	

Excellent	Satisfactory	Needs Practice	SKILL 5-17 **Administering Ear Drops** *(Continued)*	Comments
____	____	____	27. If ordered, loosely insert a cotton ball into the ear canal.	
____	____	____	28. Instruct patient to remain lying down with the affected ear upward for 5 minutes.	
____	____	____	29. Replace cap on medication bottle. Remove gloves and additional PPE, if used. Perform hand hygiene.	
____	____	____	30. Document the administration of the medication immediately after administration.	
____	____	____	31. Evaluate the patient's response to medication within an appropriate time frame.	

Skill Checklists for Taylor's Clinical Nursing Skills.
A Nursing Process Approach, 5th edition

Name ______________________ Date ______________

Unit ______________________ Position ______________

Instructor/Evaluator: ______________________ Position ______________

Excellent	Satisfactory	Needs Practice	SKILL 5-18 **Administering an Ear Irrigation** **Goal:** The irrigation is administered successfully and the patient experiences the intended effect of the medication.	**Comments**
___	___	___	1. Gather equipment. Check medication order against the original order in the health record, according to facility policy. Clarify any inconsistencies. Check the patient's health record for allergies.	
___	___	___	2. Know the actions, special nursing considerations, safe dose ranges, purpose of administration, and adverse effects of the medication to be administered. Consider the appropriateness of the medication for this patient.	
___	___	___	3. Perform hand hygiene.	
___	___	___	4. Move the medication supply system to the outside of the patient's room or prepare for administration at the medication supply system in the medication area. Alternatively, access the medication administration supply system at or inside the patient's room.	
___	___	___	5. Unlock the medication supply system or drawer. Enter pass code and scan employee identification, if required.	
___	___	___	6. ***Prepare medications for one patient at a time.***	
___	___	___	7. Read the eMAR/MAR and select the proper medication from medication supply system or the patient's medication drawer.	
___	___	___	8. Compare the label with the eMAR/MAR. Check expiration dates and perform calculations, if necessary. Scan the bar code on the package, if required.	
___	___	___	9. ***Depending on facility policy, the third check of the label may occur at this point. If so, when all medications for one patient have been prepared, recheck the labels with the eMAR/MAR before taking the medications to the patient. However, many facilities require the third check to occur at the bedside, after identifying the patient.***	
___	___	___	10. ***Lock the medication supply system before leaving it.***	
___	___	___	11. Transport medications to the patient's bedside carefully, and keep the medications in sight at all times.	
___	___	___	12. ***Ensure that the patient receives the medications at the correct time.***	
___	___	___	13. Perform hand hygiene and put on PPE, if indicated.	

SKILL 5-18

Administering an Ear Irrigation *(Continued)*

Excellent	Satisfactory	Needs Practice		Comments
___	___	___	14. ***Identify the patient. Compare the information with the eMAR/MAR. The patient should be identified using at least two of the following methods*** (The Joint Commission, 2018):	
___	___	___	a. Check the name on the patient's identification band.	
___	___	___	b. Check the identification number on the patient's identification band.	
___	___	___	c. Check the birth date on the patient's identification band.	
___	___	___	d. Ask the patient to state his or her name and birth date, based on facility policy.	
___	___	___	15. Explain the procedure to the patient.	
___	___	___	16. Scan the patient's bar code on the identification band, if required.	
___	___	___	17. Assemble equipment at patient's bedside.	
___	___	___	18. Put on gloves.	
___	___	___	19. Have the patient sit up or lie with head tilted slightly toward side of the affected ear. Protect the patient and bed with a waterproof pad. Have the patient support the basin under the ear to receive the irrigating solution.	
___	___	___	20. Cleanse external ear of any drainage with cotton ball or washcloth moistened with normal saline or water.	
___	___	___	21. Pretreat the ear with 2 to 4 drops of warm water or irrigating solution and wait 15 minutes.	
___	___	___	22. Fill irrigating or bulb syringe with warmed solution. If an irrigating container is used, prime the tubing.	
___	___	___	23. Straighten the auditory canal by pulling the cartilaginous portion of pinna up and back for an adult.	
___	___	___	24. Point the syringe tip superiorly and posteriorly toward the upper back to the ear canal wall. Use a gentle squirting motion to ***direct a steady, slow stream of solution against the roof of the auditory canal, using only enough force to remove secretions. Do not occlude the auditory canal with the irrigating nozzle.*** Allow solution to flow out unimpeded.	
___	___	___	25. When irrigation is complete, place a cotton ball loosely in the auditory meatus and have the patient lie on side of affected ear on a towel or absorbent pad.	
___	___	___	26. Remove gloves and any additional PPE, if used. Perform hand hygiene.	

Excellent	Satisfactory	Needs Practice	SKILL 5-18 **Administering an Ear Irrigation** *(Continued)*	Comments
___	___	___	27. Document the administration of the medication immediately after administration.	
___	___	___	28. Evaluate the patient's response to the procedure. Return in 10 to 15 minutes and remove cotton ball and assess drainage. Evaluate the patient's response to the medication within an appropriate time frame.	

Skill Checklists for Taylor's Clinical Nursing Skills.
A Nursing Process Approach, 5th edition

Name ______________________ Date ______________________

Unit ______________________ Position ______________________

Instructor/Evaluator: ______________________ Position ______________________

Excellent	Satisfactory	Needs Practice	SKILL 5-19 **Administering a Nasal Spray** **Goal:** The medication is administered successfully into the nose and the patient experiences the intended effect of the medication.	**Comments**
___	___	___	1. Gather equipment. Check medication order against the original order in the health record, according to facility policy. Clarify any inconsistencies. Check the patient's health record for allergies.	
___	___	___	2. Know the actions, special nursing considerations, safe dose ranges, purpose of administration, and adverse effects of the medication to be administered. Consider the appropriateness of the medication for this patient.	
___	___	___	3. Perform hand hygiene.	
___	___	___	4. Move the medication supply system to the outside of the patient's room or prepare for administration at the medication supply system in the medication area. Alternatively, access the medication administration supply system at or inside the patient's room.	
___	___	___	5. Unlock the medication supply system or drawer. Enter pass code and scan employee identification, if required.	
___	___	___	6. ***Prepare medications for one patient at a time.***	
___	___	___	7. Read the eMAR/MAR and select the proper medication from the patient's medication drawer or medication supply system.	
___	___	___	8. Compare the label with the eMAR/MAR. Check expiration dates and perform calculations, if necessary. Scan the bar code on the package, if required.	
___	___	___	9. ***Depending on facility policy, the third check of the label may occur at this point. If so, when all medications for one patient have been prepared, recheck the labels with the eMAR/MAR before taking the medications to the patient. However, many facilities require the third check to occur at the bedside, after identifying the patient.***	
___	___	___	10. ***Lock the medication supply system before leaving it.***	
___	___	___	11. Transport medications to the patient's bedside carefully, and keep the medications in sight at all times.	
___	___	___	12. ***Ensure that the patient receives the medications at the correct time.***	
___	___	___	13. Perform hand hygiene and put on PPE, if indicated.	

Excellent	Satisfactory	Needs Practice	SKILL 5-19 **Administering a Nasal Spray** *(Continued)*	Comments
___	___	___	14. ***Identify the patient. Compare the information with the eMAR/MAR. The patient should be identified using at least two of the following methods*** (The Joint Commission, 2018):	
___	___	___	a. Check the name on the patient's identification band.	
___	___	___	b. Check the identification number on the patient's identification band.	
___	___	___	c. Check the birth date on the patient's identification band.	
___	___	___	d. Ask the patient to state his or her name and birth date, based on facility policy.	
___	___	___	15. ***Complete necessary assessments before administering medications. Check the patient's allergy bracelet or ask the patient about allergies. Explain the purpose and action of each medication to the patient.***	
___	___	___	16. Scan the patient's bar code on the identification band, if required.	
___	___	___	17. ***Based on facility policy, the third check of the label may occur at this point. If so, recheck the labels with the eMAR/MAR before administering the medications to the patient.***	
___	___	___	18. Put on gloves.	
___	___	___	19. Provide patient with paper tissues and ask the patient to blow his or her nose.	
___	___	___	20. Have the patient sit up with head tilted back. ***Tilting the patient's head should be avoided if the patient has a cervical spine injury or other condition resulting in limited range of notion.***	
___	___	___	21. Instruct the patient that it is necessary to inhale gently through the nose as the spray is being administered or not to inhale gently as the spray is being administered. Your instruction to the patient will depend on the medication being administered. Consult the manufacturer's instructions for each medication.	
___	___	___	22. Agitate the bottle gently, if required for specific medication. Insert the tip of the nosepiece of the bottle into one nostril. Close the opposite nostril with a finger. Instruct the patient to breathe in gently through the nostril, if required. Compress or activate the bottle to release one spray at the same time the patient breathes in.	

Excellent	Satisfactory	Needs Practice	SKILL 5-19 **Administering a Nasal Spray** *(Continued)*	Comments
___	___	___	23. Keep the medication container compressed and remove it from the nostril. Release the container from the compressed state. Do not allow the container to return to its original position until it is removed from the patient's nose.	
___	___	___	24. Have the patient hold his or her breath for a few seconds, and then breathe out slowly through the mouth. Repeat in the other nostril, as prescribed or indicated.	
___	___	___	25. Wipe the outside of the bottle nose piece with a clean, dry tissue or cloth and replace the cap. Instruct the patient to avoid blowing his or her nose for 5 to 10 minutes, depending on the medication.	
___	___	___	26. Remove gloves. Assist the patient to a comfortable position.	
___	___	___	27. Remove additional PPE, if used. Perform hand hygiene.	
___	___	___	28. Document the administration of the medication immediately after administration.	
___	___	___	29. Evaluate the patient's response to the procedure and medication within an appropriate time frame.	

Skill Checklists for Taylor's Clinical Nursing Skills. A Nursing Process Approach, 5th edition

Name ______________________ Date ______________________

Unit ______________________ Position ______________________

Instructor/Evaluator: ______________________ Position ______________________

SKILL 5-20

Administering a Vaginal Cream

Goal: The medication is administered successfully into the vagina and the patient experiences the intended effect of the medication.

Excellent	Satisfactory	Needs Practice		Comments
___	___	___	1. Gather equipment. Check medication order against the original order in the health record, according to facility policy. Clarify any inconsistencies. Check the patient's health record for allergies.	
___	___	___	2. Know the actions, special nursing considerations, safe dose ranges, purpose of administration, and adverse effects of the medication to be administered. Consider the appropriateness of the medication for this patient.	
___	___	___	3. Perform hand hygiene.	
___	___	___	4. Move the medication supply system to the outside of the patient's room or prepare for administration at the medication supply system in the medication area. Alternatively, access the medication administration supply system at or inside the patient's room.	
___	___	___	5. Unlock the medication supply system or drawer. Enter pass code and scan employee identification, if required.	
___	___	___	6. ***Prepare medications for one patient at a time.***	
___	___	___	7. Read the eMAR/MAR and select the proper medication from medication supply system or the patient's medication drawer.	
___	___	___	8. Compare the label with the eMAR/MAR. Check expiration dates and perform calculations, if necessary. Scan the bar code on the package, if required.	
___	___	___	9. ***Depending on facility policy, the third check of the label may occur at this point. If so, when all medications for one patient have been prepared, recheck the labels with the eMAR/MAR before taking the medications to the patient. However, many facilities require the third check to occur at the bedside, after identifying the patient.***	
___	___	___	10. ***Lock the medication supply system before leaving it.***	
___	___	___	11. Transport medications to the patient's bedside carefully, and keep the medications in sight at all times.	
___	___	___	12. ***Ensure that the patient receives the medications at the correct time.***	
___	___	___	13. Perform hand hygiene and put on PPE, if indicated.	

Excellent	Satisfactory	Needs Practice	SKILL 5-20 **Administering a Vaginal Cream** *(Continued)*	Comments
___	___	___	14. ***Identify the patient. Compare the information with the eMAR/MAR. The patient should be identified using at least two of the following methods*** (The Joint Commission, 2018):	
___	___	___	a. Check the name on the patient's identification band.	
___	___	___	b. Check the identification number on the patient's identification band.	
___	___	___	c. Check the birth date on the patient's identification band.	
___	___	___	d. Ask the patient to state his or her name and birth date, based on facility policy.	
___	___	___	15. ***Complete necessary assessments before administering medications. Check the patient's allergy bracelet or ask the patient about allergies. Explain the purpose and action of each medication to the patient.***	
___	___	___	16. Scan the patient's bar code on the identification band, if required.	
___	___	___	17. ***Based on facility policy, the third check of the label may occur at this point. If so, recheck the labels with the eMAR/MAR before administering the medications to the patient.***	
___	___	___	18. Ask the patient to void before inserting the medication.	
___	___	___	19. Put on gloves.	
___	___	___	20. Position the patient so that she is lying on her back with the knees flexed. Maintain privacy with draping. Provide adequate light to visualize the vaginal opening.	
___	___	___	21. Perform perineal care. Spread labia with fingers, and cleanse area at vaginal orifice with disposable washcloth or washcloth and warm water, using a different corner of the washcloth with each stroke. Wipe from above the vaginal orifice downward toward the sacrum (front to back).	
___	___	___	22. Remove gloves and put on new gloves.	
___	___	___	23. Fill vaginal applicator with prescribed amount of cream.	
___	___	___	24. Lubricate applicator with the lubricant, as necessary.	
___	___	___	25. Spread the labia with your nondominant hand and gently introduce the applicator with your dominant hand, in a rolling manner, while directing it downward and backward.	
___	___	___	26. After the applicator is properly positioned, labia may be allowed to fall in place if necessary to free the hand for manipulating the plunger. Push the plunger to its full length and then gently remove applicator with plunger depressed.	

SKILL 5-20

Administering a Vaginal Cream *(Continued)*

Excellent	Satisfactory	Needs Practice		Comments
___	___	___	27. ***Ask the patient to remain in the supine position for a minimum of 5 to 10 minutes after insertion. Some medications are administered prior to lying down to go to bed.*** Offer the patient a perineal pad to collect drainage.	
___	___	___	28. Dispose of the applicator in an appropriate receptacle or clean the nondisposable applicator according to manufacturer's directions.	
___	___	___	29. Remove gloves and additional PPE, if used. Perform hand hygiene.	
___	___	___	30. Document the administration of the medication immediately after administration.	
___	___	___	31. Evaluate the patient's response to the medication within an appropriate time frame.	

Skill Checklists for Taylor's Clinical Nursing Skills. A Nursing Process Approach, 5th edition

Name ______________________ Date ______________________

Unit ______________________ Position ______________________

Instructor/Evaluator: ______________________ Position ______________________

SKILL 5-21

Administering a Rectal Suppository

Goal: The medication is administered successfully into the rectum and the patient experiences the intended effect of the medication.

Excellent	Satisfactory	Needs Practice		Comments
___	___	___	1. Gather equipment. Check medication order against the original order in the health record, according to facility policy. Clarify any inconsistencies. Check the patient's health record for allergies.	
___	___	___	2. Know the actions, special nursing considerations, safe dose ranges, purpose of administration, and adverse effects of the medication to be administered. Consider the appropriateness of the medication for this patient.	
___	___	___	3. Perform hand hygiene.	
___	___	___	4. Move the medication supply system to the outside of the patient's room or prepare for administration at the medication supply system in the medication area. Alternatively, access the medication administration supply system at or inside the patient's room.	
___	___	___	5. Unlock the medication supply system or drawer. Enter pass code and scan employee identification, if required.	
___	___	___	6. *Prepare medications for one patient at a time.*	
___	___	___	7. Read the eMAR/MAR and select the proper medication from medication supply system or the patient's medication drawer.	
___	___	___	8. Compare the label with the eMAR/MAR. Check expiration dates and perform calculations, if necessary. Scan the bar code on the package, if required.	
___	___	___	9. *Depending on facility policy, the third check of the label may occur at this point. If so, when all medications for one patient have been prepared, recheck the labels with the eMAR/MAR before taking the medications to the patient. However, many facilities require the third check to occur at the bedside, after identifying the patient.*	
___	___	___	10. *Lock the medication supply system before leaving it.*	
___	___	___	11. Transport medications to the patient's bedside carefully, and keep the medications in sight at all times.	
___	___	___	12. *Ensure that the patient receives the medications at the correct time.*	
___	___	___	13. Perform hand hygiene and put on PPE, if indicated.	

Excellent	Satisfactory	Needs Practice	SKILL 5-21 **Administering a Rectal Suppository** *(Continued)*	Comments
___	___	___	14. ***Identify the patient. Compare the information with the eMAR/MAR. The patient should be identified using at least two of the following methods*** (The Joint Commission, 2018):	
___	___	___	a. Check the name on the patient's identification band.	
___	___	___	b. Check the identification number on the patient's identification band.	
___	___	___	c. Check the birth date on the patient's identification band.	
___	___	___	d. Ask the patient to state his or her name and birth date, based on facility policy.	
___	___	___	15. ***Complete necessary assessments before administering medications. Check the patient's allergy bracelet or ask the patient about allergies. Explain the purpose and action of each medication to the patient.***	
___	___	___	16. Scan the patient's bar code on the identification band, if required.	
___	___	___	17. ***Based on facility policy, the third check of the label may occur at this point. If so, recheck the labels with the eMAR/MAR before administering the medications to the patient.***	
___	___	___	18. Put on gloves.	
___	___	___	19. Assist the patient to his or her left side in a Sims' position. Drape accordingly to expose only the buttocks.	
___	___	___	20. Remove the suppository from its wrapper. Apply lubricant to the rounded end. Lubricate the index finger of your dominant hand.	
___	___	___	21. Separate the buttocks with your nondominant hand and instruct the patient to breathe slowly and deeply through his or her mouth while the suppository is being inserted.	
___	___	___	22. Using your index finger, insert the suppository, round end first, *along the rectal wall.* Insert about 3 to 4 in.	
___	___	___	23. Use toilet tissue to clean any stool or lubricant from around the anus. Release the buttocks. Encourage the patient to remain on his or her side for at least 5 minutes and retain the suppository for the appropriate amount of time for the specific medication.	
___	___	___	24. Remove gloves and any additional PPE, if used. Perform hand hygiene.	
___	___	___	25. Document the administration of the medication immediately after administration.	
___	___	___	26. Evaluate the patient's response to the medication within an appropriate time frame.	

Skill Checklists for Taylor's Clinical Nursing Skills. A Nursing Process Approach, 5th edition

Name ______________________ Date ______________________

Unit ______________________ Position ______________________

Instructor/Evaluator: ______________________ Position ______________________

SKILL 5-22

Administering Medication via a Metered-Dose Inhaler (MDI)

Goal: The medication is administered and breathed in by the patient and the patient experiences the intended effect of the medication.

Excellent	Satisfactory	Needs Practice		Comments
____	____	____	1. Gather equipment. Check each medication order against the original order in the health record, according to facility policy. Clarify any inconsistencies. Check the patient's health record for allergies.	
____	____	____	2. Know the actions, special nursing considerations, safe dose ranges, purpose of administration, and adverse effects of the medications to be administered. Consider the appropriateness of the medication for this patient.	
____	____	____	3. Perform hand hygiene.	
____	____	____	4. Move the medication supply system to the outside of the patient's room or prepare for administration at the medication supply system in the medication area. Alternatively, access the medication administration supply system at or inside the patient's room.	
____	____	____	5. Unlock the medication supply system or drawer. Enter pass code and scan employee identification, if required.	
____	____	____	6. ***Prepare medications for one patient at a time.***	
____	____	____	7. Read the eMAR/MAR and select the proper medication from the patient's medication drawer or medication supply system.	
____	____	____	8. Compare the label with the eMAR/MAR. Check expiration dates and perform calculations, if necessary. Scan the bar code on the package, if required.	
____	____	____	9. ***Depending on facility policy, the third check of the label may occur at this point. If so, when all medications for one patient have been prepared, recheck the labels with the eMAR/MAR before taking the medications to the patient. However, many facilities require the third check to occur at the bedside, after identifying the patient.***	
____	____	____	10. ***Lock the medication supply system before leaving it.***	
____	____	____	11. Transport medications to the patient's bedside carefully, and keep the medications in sight at all times.	
____	____	____	12. ***Ensure that the patient receives the medications at the correct time.***	
____	____	____	13. Perform hand hygiene and put on PPE, if indicated.	

Excellent	Satisfactory	Needs Practice	SKILL 5-22 **Administering Medication via a Metered-Dose Inhaler (MDI)** *(Continued)*	Comments
___	___	___	14. ***Identify the patient. Compare the information with the eMAR/MAR. The patient should be identified using at least two of the following methods*** (The Joint Commission, 2018):	
___	___	___	a. Check the name on the patient's identification band.	
___	___	___	b. Check the identification number on the patient's identification band.	
___	___	___	c. Check the birth date on the patient's identification band.	
___	___	___	d. Ask the patient to state his or her name and birth date, based on facility policy.	
___	___	___	15. ***Complete necessary assessments before administering medications. Check the patient's allergy bracelet or ask the patient about allergies. Explain what you are going to do and the reason for doing it to the patient.***	
___	___	___	16. Scan the patient's bar code on the identification band, if required.	
___	___	___	17. ***Based on facility policy, the third check of the label may occur at this point. If so, recheck the labels with the eMAR/MAR before administering the medications to the patient.***	
___	___	___	18. Shake the inhaler well.	
___	___	___	19. Remove the mouthpiece cover from the MDI and the spacer. Attach the MDI to the spacer by inserting in the open end of the spacer, opposite the mouthpiece.	
___	___	___	20. Have patient place the spacer's mouthpiece into mouth, grasping securely with teeth and sealing the lips tightly around the mouthpiece. Have patient breathe normally through the spacer.	
___	___	___	21. The patient should breathe out completely, then depress the canister once, releasing one puff into the spacer, then inhale slowly and deeply through the mouth.	
___	___	___	22. ***Instruct patient to hold his or her breath for 5 to 10 seconds, or as long as possible, and then to exhale slowly through pursed lips.***	
___	___	___	23. Wait 1 to 5 minutes, as prescribed, before administering the next puff, as prescribed.	
___	___	___	24. After the prescribed number of puffs has been administered, have the patient remove the MDI from the spacer and replace the caps on both MDI and spacer.	

SKILL 5-22

Administering Medication via a Metered-Dose Inhaler (MDI) *(Continued)*

Excellent	Satisfactory	Needs Practice		Comments
___	___	___	25. Have the patient gargle and rinse with tap water after using an MDI, as necessary. Clean the MDI according to the manufacturer's directions.	
___	___	___	26. Remove PPE, if used. Perform hand hygiene.	
___	___	___	27. Document the administration of the medication immediately after administration.	
___	___	___	28. Evaluate the patient's response to the medication within an appropriate time frame. Reassess lung sounds, oxygen saturation level, and respirations, as indicated.	

Skill Checklists for Taylor's Clinical Nursing Skills.
A Nursing Process Approach, 5th edition

Name ______________________ Date ______________________

Unit ______________________ Position ______________________

Instructor/Evaluator: ______________________ Position ______________________

SKILL 5-23

Administering Medication via a Dry Powder Inhaler

Excellent	Satisfactory	Needs Practice	**Goal:** The medication is administered and breathed in by the patient and the patient experiences the intended effect of the medication.	**Comments**
____	____	____	1. Gather equipment. Check each medication order against the original order in the health record, according to facility policy. Clarify any inconsistencies. Check the patient's health record for allergies.	
____	____	____	2. Know the actions, special nursing considerations, safe dose ranges, purpose of administration, and adverse effects of the medications to be administered. Consider the appropriateness of the medication for this patient.	
____	____	____	3. Perform hand hygiene.	
____	____	____	4. Move the medication supply system to the outside of the patient's room or prepare for administration at the medication supply system in the medication area. Alternatively, access the medication administration supply system at or inside the patient's room.	
____	____	____	5. Unlock the medication supply system or drawer. Enter pass code and scan employee identification, if required.	
____	____	____	6. ***Prepare medications for one patient at a time.***	
____	____	____	7. Read the eMAR/MAR and select the proper medication from the patient's medication drawer or medication supply system.	
____	____	____	8. Compare the label with the eMAR/MAR. Check expiration dates and perform calculations, if necessary. Scan the bar code on the package, if required.	
____	____	____	9. ***Depending on facility policy, the third check of the label may occur at this point. If so, when all medications for one patient have been prepared, recheck the labels with the eMAR/MAR before taking the medications to the patient. However, many facilities require the third check to occur at the bedside, after identifying the patient.***	
____	____	____	10. ***Lock the medication supply system before leaving it.***	
____	____	____	11. Transport medications to the patient's bedside carefully, and keep the medications in sight at all times.	
____	____	____	12. ***Ensure that the patient receives the medications at the correct time.***	
____	____	____	13. Perform hand hygiene and put on PPE, if indicated.	

Excellent	Satisfactory	Needs Practice	SKILL 5-23 **Administering Medication via a Dry Powder Inhaler** *(Continued)*	Comments
___	___	___	14. ***Identify the patient. Compare the information with the eMAR/MAR. The patient should be identified using at least two of the following methods*** (The Joint Commission, 2018):	
___	___	___	a. Check the name on the patient's identification band.	
___	___	___	b. Check the identification number on the patient's identification band.	
___	___	___	c. Check the birth date on the patient's identification band.	
___	___	___	d. Ask the patient to state his or her name and birth date, based on facility policy.	
___	___	___	15. ***Complete necessary assessments before administering medications. Check the patient's allergy bracelet or ask the patient about allergies. Explain what you are going to do, and the reason for doing it, to the patient.***	
___	___	___	16. Scan the patient's bar code on the identification band, if required.	
___	___	___	17. ***Based on facility policy, the third check of the label may occur at this point. If so, recheck the labels with the eMAR/MAR before administering the medications to the patient.***	
___	___	___	18. Remove the mouthpiece cover or remove the device from storage container. Load a dose into the device as directed by the manufacturer, if necessary. Alternatively, activate the inhaler, if necessary, according to manufacturer's directions.	
___	___	___	19. Have the patient breathe out slowly and completely, without breathing into the DPI.	
___	___	___	20. Instruct the patient to place teeth over, and seal lips around, the mouthpiece. ***It is important to not block the opening with the tongue or teeth.***	
___	___	___	21. ***Instruct patient to breathe in strong, steady and deeply through the mouth, for longer than 2 to 3 seconds.***	
___	___	___	22. Remove inhaler from mouth. Instruct patient to hold the breath for 5 to 10 seconds, or as long as possible, and then to exhale slowly through pursed lips.	
___	___	___	23. Wait 1 to 5 minutes, as prescribed, before administering the next puff.	
___	___	___	24. After the prescribed number of puffs has been administered, have the patient replace the cap or storage container.	

Excellent	Satisfactory	Needs Practice	SKILL 5-23 **Administering Medication via a Dry Powder Inhaler** *(Continued)*	Comments
____	____	____	25. Have the patient gargle and rinse with tap water after using DPI, as necessary. Clean the DPI according to the manufacturer's directions.	
____	____	____	26. Remove gloves and additional PPE, if used. Perform hand hygiene.	
____	____	____	27. Document the administration of the medication immediately after administration.	
____	____	____	28. Evaluate patient's response to the medication within an appropriate time frame. Reassess lung sounds, oxygen saturation level, and respirations, as indicated.	

Skill Checklists for Taylor's Clinical Nursing Skills. A Nursing Process Approach, 5th edition

Name ______________________ Date ______________________

Unit ______________________ Position ______________________

Instructor/Evaluator: ______________________ Position ______________________

SKILL 5-24

Administering Medication via a Small-Volume Nebulizer

Excellent	Satisfactory	Needs Practice	**Goal:** The medication is administered and breathed in by the patient and the patient experiences the intended effect of the medication.	**Comments**
___	___	___	1. Gather equipment. Check each medication order against the original order in the health record, according to facility policy. Clarify any inconsistencies. Check the patient's health record for allergies.	
___	___	___	2. Know the actions, special nursing considerations, safe dose ranges, purpose of administration, and adverse effects of the medications to be administered. Consider the appropriateness of the medication for this patient.	
___	___	___	3. Perform hand hygiene.	
___	___	___	4. Move the medication supply system to the outside of the patient's room or prepare for administration at the medication supply system in the medication area. Alternatively, access the medication administration supply system at or inside the patient's room.	
___	___	___	5. Unlock the medication supply system or drawer. Enter pass code and scan employee identification, if required.	
___	___	___	6. *Prepare medications for one patient at a time.*	
___	___	___	7. Read the eMAR/MAR and select the proper medication from medication supply system or the patient's medication drawer.	
___	___	___	8. Compare the label with the eMAR/MAR. Check expiration dates and perform calculations, if necessary. Scan the bar code on the package, if required.	
___	___	___	9. *Depending on facility policy, the third check of the label may occur at this point. If so, when all medications for one patient have been prepared, recheck the labels with the eMAR/MAR before taking the medications to the patient. However, many facilities require the third check to occur at the bedside, after identifying the patient.*	
___	___	___	10. *Lock the medication supply system before leaving it.*	
___	___	___	11. Transport medications to the patient's bedside carefully, and keep the medications in sight at all times.	
___	___	___	12. *Ensure that the patient receives the medications at the correct time.*	
___	___	___	13. Perform hand hygiene and put on PPE, if indicated.	

Excellent	Satisfactory	Needs Practice	SKILL 5-24 **Administering Medication via a Small-Volume Nebulizer** *(Continued)*	Comments
___	___	___	14. ***Identify the patient. Compare the information with the eMAR/MAR. The patient should be identified using at least two of the following methods*** (The Joint Commission, 2018):	
___	___	___	a. Check the name on the patient's identification band.	
___	___	___	b. Check the identification number on the patient's identification band.	
___	___	___	c. Check the birth date on the patient's identification band.	
___	___	___	d. Ask the patient to state his or her name and birth date, based on facility policy.	
___	___	___	15. ***Complete necessary assessments before administering medications. Check the patient's allergy bracelet or ask the patient about allergies. Explain what you are going to do, and the reason for doing it, to the patient.***	
___	___	___	16. Scan the patient's bar code on the identification band, if required.	
___	___	___	17. ***Based on facility policy, the third check of the label may occur at this point. If so, recheck the labels with the eMAR/MAR before administering the medications to the patient.***	
___	___	___	18. Remove the nebulizer cup from the device and open it. Place premeasured unit-dose medication in the bottom section of the cup or use a dropper to place a concentrated dose of medication in the cup. Add prescribed diluent (usually saline), if required.	
___	___	___	19. Screw the top portion of the nebulizer cup back in place and attach the cup to the nebulizer. Attach one end of tubing to the stem on the bottom of the nebulizer cuff and the other end to the air compressor or oxygen source.	
___	___	___	20. Turn on the air compressor or oxygen. Check that a fine medication mist is produced by opening the valve. Have the patient place the mouthpiece into the mouth and grasp securely with teeth and lips.	
___	___	___	21. ***Instruct the patient to inhale slowly and deeply through the mouth. A nose clip may be necessary if the patient is also breathing through the nose. Hold each breath for a slight pause, before exhaling.***	
___	___	___	22. Continue this inhalation technique until all medication in the nebulizer cup has been aerosolized (usually about 15 minutes). Once the fine mist decreases in amount, gently flick the sides of the nebulizer cup.	

Excellent	Satisfactory	Needs Practice	SKILL 5-24 **Administering Medication via a Small-Volume Nebulizer** *(Continued)*	Comments
___	___	___	23. When the medication in the nebulizer cup has been completely aerosolized, the cup will be empty. Have the patient remove the nebulizer from the mouth and gargle and rinse with tap water, as indicated. Clean and store the nebulizer and equipment according to the manufacturer's directions and facility policy.	
___	___	___	24. Remove gloves and additional PPE, if used. Perform hand hygiene.	
___	___	___	25. Document the administration of the medication immediately after administration.	
___	___	___	26. Evaluate patient's response to the medication within an appropriate time frame. Reassess lung sounds, oxygen saturation level, and respirations, as indicated.	

Skill Checklists for Taylor's Clinical Nursing Skills. A Nursing Process Approach, 5th edition

Name ______________________ Date ______________________

Unit ______________________ Position ______________________

Instructor/Evaluator: ______________________ Position ______________________

SKILL 6-1

Teaching Deep-Breathing Exercises, Coughing, and Splinting

Excellent	Satisfactory	Needs Practice	**Goal:** The patient and/or significant other verbalizes an understanding of the instructions and is able to demonstrate the activities.	**Comments**
___	___	___	1. Check the patient's health record for the type of surgery and review the prescribed orders. Gather the necessary supplies.	
___	___	___	2. Perform hand hygiene and put on PPE, if indicated.	
___	___	___	3. Identify the patient.	
___	___	___	4. Close curtains around the bed and close the door to the room, if possible. Explain what you are going to do and why you are going to do it to the patient. Place necessary supplies on the bedside stand, overbed table, or other surface within easy reach.	
___	___	___	5. Identify the patient's learning needs and the patient's level of knowledge regarding deep-breathing exercises, coughing, and splinting of the incision. If the patient has had surgery before, ask about this experience.	
___	___	___	6. Explain the rationale for performing deep-breathing exercises, coughing, and splinting of the incision.	
___	___	___	7. Teach the patient how to perform deep-breathing exercises and explain their importance.	
___	___	___	a. Assist or ask the patient to sit up (semi- or high-Fowler's position), with the neck and shoulders supported. Ask the patient to place the palms of both hands along the lower anterior rib cage.	
___	___	___	b. Ask the patient to exhale gently and completely.	
___	___	___	c. Instruct the patient to breathe in through the nose as deeply as possible and hold breath for 3 to 5 seconds.	
___	___	___	d. Instruct the patient to exhale through the mouth, pursing the lips like when whistling.	
___	___	___	e. Have the patient practice the breathing exercise three times. Instruct the patient that this exercise should be performed every 1 to 2 hours for the first 24 hours after surgery, and as necessary thereafter, depending on risk factors and pulmonary status.	

Excellent	Satisfactory	Needs Practice	SKILL 6-1 **Teaching Deep-Breathing Exercises, Coughing, and Splinting** *(Continued)*	Comments
___	___	___	8. Provide teaching regarding coughing and splinting.	
___	___	___	a. Ask the patient to sit up (semi-Fowler's position), leaning forward. Apply a folded bath blanket or small pillow against the part of the body where the incision will be (e.g., abdomen or chest).	
___	___	___	b. Ask the patient to inhale and exhale deeply and slowly through the nose three times.	
___	___	___	c. Ask the patient to take a deep breath and hold it for 3 seconds and then cough out three short times.	
___	___	___	d. Ask the patient to take a quick breath through the mouth and strongly and deeply cough again one or two times.	
___	___	___	e. Ask the patient to take another deep breath, then relax and breathe normally.	
___	___	___	f. Instruct the patient that he or she should perform these actions every 2 hours when awake after surgery.	
___	___	___	9. Validate the patient's understanding of the information. Ask the patient to give a return demonstration. Ask the patient if he or she has any questions. Encourage the patient to practice the activities and ask questions, if necessary.	
___	___	___	10. Remove PPE, if used. Perform hand hygiene.	

Skill Checklists for Taylor's Clinical Nursing Skills.
A Nursing Process Approach, 5th edition

Name ______________________ Date ______________________

Unit ______________________ Position ______________________

Instructor/Evaluator: ______________________ Position ______________________

SKILL 6-2

Teaching Leg Exercises

Goal: The patient and/or significant other verbalizes an understanding of the instructions and is able to demonstrate the activities.

Excellent	Satisfactory	Needs Practice		Comments
___	___	___	1. Check the patient's health record for the type of surgery and review the prescribed orders. Gather the necessary supplies.	
___	___	___	2. Perform hand hygiene and put on PPE, if indicated.	
___	___	___	3. Identify the patient.	
___	___	___	4. Close the curtains around the bed and close the door to the room, if possible. Explain what you are going to do and why you are going to do it to the patient. Place necessary supplies on the bedside stand, overbed table, or other surface within easy reach.	
___	___	___	5. Identify the patient's learning needs. Identify the patient's level of knowledge regarding leg exercises. If the patient has had surgery before, ask about this experience.	
___	___	___	6. Explain the rationale for performing leg exercises.	
___	___	___	7. Teach leg exercises and explain their purpose.	
___	___	___	a. Assist or ask the patient to sit up (semi-Fowler's position) and explain to the patient that you will first demonstrate, and then coach him or her to exercise one leg at a time.	
___	___	___	b. Bend the patient's knee, raise the foot, and keep it elevated for a few seconds. Then, extend the lower leg, and hold this position for a few seconds. Lower the entire leg. Practice this exercise with the other leg.	
___	___	___	c. Assist or ask the patient to point the toes of both legs toward the foot of the bed, then relax them. Next, flex or pull the toes toward the chin.	
___	___	___	d. Assist or ask the patient to keep legs extended and to make circles with both ankles, first circling to the left and then to the right. Instruct the patient to repeat these exercises three to five times with each leg. Instruct the patient to perform leg exercises every 2 to 4 hours when awake after surgery.	

Excellent	Satisfactory	Needs Practice	SKILL 6-2 **Teaching Leg Exercises** *(Continued)*	Comments
___	___	___	8. Validate the patient's understanding of the information. Ask the patient for a return demonstration. Ask the patient if he or she has any questions. Encourage the patient to practice the activities and ask questions, if necessary.	
___	___	___	9. Remove PPE, if used. Perform hand hygiene.	

Skill Checklists for Taylor's Clinical Nursing Skills. A Nursing Process Approach, 5th edition

Name ______________________ Date ______________________

Unit ______________________ Position ______________________

Instructor/Evaluator: ______________________ Position ______________________

SKILL 6-3

Providing Preoperative Patient Care

Excellent	Satisfactory	Needs Practice	**Goal:** The patient will proceed to surgery.	**Comments**
___	___	___	1. Check the patient's health record for the type of surgery and review the prescribed orders. Review the nursing database, history, and physical examination. Check that the baseline data are recorded; report those that are abnormal.	
___	___	___	2. ***Check that all diagnostic testing has been completed and results are available; identify and report abnormal results.*** Gather the necessary supplies.	
___	___	___	3. Perform hand hygiene and put on PPE, if indicated.	
___	___	___	4. Identify the patient.	
___	___	___	5. Close the curtains around the bed and close the door to the room, if possible. Explain what you are going to do and why you are going to do it to the patient and significant other. Place necessary supplies on the bedside stand, overbed table, or other surface within easy reach.	
___	___	___	6. Explore the psychological needs of the patient and family related to the surgery.	
___	___	___	a. Establish a therapeutic relationship, encouraging the patient to verbalize concerns or fears.	
___	___	___	b. Use active listening skills, answering questions and clarifying any misinformation.	
___	___	___	c. Use touch, as appropriate, to convey genuine empathy.	
___	___	___	d. Offer to contact spiritual counselor (e.g., priest, minister, rabbi) to meet spiritual needs.	
___	___	___	7. ***Identify learning needs of patient and family.*** Ensure that the informed consent of the patient for the surgery has been signed, timed, dated, and witnessed. Inquire if the patient has any questions regarding the surgical procedure. Check the patient's record to determine if an advance directive has been completed. If an advance directive has not been completed, discuss with the patient the possibility of completing it, as appropriate. If patient has had surgery before, ask about this experience.	
___	___	___	8. Teach deep-breathing exercises.	
___	___	___	9. Teach coughing and splinting.	

SKILL 6-3

Providing Preoperative Patient Care *(Continued)*

Excellent	Satisfactory	Needs Practice		Comments
___	___	___	10. Teach use of incentive spirometer, as prescribed or indicated.	
___	___	___	11. Teach leg exercises, as appropriate.	
___	___	___	12. Teach about early ambulation, as appropriate.	
___	___	___	13. Assist the patient in putting on graduated compression stockings. Demonstrate how the pneumatic compression device operates.	
___	___	___	14. Teach about turning in the bed.	
___	___	___	a. Instruct the patient to use a pillow or bath blanket to splint where the incision will be. Ask the patient to raise his or her left knee and reach across to grasp the right side rail of the bed. If the patient is turning to the left side, he or she will bend the right knee and grasp the left side rail.	
___	___	___	b. When turning the patient onto the right side, ask the patient to push with bent left leg and pull on the right side rail. Explain to the patient that you will place a pillow behind his/her back to provide support, and that the call bell will be placed within easy reach.	
___	___	___	c. Explain to the patient that position change is recommended every 2 hours.	
___	___	___	15. Provide individualized, developmentally appropriate teaching about pain management options, plans and goals.	
___	___	___	a. Discuss past experiences with pain and interventions that the patient has used to reduce pain.	
___	___	___	b. Discuss the availability of analgesic medication postoperatively.	
___	___	___	c. Discuss the use of PCA, as appropriate.	
___	___	___	d. Explore the use of other alternative and nonpharmacologic methods to reduce pain, such as position change, massage, relaxation/diversion, guided imagery, and meditation.	
___	___	___	16. Review equipment that may be used after surgery.	
___	___	___	a. Show the patient various equipment, such as IV infusion devices, electronic blood pressure cuff, tubes, urinary catheters, and surgical drains.	
___	___	___	17. Provide skin preparation.	
___	___	___	a. ***Ask the patient to bathe or shower with the antibacterial soap or solution. Remind the patient to clean the surgical site.***	

Excellent	Satisfactory	Needs Practice	SKILL 6-3 **Providing Preoperative Patient Care** *(Continued)*	Comments
___	___	___	18. Provide teaching about and follow dietary/fluid restrictions. ***Explain to the patient that both food and fluid will be restricted before surgery to ensure that the stomach contains a minimal amount of gastric secretions. This restriction is important to reduce the risk of aspiration. Emphasize to the patient the importance of avoiding food and fluids during the prescribed time period, because failure to adhere may necessitate cancellation of the surgery.***	
___	___	___	19. Provide intestinal preparation, as appropriate. In certain situations, such as surgery of the lower gastrointestinal tract, the bowel will need to be prepared by administering enemas or laxatives.	
___	___	___	a. As needed, explain the purpose of enemas or laxatives before surgery. If the patient will be administered an enema, clarify the steps as needed.	
___	___	___	20. ***Check administration of regularly scheduled medications.*** Review with the patient routine medications, over-the-counter medications, and herbal supplements that are taken regularly. Check the medical orders and review with the patient which medications he or she will be permitted to take the day of surgery.	
___	___	___	21. Provide information to the patient and family regarding timing of surgical events and potential sensations that may be experienced. Explain to patients and their families how long the surgery and postanesthesia care will last, as well as what will be done before, during, and after surgery (e.g., procedures, medications, equipment). Explain to patients that they may not drive themselves home or take public transportation alone if they have had any anesthesia or sedation.	
___	___	___	22. Remove PPE, if used. Perform hand hygiene.	

Skill Checklists for Taylor's Clinical Nursing Skills.
A Nursing Process Approach, 5th edition

Name ______________________ Date ______________________

Unit ______________________ Position ______________________

Instructor/Evaluator: ______________________ Position ______________________

SKILL 6-4

Providing Preoperative Patient Care: Day of Surgery

Excellent	Satisfactory	Needs Practice	**Goal:** The patient will proceed to surgery.	**Comments**
___	___	___	1. Check the patient's health record for the type of surgery and review the prescribed orders. Review the nursing database, history, and physical examination. Check that the baseline data are recorded; report those that are abnormal. Gather the necessary supplies.	
___	___	___	2. Perform hand hygiene and put on PPE, if indicated.	
___	___	___	3. Identify the patient.	
___	___	___	4. Close the curtains around the bed and close the door to the room, if possible. Explain what you are going to do and why you are going to do it to the patient and significant other. Place necessary supplies on the bedside stand or overbed table, within easy reach.	
___	___	___	5. Check that preoperative consent forms are signed, witnessed, and correct; that advance directives are in the health record (as applicable); and that the patient's health record is in order.	
___	___	___	6. Measure vital signs. Notify the primary care provider and surgeon of any pertinent changes (e.g., rise or drop in blood pressure, elevated temperature, cough, symptoms of infection).	
___	___	___	7. Provide hygiene and oral care. Assess for loose teeth and caps. Remind the patient of food and fluid restrictions before surgery.	
___	___	___	8. Instruct the patient to remove all personal clothing, including underwear, and to put on a hospital gown.	
___	___	___	9. Ask the patient to remove cosmetics, jewelry including body-piercing, nail polish, and prostheses (e.g., contact lenses, false eyelashes, dentures, and so forth). Some facilities allow a wedding band to be left in place depending on the type of surgery, provided it is secured to the finger with tape.	
___	___	___	10. If possible, give valuables to a family member or place them in an appropriate area, such as the hospital safe, if this is not possible. They should not be placed in the narcotics drawer.	

Excellent	Satisfactory	Needs Practice	SKILL 6-4 **Providing Preoperative Patient Care: Day of Surgery** *(Continued)*	Comments
___	___	___	11. Have patient empty bladder and bowel before surgery.	
___	___	___	12. Attend to any special preoperative orders, such as starting an IV line.	
___	___	___	13. Complete preoperative checklist and record of patient's preoperative preparation.	
___	___	___	14. Question patient regarding the location of the operative site. Document the location in the health record according to facility policy. The actual site will be marked on the patient when the patient arrives in the preoperative holding area by the licensed independent practitioner who will be directly involved in the procedure (The Joint Commission, n.d., 2017).	
___	___	___	15. Administer preoperative medication as prescribed.	
___	___	___	16. Raise side rails of bed, based on facility policy; place bed in lowest position. Instruct the patient to remain in bed or on stretcher. If necessary, use a safety belt.	
___	___	___	17. Help move the patient from the bed to the transport stretcher, if necessary. Reconfirm patient identification and ensure that all preoperative events and measures are documented.	
___	___	___	18. Tell the patient's family where the patient will be taken after surgery and the location of the waiting area where the surgeon will come to explain the outcome of the surgery. If possible, take the family to the waiting area.	
___	___	___	19. After the patient leaves for the OR, prepare the room for patients returning to a room on a hospital patient care unit and make a postoperative bed for the patient. Anticipate any necessary equipment based on the type of surgery and the patient's history.	
___	___	___	20. Remove PPE, if used. Perform hand hygiene.	

Skill Checklists for Taylor's Clinical Nursing Skills.
A Nursing Process Approach, 5th edition

Name ______________________ Date ______________________

Unit ______________________ Position ______________________

Instructor/Evaluator: ______________________ Position ______________________

SKILL 6-5

Providing Postoperative Care

Excellent	Satisfactory	Needs Practice	**Goal:** The patient will recover from the surgery.	**Comments**
			Immediate Care	
___	___	___	1. When patient returns from the PACU, participate in hand-off report from the PACU nurse and review the OR and PACU data. Gather the necessary supplies.	
___	___	___	2. Perform hand hygiene and put on PPE, if indicated.	
___	___	___	3. Identify the patient.	
___	___	___	4. Close the curtains around the bed and close the door to the room, if possible. Explain what you are going to do and why you are going to do it to the patient or significant other. Place necessary supplies on the bedside stand, overbed table, or other surface within easy reach.	
___	___	___	5. ***Place patient in safe position (semi- or high-Fowler's or side-lying). Note level of consciousness.***	
___	___	___	6. ***Obtain vital signs. Monitor and record vital signs frequently.*** Assessment order may vary, but usual frequency includes taking vital signs every 15 minutes the first hour, every 30 minutes the next 2 hours, every hour for 4 hours, and finally every 4 hours.	
___	___	___	7. Assess the patient's respiratory status. Measure the patient's oxygen saturation level. If oxygen is ordered, ensure accurate delivery device and flow rate.	
___	___	___	8. Assess the patient's cardiovascular status.	
___	___	___	9. Assess the patient's neurovascular status, based on the type of surgery performed.	
___	___	___	10. Provide for warmth, using heated or extra blankets, or forced-air warming device as necessary. Assess skin color and condition.	
___	___	___	11. Put on gloves. Assess the surgical site. Check dressings for color, odor, presence of drains, and amount of drainage. Mark the drainage on the dressing by circling the amount, and include the time. Assess dependent areas, such as turning the patient to assess visually under the patient, for bleeding from the surgical site.	

SKILL 6-5

Providing Postoperative Care *(Continued)*

Excellent	Satisfactory	Needs Practice		Comments
___	___	___	12. Verify that all tubes and drains are patent and the equipment is working; note the amount of drainage in collection device. If an indwelling urinary catheter is in place, note urinary output.	
___	___	___	13. Verify and maintain IV infusion at prescribed rate.	
___	___	___	14. Assess for pain. Check health record to verify if analgesic medication was administered in the PACU. Administer analgesics as indicated, prescribed/ordered and appropriate. If the patient has been instructed in the use of PCA for pain management, review its use. Institute nonpharmacologic pain management interventions as appropriate and indicated.	
___	___	___	15. Assess for nausea and vomiting. Administer antiemetic medication as indicated, prescribed/ordered, and appropriate.	
___	___	___	16. Provide for a safe environment. Keep bed in low position with side rails up, based on facility policy. Have call bell within patient's reach.	
___	___	___	17. Remove PPE, if used. Perform hand hygiene.	
			Ongoing Care	
___	___	___	18. Promote optimal respiratory function.	
___	___	___	a. Assess respiratory rate, depth, quality, color, and capillary refill. Ask if the patient is experiencing any difficulty breathing.	
___	___	___	b. Assist with coughing and deep-breathing exercises.	
___	___	___	c. Assist with incentive spirometry, as indicated/ordered.	
___	___	___	d. Assist with early ambulation.	
___	___	___	e. Provide frequent position changes.	
___	___	___	f. Administer oxygen, as ordered.	
___	___	___	g. Monitor pulse oximetry.	
___	___	___	19. Promote optimal cardiovascular function:	
___	___	___	a. Assess apical rate, rhythm, and quality and compare with peripheral pulses, color, and blood pressure. Ask if the patient has any chest pains or shortness of breath.	
___	___	___	b. Provide frequent position changes.	
___	___	___	c. Assist with early ambulation.	
___	___	___	d. Apply graduated compression stockings or pneumatic compression devices, if ordered and not in place. If in place, assess for integrity.	
___	___	___	e. Provide leg and range-of-motion exercises if not contraindicated.	

Excellent	Satisfactory	Needs Practice	SKILL 6-5 **Providing Postoperative Care** *(Continued)*	Comments
___	___	___	20. Promote optimal neurologic function:	
___	___	___	a. Assess level of consciousness, movement, and sensation.	
___	___	___	b. Determine the level of orientation to person, place, and time.	
___	___	___	c. Test motor ability by asking the patient to move each extremity.	
___	___	___	d. Evaluate sensation by asking the patient if he or she can feel your touch on an extremity.	
___	___	___	21. Promote optimal renal and urinary function and fluid and electrolyte status. Assess intake and output, evaluate for urinary retention and monitor serum electrolyte levels.	
___	___	___	a. Promote voiding by offering bedpan/bedside commode, or assistance to bathroom at regular intervals, noting the frequency, amount, and if any burning or urgency symptoms.	
___	___	___	b. Monitor urinary catheter drainage if present.	
___	___	___	c. Measure intake and output.	
___	___	___	22. Promote optimal gastrointestinal function and meet nutritional needs:	
___	___	___	a. Assess abdomen for distention and firmness. Ask if patient feels nauseated, any vomiting, and if passing flatus.	
___	___	___	b. Auscultate for bowel sounds.	
___	___	___	c. Assist with diet progression; encourage fluid intake; monitor intake.	
___	___	___	d. Medicate for nausea and vomiting, as ordered.	
___	___	___	23. Promote optimal wound healing.	
___	___	___	a. Assess condition of wound for presence of drains and any drainage.	
___	___	___	b. Use surgical asepsis for dressing changes and drain care.	
___	___	___	c. Inspect all skin surfaces for beginning signs of pressure injury and use pressure-relieving supports to minimize potential skin breakdown.	

SKILL 6-5

Providing Postoperative Care *(Continued)*

Excellent	Satisfactory	Needs Practice		Comments
___	___	___	24. Promote optimal comfort and relief from pain.	
___	___	___	a. Assess for pain (location and intensity using pain scale).	
___	___	___	b. Provide for rest and comfort; provide extra blankets, as needed, for warmth.	
___	___	___	c. Administer analgesics, as needed, and/or initiate nonpharmacologic methods, as appropriate.	
___	___	___	25. Promote optimal meeting of psychosocial needs:	
___	___	___	a. Provide emotional support to patient and family, as needed.	
___	___	___	b. Explain procedures and offer explanations regarding postoperative recovery, as needed, to both patient and family members.	

Skill Checklists for Taylor's Clinical Nursing Skills. A Nursing Process Approach, 5th edition

Name ______________________ Date ______________________

Unit ______________________ Position ______________________

Instructor/Evaluator: ______________________ Position ______________________

SKILL 6-6

Applying a Forced-Air Warming Device

Goal: The patient returns to and maintains a temperature of 97.7°F to 99.5°F (36.5°C to 37.5°C).

Excellent	Satisfactory	Needs Practice		Comments
___	___	___	1. Check the patient's health record for the order for the use of a forced-air warming device. Gather the necessary supplies.	
___	___	___	2. Perform hand hygiene and put on PPE, if indicated.	
___	___	___	3. Identify the patient.	
___	___	___	4. Close the curtains around the bed and close the door to the room, if possible. Explain what you are going to do and why you are going to do it to the patient or significant other. Place necessary supplies on the bedside stand, overbed table, or other surface within easy reach.	
___	___	___	5. ***Assess the patient's temperature.***	
___	___	___	6. Plug forced-air warming device into electrical outlet. Place forced-air blanket over patient, with plastic side up. Keep air-hose inlet at foot of bed.	
___	___	___	7. Securely insert air hose into inlet. Place a lightweight fabric blanket over the forced-air blanket, according to manufacturer's instructions. Turn the machine on and adjust temperature of air to desired effect.	
___	___	___	8. Remove PPE, if used. Perform hand hygiene.	
___	___	___	9. ***Monitor the patient's temperature at least every 30 minutes while using the forced-air device. If rewarming a patient with hypothermia, do not raise the temperature more than 1°C/hr to prevent a rapid vasodilation effect.***	
___	___	___	10. Discontinue use of the forced-air device once patient's temperature is adequate and the patient can maintain the temperature without assistance.	
___	___	___	11. Remove device and clean according to facility policy and manufacturer's instructions.	

Skill Checklists for Taylor's Clinical Nursing Skills. A Nursing Process Approach, 5th edition

Name ______________________ Date ______________________

Unit ______________________ Position ______________________

Instructor/Evaluator: ______________________ Position ______________________

SKILL 7-1

Assisting With a Shower or Tub Bath

Goal: The patient will be clean and fresh, and without injury.

Excellent	Satisfactory	Needs Practice		Comments
___	___	___	1. Review the patient's health record for any limitations in physical activity. Check presence of medical order for clearing the patient to shower, if required by facility policy.	
___	___	___	2. Check to see that the bathroom is available, clean, and safe. Make sure showers and tubs have mats or nonskid strips to prevent patients from falling. Place a mat or towel on the floor in front of the shower or tub. Put a shower or tub chair in place, as appropriate. Place "occupied" sign on door of room, as appropriate for setting.	
___	___	___	3. Gather necessary hygienic and toiletry items, and linens. Place within easy reach of shower or tub.	
___	___	___	4. Perform hand hygiene.	
___	___	___	5. Identify the patient. Discuss the procedure with the patient and assess the patient's ability to assist in the bathing process, as well as personal hygiene preferences.	
___	___	___	6. Assist the patient to bathroom to void or defecate, if appropriate.	
___	___	___	7. Assist the patient to put on a robe and slippers or nonskid socks. Cover IV access site(s) according to facility policy.	
___	___	___	8. Assist the patient to the shower or tub.	
___	___	___	9. Close the curtains around the shower or tub, as appropriate, and close the door to the bathroom. Adjust the room temperature, if necessary. Shower: Turn shower on. Check to see that the water temperature is safe and comfortable. Tub: Fill tub halfway with water. Check to see that the water temperature is safe and comfortable. Adjust water temperature, if appropriate, based on patient preference. ***Water temperature should be adjusted to 100°F to less than 120° to 125°F, with the lower temperature limit suggested for children and older adults*** (Burn Foundation, 2016).	
___	___	___	10. Explain the use of the call device and ensure that it is within the reach of the shower or tub.	

Excellent	Satisfactory	Needs Practice	SKILL 7-1 **Assisting With a Shower or Tub Bath** *(Continued)*	Comments
___	___	___	11. Put on gloves, as indicated. Help the patient get in and out of the shower or tub, as necessary. Use safety bars. For a tub: Have the patient grasp the handrails at the side of the tub, or place a chair at the side of the tub. The patient sits on the chair and eases to the edge of the tub. After putting both feet into the tub, have the patient reach to the opposite side and ease down into the tub. The patient may kneel first in the tub and then sit in it.	
___	___	___	12. If necessary, use a hydraulic lift, when available, to lower patients who are unable to maneuver safely or completely bear their own weight. Some community-based settings have walk-in tubs available.	
___	___	___	13. Keep room door unlocked. Remain in room with the patient to offer assistance, as appropriate. If assistance is needed with bathing, put on gloves. Otherwise, check on the patient every 5 minutes. ***Never leave young children or confused patients alone in the bathroom.***	
___	___	___	14. Assist the patient out of the shower or tub when bathing is complete. Obtain the assistance of additional personnel, as appropriate. Use safety bars. For a tub: Drain the water from the tub. Have the patient grasp the handrails at the side of the tub. Assist the patient to the edge of the tub. Have the patient ease to a chair placed at the side of the tub, then remove feet out of tub. The patient may kneel first in the tub and then move to the side of the tub.	
___	___	___	15. If necessary, use a hydraulic lift, when available, to raise patients who are unable to maneuver safely or completely bear their own weight.	
___	___	___	16. Put on gloves, as indicated. Assist the patient with drying, application of emollients, and dressing, as appropriate or necessary. Remove cover from IV access site.	
___	___	___	17. Remove gloves, if used. Assist the patient to the room and into a position of comfort.	
___	___	___	18. Clean shower or tub according to facility policy. Dispose of soiled linens according to facility policy. Remove "occupied" sign from door of bathroom.	
___	___	___	19. Perform hand hygiene.	

Skill Checklists for Taylor's Clinical Nursing Skills. A Nursing Process Approach, 5th edition

Name ______________________ Date ______________________

Unit ______________________ Position ______________________

Instructor/Evaluator: ______________________ Position ______________________

SKILL 7-2

Providing a Bed Bath

Excellent	Satisfactory	Needs Practice	**Goal:** The patient will be clean and fresh.	**Comments**
___	___	___	1. Review the patient's health record for any limitations in physical activity.	
___	___	___	2. Perform hand hygiene and put on gloves and/or other PPE, if indicated.	
___	___	___	3. Identify the patient. Discuss the procedure with the patient and assess the patient's ability to assist in the bathing process, as well as personal hygiene preferences.	
___	___	___	4. Assemble equipment on the overbed table or other surface within reach.	
___	___	___	5. Close the curtains around the bed and close the door to the room, if possible. Adjust the room temperature, if necessary.	
___	___	___	6. Adjust the bed to a comfortable working height; usually elbow height of the caregiver (VHACEOSH, 2016).	
___	___	___	7. Remove sequential compression devices and antiembolism stockings from lower extremities according to facility protocol.	
___	___	___	8. Put on gloves. Offer the patient a bedpan or urinal.	
___	___	___	9. Remove gloves and perform hand hygiene.	
___	___	___	10. Put on a clean pair of gloves. Lower the side rail nearest to you and assist the patient to the side of bed where you will work. Have the patient lie on his or her back.	
___	___	___	11. Loosen top covers and remove all except the top sheet. Place a bath blanket over the patient and then remove the top sheet while the patient holds the bath blanket in place. If linen is to be reused, fold it over a chair. Place soiled linen in laundry bag. Take care to prevent linen from coming in contact with your clothing.	
___	___	___	12. Remove the patient's gown or clothing and keep the bath blanket in place. If the patient has an IV line and is not wearing a gown with snap sleeves, remove gown from other arm first. Lower the IV container and pass the gown over the tubing and the container. ***Rehang the container and check the drip rate.***	

Excellent	Satisfactory	Needs Practice	SKILL 7-2 **Providing a Bed Bath** *(Continued)*	Comments
___	___	___	13. *Raise side rails.* Fill basin with a sufficient amount of comfortably warm water (100°F to less than 120° to 125°F). Add the skin cleanser, if appropriate, according to manufacturer's directions. Change, as necessary, throughout the bath. Lower the side rail nearest to you when you return to the bedside to begin the bath.	
___	___	___	14. Put on gloves, if indicated. Lay a towel across the patient's chest and on top of bath blanket.	
___	___	___	15. With no cleanser on the washcloth, wipe one eye from the inner part of the eye, near the nose, to the outer part. Rinse or turn the cloth before washing the other eye.	
___	___	___	16. Bathe the patient's face, neck, and ears. Apply appropriate emollient.	
___	___	___	17. Expose the patient's far arm and place towel lengthwise under it. Using firm strokes, wash hand, arm, and axilla, lifting the arm as necessary to access axillary region. Rinse, if necessary, and dry. Apply appropriate emollient. Cover the area with the bath blanket.	
___	___	___	18. Repeat Action 17 for the arm nearest you. Another option might be to bathe one side of the patient first and then move to the other side of the bed to complete the bath.	
___	___	___	19. Spread a towel across the patient's chest. Lower the bath blanket to the patient's umbilical area. Wash, rinse, if necessary, and dry chest. Keep chest covered with towel between the wash and rinse. Pay special attention to the folds of skin under the breasts. Apply appropriate emollient.	
___	___	___	20. Lower the bath blanket to the perineal area. Place a towel over the patient's chest.	
___	___	___	21. Wash, rinse, if necessary, and dry abdomen. Carefully inspect and clean umbilical area and any abdominal folds or creases. Apply appropriate emollient.	
___	___	___	22. Return bath blanket to original position and expose far leg. Place towel under far leg. Using firm strokes, wash, rinse, if necessary, and dry leg from ankle to knee and knee to groin. Apply appropriate emollient.	
___	___	___	23. Wash, rinse if necessary, and dry the foot. Pay particular attention to the areas between toes. Apply appropriate emollient.	
___	___	___	24. Repeat Actions 22 and 23 for the other leg and foot.	
___	___	___	25. Make sure the patient is covered with bath blanket. Change water and washcloth at this point or earlier, if necessary.	

Excellent	Satisfactory	Needs Practice	SKILL 7-2 **Providing a Bed Bath** *(Continued)*	Comments
____	____	____	26. Assist the patient to a prone or side-lying position. Put on gloves, if not applied earlier. Position bath blanket and towel to expose only the back and buttocks.	
____	____	____	27. Wash, rinse, if necessary, and dry back and buttocks area. ***Pay particular attention to cleansing between gluteal folds, and observe for any redness or skin breakdown in the sacral area.***	
____	____	____	28. If not contraindicated, give the patient a backrub. Alternatively, back massage may be given after perineal care. Apply appropriate emollient and/or skin barrier product.	
____	____	____	29. Raise the side rail. Refill basin with clean water. Discard washcloth and towel. Remove gloves and put on clean gloves.	
____	____	____	30. Clean perineal area or set the patient up so that he or she can complete perineal self-care. If the patient is unable to do so, lower the side rail and complete perineal care. Apply skin barrier, as indicated. Raise the side rail, remove gloves, and perform hand hygiene.	
____	____	____	31. Help the patient put on a clean gown or clothing and assist with the use of other personal toiletries, such as deodorant or cosmetics.	
____	____	____	32. Protect pillow with towel, and groom the patient's hair.	
____	____	____	33. ***When finished, make sure the patient is comfortable, with the side rails up and the bed in the lowest position.***	
____	____	____	34. Change bed linens. Dispose of soiled linens according to facility policy. Clean bath basin according to facility policy before returning to storage at bedside. Remove gloves and any other PPE, if used. Perform hand hygiene.	

Skill Checklists for Taylor's Clinical Nursing Skills.
A Nursing Process Approach, 5th edition

Name ______________________ Date ______________________

Unit ______________________ Position ______________________

Instructor/Evaluator: ______________________ Position ______________________

SKILL 7-3

Assisting the Patient With Oral Care

Goal: The patient has a clean mouth and clean teeth, exhibits a positive body image, and verbalizes the importance of oral care.

Excellent	Satisfactory	Needs Practice		Comments
___	___	___	1. Perform hand hygiene and put on gloves if assisting with oral care, and/or other PPE, if indicated.	
___	___	___	2. Identify the patient. Explain the procedure to the patient.	
___	___	___	3. Assemble equipment on overbed table or other surface within the patient's reach.	
___	___	___	4. Close the room door or curtains. Place the bed at an appropriate and comfortable working height; usually elbow height of the caregiver (VHACEOSH, 2016).	
___	___	___	5. Lower the side rail and assist the patient to a sitting position, if permitted, or turn the patient onto side. Place towel across the patient's chest.	
___	___	___	6. Encourage the patient to brush own teeth according to the following guidelines. Assist, if necessary.	
___	___	___	a. Moisten toothbrush and apply toothpaste to bristles.	
___	___	___	b. Place brush at a 45-degree angle to gum line and brush from gum line to crown of each tooth. Brush outer and inner surfaces. Brush back and forth across biting surface of each tooth.	
___	___	___	c. Brush tongue gently with toothbrush.	
___	___	___	d. Have the patient rinse vigorously with water and spit into emesis basin. Repeat until clear. Suction may be used as an alternative for removal of fluid and secretions from the mouth.	

Excellent	Satisfactory	Needs Practice	SKILL 7-3 **Assisting the Patient With Oral Care** *(Continued)*	Comments
____	____	____	7. Assist patient to floss teeth, if appropriate:	
____	____	____	a. Remove approximately 18 in of dental floss from container or use a plastic floss holder. Wrap most of the floss around one of the middle fingers. Wind the remaining floss around the same finger of the opposite hand, keeping about 1 to 1.5 in of floss taut between the fingers.	
____	____	____	b. Insert floss gently between teeth, moving it back and forth downward to the gums.	
____	____	____	c. Move the floss up and down, first on one side of a tooth and then on the side of the other tooth, until the surfaces are clean. Repeat in the spaces between all teeth and the backside of the last teeth.	
____	____	____	d. Instruct the patient to rinse mouth well with water after flossing.	
____	____	____	8. Offer a mouth rinse if the patient prefers or if use has been recommended.	
____	____	____	9. Offer lip balm or petroleum jelly.	
____	____	____	10. Remove equipment. Remove gloves and discard. Raise the side rail and lower the bed. Assist the patient to a position of comfort.	
____	____	____	11. Remove any other PPE, if used. Perform hand hygiene.	

Skill Checklists for Taylor's Clinical Nursing Skills. A Nursing Process Approach, 5th edition

Name ______________________ Date ______________________

Unit ______________________ Position ______________________

Instructor/Evaluator: ______________________ Position ______________________

SKILL 7-4

Providing Oral Care for the Dependent Patient

Goal: The patient has a clean mouth and clean teeth; is free from impaired oral mucous membranes; and verbalizes, if able, anunderstanding about the importance of oral care.

Excellent	Satisfactory	Needs Practice		Comments
___	___	___	1. Perform hand hygiene and put on PPE, if indicated.	
___	___	___	2. Identify the patient. Explain the procedure to the patient.	
___	___	___	3. Assemble equipment on overbed table or other surface within reach.	
___	___	___	4. Close the room door or curtains. Place the bed at an appropriate and comfortable working height, usually elbow height of the caregiver (VHACEOSH, 2016). Lower one side rail and position the patient on the side, with head tilted forward. Place towel across the patient's chest and emesis basin in position under chin. Depending on equipment in use, connect the suction toothbrush or suction catheter to suction tubing and turn on suction. Put on gloves.	
___	___	___	5. Gently open the patient's mouth by applying pressure to the lower jaw at the front of the mouth. Do not use fingers to hold the patient's mouth open. Use another toothbrush or mouth prop to keep the mouth open (Johnson & Chalmers, 2011). Remove dentures, if present.	
___	___	___	6. If using a regular toothbrush and suction catheter, one care giver provides oral cleaning and the other removes secretions with the suction catheter.	
___	___	___	7. Brush the teeth and gums carefully with toothbrush and paste or other oral cleanser. Lightly brush the tongue.	
___	___	___	8. Moisten toothbrush with water to rinse the oral cavity. ***Position the patient's head to allow for return of water. If using regular toothbrush, use suction catheter to remove the water and cleanser from oral cavity.***	
___	___	___	9. Using the suction swab, apply a therapeutic antiseptic mouth rinse as indicated. Apply oral moisturizer as indicated.	
___	___	___	10. Clean the dentures before replacing.	
___	___	___	11. Apply lubricant to the patient's lips.	
___	___	___	12. Remove equipment and return the patient to a position of comfort. Remove gloves. Raise the side rail and lower the bed.	
___	___	___	13. Remove additional PPE, if used. Perform hand hygiene.	

Skill Checklists for Taylor's Clinical Nursing Skills. A Nursing Process Approach, 5th edition

Name ______________________ Date ______________________

Unit ______________________ Position ______________________

Instructor/Evaluator: ______________________ Position ______________________

SKILL 7-5

Providing Denture Care

Goal: The patient will have a clean mouth and clean dentures, exhibit a positive body image, and verbalize the importance of oral care.

Excellent	Satisfactory	Needs Practice		Comments
___	___	___	1. Perform hand hygiene and put on PPE, if indicated.	
___	___	___	2. Identify the patient. Explain the procedure to the patient.	
___	___	___	3. Assemble equipment on overbed table or other surface within reach.	
___	___	___	4. Provide privacy for the patient.	
___	___	___	5. Lower the side rail and assist the patient to a sitting position, if permitted, or turn the patient onto the side. Place a towel across the patient's chest. Raise the bed to a comfortable working position, usually elbow height of the caregiver (VHACEOSH, 2016). Put on gloves.	
___	___	___	6. Apply gentle pressure with 4 × 4 gauze to grasp lower denture plate and remove it. If necessary, use a slight rocking motion to remove plate. Place it immediately in denture cup. Grasp upper denture with gauze and remove it. Place in denture cup.	
___	___	___	7. Place paper towels or washcloth in sink while brushing. Using the toothbrush and denture paste, brush all denture surfaces gently but thoroughly. Be sure to completely remove any denture adhesive remaining on the denture (Felton et al., 2011). If the patient prefers, add denture cleaner to cup with water and follow directions on preparation. After denture soaks, brush denture as previously described.	
___	___	___	8. Rinse thoroughly with water. Apply denture adhesive, if appropriate, following product directions.	
___	___	___	9. Use a toothbrush and toothpaste to gently clean gums, mucous membranes, and tongue. Offer water and/or mouth rinse so the patient can rinse mouth before replacing dentures.	
___	___	___	10. Insert upper denture in mouth and press firmly. Insert lower denture. If adhesive is used, ask the patient to bite firmly. Check that the dentures are securely in place and comfortable.	

SKILL 7-5

Providing Denture Care *(Continued)*

Excellent	Satisfactory	Needs Practice		Comments
____	____	____	11. If the patient desires, dentures can be stored in the denture cup in cold water, instead of returning to the mouth. Label the cup and place it on the patient's bedside table.	
____	____	____	12. Remove equipment and return the patient to a position of comfort. Remove your gloves. Raise the side rail and lower the bed.	
____	____	____	13. Remove additional PPE, if used. Perform hand hygiene.	

Skill Checklists for Taylor's Clinical Nursing Skills. A Nursing Process Approach, 5th edition

Name ______________________ Date ______________________

Unit ______________________ Position ______________________

Instructor/Evaluator: ______________________ Position ______________________

SKILL 7-6

Removing Contact Lenses

Excellent	Satisfactory	Needs Practice	**Goal:** The lenses are removed without trauma to the eye and stored safely.	Comments
___	___	___	1. Perform hand hygiene and put on PPE, if indicated.	
___	___	___	2. Identify the patient. Explain the procedure to the patient.	
___	___	___	3. Assemble equipment on overbed table or other surface within reach.	
___	___	___	4. Close the curtains around the bed and close the door to the room, if possible.	
___	___	___	5. Assist the patient to a supine position. Raise the bed to a comfortable working position, usually elbow height of the caregiver (VHACEOSH, 2016). Lower the side rail closest to you.	
___	___	___	6. If containers are not already labeled, do so now. Place 5 mL of normal saline or appropriate contact disinfecting solution in each container.	
___	___	___	7. Put on gloves. Remove soft contact lens:	
___	___	___	a. Have the patient look forward. Retract the lower lid with one hand. Using the pad of the index finger of the other hand, move the lens down to the sclera.	
___	___	___	b. Using the pads of the thumb and index finger, grasp the lens with a gentle pinching motion and remove it.	
___	___	___	8. Place the first lens in its designated cup in the storage case before removing the second lens.	
___	___	___	9. Repeat actions to remove other contact lens.	
___	___	___	10. If the patient is awake and has glasses at bedside, offer the patient glasses.	
___	___	___	11. Remove equipment and return the patient to a position of comfort. Remove your gloves. Raise the side rail and lower the bed.	
___	___	___	12. Remove additional PPE, if used. Perform hand hygiene.	

Skill Checklists for Taylor's Clinical Nursing Skills. A Nursing Process Approach, 5th edition

Name ______________________ Date ______________

Unit ______________________ Position ______________

Instructor/Evaluator: ______________________ Position ______________

SKILL 7-7

Shampooing a Patient's Hair in Bed

Excellent	Satisfactory	Needs Practice	**Goal:** The patient's hair will be clean.	**Comments**
___	___	___	1. Review the health record for any limitations in physical activity, or contraindications to the procedure. Confirm the presence of a medical order for shampooing the patient's hair, if required by facility policy.	
___	___	___	2. Perform hand hygiene. Put on PPE, as indicated.	
___	___	___	3. Identify the patient. Explain the procedure to the patient.	
___	___	___	4. Assemble equipment on overbed table or other surface within reach.	
___	___	___	5. Close the curtains around the bed and close the door to the room, if possible.	
___	___	___	6. Lower the head of the bed. Raise the bed to a comfortable working position, usually the elbow height of the caregiver (VHACEOSH, 2016). Lower the side rail. Remove the pillow and place a protective pad under the patient's head and shoulders.	
___	___	___	7. ***Fill the pitcher with comfortably warm water (100°F to less than 120° to 125°F).*** Position the patient at the top of the bed, in a supine position. Have the patient lift his or her head and place the shampoo board underneath the patient's head. If necessary, pad the edge of the board with a small towel.	
___	___	___	8. Place a drain container underneath the drain of the shampoo board.	
___	___	___	9. Put on gloves. If the patient is able, have him or her hold a folded washcloth at the forehead. Pour a pitcher of warm water slowly over the patient's head, making sure that all hair is saturated. Refill pitcher, if needed.	
___	___	___	10. Apply a small amount of shampoo to the patient's hair. Lather shampoo. Massage deep into the scalp, avoiding any cuts, lesions, or sore spots.	
___	___	___	11. Rinse with comfortably warm water until all shampoo is out of hair. Repeat shampoo, if necessary.	
___	___	___	12. If the patient has thick hair or requests it, apply a small amount of conditioner to the hair and massage throughout. Avoid any cuts, lesions, or sore spots.	

Excellent	Satisfactory	Needs Practice	SKILL 7-7 **Shampooing a Patient's Hair in Bed** *(Continued)*	Comments
____	____	____	13. If drain container is small, empty before rinsing hair. Rinse with comfortably warm water until all conditioner is out of hair.	
____	____	____	14. Remove shampoo board. Place towel around the patient's hair.	
____	____	____	15. Pat hair dry, avoiding any cuts, lesions, or sore spots. Remove protective padding, but keep one dry protective pad under the patient's hair.	
____	____	____	16. Gently brush hair, removing tangles, as needed.	
____	____	____	17. Blow-dry hair on a cool setting, if allowed and if the patient wishes. If not, consider covering the patient's head with a dry towel, until hair is dry.	
____	____	____	18. Change the patient's gown and remove protective pad. Replace pillow.	
____	____	____	19. Remove the equipment and return the patient to a position of comfort. Remove your gloves. Raise the side rail and lower the bed.	
____	____	____	20. Remove additional PPE, if used. Perform hand hygiene.	

Skill Checklists for Taylor's Clinical Nursing Skills. A Nursing Process Approach, 5th edition

Name ______________________ Date ______________________

Unit ______________________ Position ______________________

Instructor/Evaluator: ______________________ Position ______________________

SKILL 7-8

Assisting the Patient to Shave

Goal: The patient will be clean, without evidence of hair growth or trauma to the skin.

Excellent	Satisfactory	Needs Practice		Comments
___	___	___	1. Review the health record for any limitations in physical activity, or contraindications to the procedure. Confirm the presence of a medical order for shaving the patient, if required by facility policy.	
___	___	___	2. Perform hand hygiene. Put on PPE, as indicated.	
___	___	___	3. Identify the patient. Explain the procedure to the patient.	
___	___	___	4. Assemble equipment on overbed table or other surface within reach.	
___	___	___	5. Close the curtains around the bed and close the door to the room, if possible.	
___	___	___	6. Raise the bed to a comfortable working position, usually elbow height of the caregiver (VHACEOSH, 2016). Lower the side rail. Cover the patient's chest with a towel or waterproof pad. Fill bath basin with comfortably warm (100°F to less than 120° to 125°F) water. Put on gloves. Wet a washcloth in the basin of water. Press the warm washcloth on the area to be shaved.	
___	___	___	7. Dispense shaving cream or gel into the palm of the hand. Apply cream to the area to be shaved in a layer about 0.5 in thick. Allow to remain on the skin for a few minutes.	
___	___	___	8. With one hand, hold the skin steady at the area to be shaved. Using a smooth stroke, begin shaving. If shaving the face, shave with the direction of hair growth in short strokes. If shaving a leg, shave against the hair in upward, short strokes. If shaving an underarm, hold skin steady and use short, upward strokes.	
___	___	___	9. Remove residual shaving cream with wet washcloth.	
___	___	___	10. If the patient requests, apply aftershave or lotion to the area shaved.	
___	___	___	11. Remove equipment and return the patient to a position of comfort. Remove your gloves. Raise the side rail and lower the bed.	
___	___	___	12. Remove additional PPE, if used. Perform hand hygiene.	

Skill Checklists for Taylor's Clinical Nursing Skills. A Nursing Process Approach, 5th edition

Name ______________________ Date ______________

Unit ______________________ Position ______________

Instructor/Evaluator: ______________________ Position ______________

SKILL 7-9

Providing Nail Care

Goal: Nails are trimmed and clean with smooth edges and intact cuticles, without evidence of trauma to nails or surrounding skin.

Excellent	Satisfactory	Needs Practice		Comments
___	___	___	1. Review health record for any limitations in physical activity, or contraindications to the procedure. Confirm presence of medical order for nail care, if required by facility policy.	
___	___	___	2. Perform hand hygiene. Put on PPE, as indicated.	
___	___	___	3. Identify the patient. Explain the procedure to the patient.	
___	___	___	4. Assemble equipment on overbed table or other surface within reach.	
___	___	___	5. Close the curtains around the bed and close the door to the room, if possible.	
___	___	___	6. Raise bed to a comfortable working position, usually elbow height of the caregiver (VHACEOSH, 2016). Lower the side rail. Place a towel or waterproof pad under the patient's hand or foot.	
___	___	___	7. Put on gloves. Wash the patient's hands or feet, depending on the care to be given.	
___	___	___	8. Gently clean under the nails using the cuticle or orangewood stick. Wash hand or foot.	
___	___	___	9. Clip nails, if necessary. Avoid cutting the whole nail in one attempt. Use the tip of the nail clipper and take small cuts. Cut the nail straight across. Do not trim so far down on the sides that the skin and cuticle are injured. ***Only file, do not cut, the nails of patients with diabetes or circulatory problems.***	
___	___	___	10. File the nail straight across, then round the tips in a gentle curve, to shape the nail. Do not trim so far down on the sides that the skin and cuticle are injured. ***Only file, do not cut, the nails of patients with diabetes or circulatory problems.***	
___	___	___	11. Remove hangnails, which are broken pieces of cuticle, by carefully trimming them off with cuticle scissors. ***Do not pull or rip off hangnails.*** Avoid injury to tissue with the cuticle scissors.	
___	___	___	12. Gently push cuticles back off the nail using the orangewood or cuticle stick or towel.	

SKILL 7-9

Providing Nail Care *(Continued)*

Excellent	Satisfactory	Needs Practice		Comments
___	___	___	13. Dry hand or foot thoroughly, taking care to be sure to dry between fingers or toes. Apply an emollient to the hand or foot, rubbing it into the nails and cuticles. ***Do not moisturize between the toes of patients with peripheral artery disease.***	
___	___	___	14. Repeat Steps 7-13 for other extremity or extremities.	
___	___	___	15. Remove equipment and return the patient to a position of comfort. Remove your gloves. Raise the side rail and lower the bed.	
___	___	___	16. Remove additional PPE, if used. Perform hand hygiene.	

Skill Checklists for Taylor's Clinical Nursing Skills.
A Nursing Process Approach, 5th edition

Name ______________________ Date ______________________

Unit ______________________ Position ______________________

Instructor/Evaluator: ______________________ Position ______________________

SKILL 7-10
Making an Unoccupied Bed

Goal: The bed linens are changed without injury to the patient or nurse.

Excellent	Satisfactory	Needs Practice		Comments
____	____	____	1. Perform hand hygiene. Put on PPE, as indicated.	
____	____	____	2. Explain to the patient what you are going to do and the reason for doing it, if the patient is present in the room.	
____	____	____	3. Assemble necessary equipment on the bedside stand, overbed table, or other surface within reach.	
____	____	____	4. Adjust the bed to a comfortable working height, usually elbow height of the caregiver (VHACEOSH, 2016). Drop the side rails.	
____	____	____	5. Disconnect call bell or any tubes from bed linens.	
____	____	____	6. Put on gloves. Loosen all linen as you move around the bed, from the head of the bed on the far side to the head of the bed on the near side.	
____	____	____	7. Fold reusable linens, such as sheets, blankets, or spread, in place on the bed in fourths and hang them over a clean chair.	
____	____	____	8. Snugly roll all the soiled linen inside the bottom sheet. Hold linen away from your body and place directly into the laundry hamper. ***Do not place on floor or furniture. Do not hold soiled linens against your clothing.***	
____	____	____	9. If possible, shift mattress up to head of bed. If mattress is soiled, clean and dry according to facility policy before applying new sheets.	
____	____	____	10. Remove your gloves, unless indicated for transmission-based precautions. Place the bottom sheet on the mattress and secure the bottom sheet over the corners at the head and foot of the mattress.	
____	____	____	11. Push the sheet open to the center of the mattress, pulling the sheet taut from the secured corners.	

SKILL 7-10

Making an Unoccupied Bed *(Continued)*

Excellent	Satisfactory	Needs Practice		Comments
___	___	___	12. If using, place the drawsheet with its centerfold in the center of the bed and positioned so it will be located under the patient's midsection. Open the drawsheet and fan-fold to the center of the mattress. If a protective pad is used, place it over the drawsheet in the proper area and open to the centerfold. Not all facilities use drawsheets routinely. The nurse may decide to use one. In some institutions, the protective pad doubles as a drawsheet. Tuck the drawsheet securely under the mattress.	
___	___	___	13. Move to the other side of the bed to secure bottom linens. Pull the bottom sheet tightly and secure over the corners at the head and foot of the mattress. Pull the drawsheet tightly and tuck it securely under the mattress.	
___	___	___	14. Place the top sheet on the bed with its centerfold in the center of the bed and with the hem even with the head of the mattress. Unfold the top sheet. Follow same procedure with top blanket or spread, placing the upper edge about 6 in below the top of the sheet.	
___	___	___	15. Tuck the top sheet and blanket under the foot of the bed on the near side. Miter the corners.	
___	___	___	16. Fold the upper 6 in of the top sheet down over the spread and make a cuff.	
___	___	___	17. Move to the other side of the bed and follow the same procedure for securing top sheets under the foot of the bed and making a cuff.	
___	___	___	18. Place the pillows on the bed. Open each pillowcase in the same manner as you opened other linens. Gather the pillowcase over one hand toward the closed end. Grasp the pillow with the hand inside the pillowcase. Keep a firm hold on the top of the pillow and pull the cover onto the pillow. Place the pillow at the head of the bed.	
___	___	___	19. Fan-fold or pie-fold the top linens.	
___	___	___	20. Secure the signal device on the bed, according to facility policy.	
___	___	___	21. Raise the side rail and lower the bed.	
___	___	___	22. Dispose of soiled linen according to facility policy.	
___	___	___	23. Remove any other PPE, if used. Perform hand hygiene.	

Skill Checklists for Taylor's Clinical Nursing Skills. A Nursing Process Approach, 5th edition

Name ______________________ Date ______________________

Unit ______________________ Position ______________________

Instructor/Evaluator: ______________________ Position ______________________

SKILL 7-11

Making an Occupied Bed

Goal: The bed linens are applied without injury to the patient or nurse.

Excellent	Satisfactory	Needs Practice		Comments
___	___	___	1. Check health care record for limitations on the patient's physical activity.	
___	___	___	2. Perform hand hygiene. Put on PPE, as indicated.	
___	___	___	3. Identify the patient. Explain what you are going to do.	
___	___	___	4. Assemble equipment on overbed table or other surface within reach.	
___	___	___	5. Close the curtains around the bed and close the door to the room, if possible.	
___	___	___	6. Adjust the bed to a comfortable working height, usually elbow height of the caregiver (VHACEOSH, 2016).	
___	___	___	7. Lower the side rail nearest you, leaving the opposite side rail up. Place the bed in a flat position unless contraindicated.	
___	___	___	8. Put on gloves. Check bed linens for the patient's personal items. ***Disconnect the call bell or any tubes/drains from bed linens.***	
___	___	___	9. Place a bath blanket over the patient. Have the patient hold on to the bath blanket while you reach under it and remove the top linens. Leave the top sheet in place if a bath blanket is not used. Fold linen that is to be reused over the back of a chair. Discard soiled linen in a laundry bag or hamper. ***Do not place on floor or furniture. Do not hold soiled linens against your clothing.***	
___	___	___	10. If possible, and another person is available to assist, grasp mattress securely and shift it up to head of bed.	
___	___	___	11. Assist the patient to turn toward the opposite side of the bed, and reposition pillow under the patient's head.	
___	___	___	12. Loosen all bottom linens from head, foot, and side of bed.	
___	___	___	13. Fan-fold or roll soiled linens as close to the patient as possible.	
___	___	___	14. Use clean linen and make the near side of the bed. Place the bottom sheet in the center of the bed. Open the sheet and pull the bottom sheet over the corners at the head and foot of the mattress. Push the sheet toward the center of the bed, pulling it taut and positioning it under the old linens.	

SKILL 7-11

Making an Occupied Bed *(Continued)*

Excellent	Satisfactory	Needs Practice		Comments
___	___	___	15. If using, place the drawsheet with its centerfold in the center of the bed and positioned so it will be located under the patient's midsection. Open the drawsheet and fan-fold it to the center of the mattress. Tuck the drawsheet securely under the mattress. If a protective pad is used, place it over the drawsheet in the proper area and open to the centerfold. Not all facilities use drawsheets routinely. The nurse may decide to use one.	
___	___	___	16. Raise the side rail. Assist the patient to roll over the folded linen in the middle of the bed toward you. Reposition pillow and bath blanket or top sheet. Move to other side of the bed and lower the side rail.	
___	___	___	17. Loosen and remove all bottom linen. Discard soiled linen in laundry bag or hamper. ***Do not place on floor or furniture. Do not hold soiled linens against your clothing.***	
___	___	___	18. Ease clean linen from under the patient. Pull the bottom sheet taut and secure at the corners at the head and foot of the mattress. Pull the drawsheet tight and smooth. Tuck the drawsheet securely under the mattress.	
___	___	___	19. Assist the patient to turn back to the center of bed. Remove pillow and change pillowcase. Open each pillowcase in the same manner as you opened other linens. Gather the pillowcase over one hand toward the closed end. Grasp the pillow with the hand inside the pillowcase. Keep a firm hold on the top of the pillow and pull the cover onto the pillow. Place the pillow under the patient's head.	
___	___	___	20. Apply top linen, sheet, and blanket, if desired, so that it is centered. Fold the top linens over at the patient's shoulders to make a cuff. Have the patient hold on to top linen and remove the bath blanket from underneath.	
___	___	___	21. Secure top linens under foot of mattress and miter corners. Loosen top linens over the patient's feet by grasping them in the area of the feet and pulling gently toward the foot of bed.	
___	___	___	22. Return the patient to a position of comfort. Remove your gloves. Raise the side rail and lower the bed. Reattach call bell.	
___	___	___	23. Dispose of soiled linens according to facility policy.	
___	___	___	24. Remove any other PPE, if used. Perform hand hygiene.	

Skill Checklists for Taylor's Clinical Nursing Skills.
A Nursing Process Approach, 5th edition

Name ______________________ Date ______________________

Unit ______________________ Position ______________________

Instructor/Evaluator: ______________________ Position ______________________

SKILL 8-1
Preventing Pressure Injury

Excellent	Satisfactory	Needs Practice	**Goal:** The patient does not experience pressure injury and/or alterations in skin integrity.	**Comments**
___	___	___	1. Perform hand hygiene and put on PPE, if indicated.	
___	___	___	2. Identify the patient.	
___	___	___	3. Discuss pressure injury prevention with the patient and/or patient caregivers. Explain what pressure injury is, the causes of pressure injuries, and the importance of a pressure injury prevention plan (WOCN, 2016).	
___	___	___	4. Assess the patient's skin at least daily, paying special attention to the skin over bony prominences and the skin in contact with medical devices (Doughty & McNichol, 2016; NPUAP, EPUAT, PPPIA, 2014a).	
___	___	___	5. Assess the patient's risk for pressure injury upon entry to a health care setting and on a regularly scheduled basis or when there is a significant change in the patient's condition, incorporating appropriate assessment tools and scales, based on facility policy (WOCN, 2016).	
___	___	___	6. Utilize appropriate support surfaces to redistribute tissue loads, based on facility policy and availability. Appropriate support surfaces may include, but are not limited to, integrated bed systems, specialized and/or low-pressure mattresses and overlays, seating surfaces and cushions, heel elevation devices, and foam positioning wedges. Note: Pressure redistribution devices should serve as adjuncts and not replacements for repositioning of patients (WOCN, 2016). ***Do not use foam rings, foam cut-outs or donut-type devices.*** The Wound, Ostomy and Continence Nurses Society (WOCN, 2016) has developed a content-validated algorithm for support surface selection.	

Excellent	Satisfactory	Needs Practice	SKILL 8-1 **Preventing Pressure Injury** *(Continued)*	Comments
___	___	___	7. Routinely reposition the patient; at least every 2 hours for bedridden patients and every hour for patients in a chair or wheelchair (Doughty & McNichol, 2016). Consider the pressure redistribution support surface in the use as well as the individual patient's status when determining the frequency of repositioning; the use of some types of support surfaces may extend the frequency (Doughty & McNichol; NPUAP, EPUAP, PPPIA, 2014a). Note: Regular repositioning may not be possible due to the patient's medical condition and alternative strategies such as a "high-specification bed" may be required (NPUAP, EPUAP, PPPIA, 2014a; WOCN, 2016).	
___	___	___	8. Use a 30-degree side-lying position (lateral tilt position) when positioning patients at risk for pressure injury in side-lying positions (WOCN, 2016).	
___	___	___	9. Encourage and provide early mobilization. Develop a schedule for progressive sitting and ambulation as rapidly as tolerated by the individual patient. Collaborate with the physical and occupational therapists to develop an individualized intervention plan.	
___	___	___	10. Maintain the head-of-bed elevation at or below 30 degrees, or at the lowest degree of elevation appropriate for the patient's medical condition.	
___	___	___	11. Consider the use of a prophylactic dressing, such as a polyurethane foam dressing, on bony prominences, such as heels and the sacrum. Replace prophylactic dressings that are damaged, displaced, loosened, or excessively moist (NPUAP, EPUAP, PPPIA, 2014a).	
___	___	___	12. Consider the use of low-friction patient care textiles, such as bed linens and patient gowns, and the use of silk-like fabrics instead of cotton or cotton-blend fabrics.	
___	___	___	13. Utilize proper lifting, positioning, and repositioning techniques (safe patient handling and movement techniques); for example, use lift/repositioning sheets and sufficient caregivers when moving a patient. Collaborate with the physical and occupational therapists to develop an individualized intervention plan.	
___	___	___	14. Utilize interventions to protect the skin from excessive exposure to moisture from wound exudate, perspiration, mucous, saliva, fistula or stoma effluent, and urinary and fecal incontinence.	

Excellent	Satisfactory	Needs Practice	SKILL 8-1 **Preventing Pressure Injury** *(Continued)*	Comments
___	___	___	15. Provide appropriate interventions to support the patient's nutritional status and ensure adequate intake. Interventions may include strategies to enhance oral intake, nutritional supplements, fortified foods, and/or enteral or parenteral feeding (Baranoski & Ayello, 2016). Collaborate with the registered dietician and dietary staff to develop an individualized nutrition intervention plan (NPUAP, EPUAP, PPPIA, 2014a).	
___	___	___	16. Implement interventions to prevent pressure injury related to the use of medical devices, based on the individual patient's situation.	
___	___	___	a. Ensure correct for patient size and application of devices in use.	
___	___	___	b. Use cushioning dressings under the device, as appropriate to the individual patient and clinical use (NPUAP, EPUAP, PPPIA, 2014a).	
___	___	___	c. Inspect the skin under the devices and observe for edema under the devices at least twice daily or more often, as indicated.	
___	___	___	d. Remove device as soon as medically feasible. Reposition or rotate any medical device daily when possible.	
___	___	___	e. Keep the skin clean and dry under medical devices.	
___	___	___	17. Provide education to the patient and caregiver(s) about the prevention plan and ways to minimize the risk of pressure injury.	
___	___	___	18. Remove gloves and additional PPE, if used. Perform hand hygiene.	
___	___	___	19. Evaluate the patient's response to interventions. Reassess and alter care plan as indicated by facility policies and procedures, as appropriate.	

Skill Checklists for Taylor's Clinical Nursing Skills. A Nursing Process Approach, 5th edition

Name ______ Date ______

Unit ______ Position ______

Instructor/Evaluator: ______ Position ______

SKILL 8-2

Cleaning a Wound and Applying a Dressing (General Guidelines)

Goal: The wound is cleaned and dressed without contaminating the wound area, causing trauma to the wound, and/or causing the patient to experience pain or discomfort.

Excellent	Satisfactory	Needs Practice		Comments
___	___	___	1. Review the patient's health record for prescribed wound care or the nursing care plan related to wound care. Gather necessary supplies.	
___	___	___	2. Perform hand hygiene and put on PPE, if indicated.	
___	___	___	3. Identify the patient.	
___	___	___	4. Assemble equipment on the overbed table or other surface within reach.	
___	___	___	5. Close the curtains around the bed and close the door to the room, if possible. Explain to the patient what you are going to do and why you are going to do it.	
___	___	___	6. Assess the patient for the possible need for nonpharmacologic pain-reducing interventions or analgesic medication before wound care dressing change. Administer appropriate prescribed analgesic. Allow enough time for the analgesic to achieve its effectiveness.	
___	___	___	7. Place a waste receptacle or bag at a convenient location for use during the procedure.	
___	___	___	8. Adjust the bed to a comfortable working height, usually elbow height of the caregiver (VHA Center for Engineering & Occupational Safety and Health [CEOSH], 2016).	
___	___	___	9. Assist the patient to a comfortable position that provides easy access to the wound area. Use the bath blanket to cover any exposed area other than the wound. Place a waterproof pad under the wound site.	

Excellent	Satisfactory	Needs Practice	SKILL 8-2 **Cleaning a Wound and Applying a Dressing (General Guidelines)** *(Continued)*	Comments
___	___	___	10. Check the position of drains, tubes, or other adjuncts before removing the dressing. Put on clean, disposable gloves and loosen the tape or adhesive edge on the old dressings by removing in the direction of hair growth and the use of a push–pull method. Push–pull method: lift a corner of the dressing away from the skin, and then gently push the skin away from the dressing/adhesive. Continue moving fingers of the opposite hand to support the skin as the product is removed (McNichol, Lund, Rose, & Gray, 2013). Carefully lift the adhesive barrier from the surrounding skin to prevent medical adhesive–related skin injury (MARSI). Remove the sides/edges first, then the center. If there is resistance, use an adhesive remover (McNichol et al., 2013).	
___	___	___	11. Carefully remove the soiled dressings. If any part of the dressing sticks to the underlying skin, use small amounts of sterile saline to help loosen and remove it.	
___	___	___	12. After removing the dressing, note the presence, amount, type, color, and odor of any drainage on the dressings. Place soiled dressings in the appropriate waste receptacle. Remove your gloves and dispose of them in an appropriate waste receptacle.	
___	___	___	13. Perform hand hygiene.	
___	___	___	14. Inspect the wound site for size, appearance, and drainage. Assess if any pain is present. Check the status of sutures, adhesive closure strips, staples, and drains or tubes, if present. Note any problems to include in your documentation.	
___	___	___	15. ***Using sterile technique, prepare a sterile work area and open the needed supplies.***	
___	___	___	16. Open the sterile cleaning solution. Depending on the amount of cleaning needed, the solution might be poured directly over gauze sponges over a container for small cleaning jobs, or into a basin for more complex or larger cleaning.	
___	___	___	17. Put on sterile gloves. Alternatively, clean gloves (clean technique) may be used when cleaning a chronic wound or pressure injury.	
___	___	___	18. Clean the wound. ***Clean from top to bottom and/or from the center to the outside.*** Use new gauze for each wipe, placing the used gauze in the waste receptacle. Alternatively, spray the wound from top to bottom with a commercially prepared wound cleanser; wound irrigation is often used to clean open wounds and may also be used for other types of wounds. Refer to Skill 8-3.	

Excellent	Satisfactory	Needs Practice	SKILL 8-2 **Cleaning a Wound and Applying a Dressing (General Guidelines)** *(Continued)*	Comments
___	___	___	19. Once the wound is cleaned, dry the area using a gauze sponge in the same manner.	
___	___	___	20. If a drain is in use at the wound location, clean around the drain. Refer to Skills 8-6, 8-7, 8-8, and 8-9.	
___	___	___	21. Remove gloves and place in the waste receptacle. Perform hand hygiene.	
___	___	___	22. Put on sterile gloves. Alternately, clean gloves (clean technique) may be used when cleaning a chronic wound or pressure injury. Apply a skin protectant or barrier to the healthy skin around the wound where the dressing adhesive or tape will be placed and where wound drainage may come in contact with the skin.	
___	___	___	23. Apply any topical medications, foams, gels, and/or gauze to the wound as prescribed; ensure products stay confined to the wound and do not impact on intact surrounding tissue/skin.	
___	___	___	24. Gently place a layer of dry, sterile dressing, or other prescribed cover dressing at the wound center and extend it at least 1 in beyond the wound in all directions. Alternately, follow the manufacturer's directions for application. Forceps may be used to apply the dressing.	
___	___	___	25. As necessary, apply a surgical or abdominal pad (ABD) over the gauze at the site of the outermost layer of the dressing, with the side of the dressing with the blue line facing away from the patient. Alternately, note the side of the dressing that contains the moisture barrier and place away from the patient, based on the dressing material in use. Note: May not be necessary or appropriate, based on the cover dressing used in step 22.	
___	___	___	26. Apply tape, Montgomery straps, or roller gauze to secure the dressings. Alternately, many commercial wound products are self-adhesive and do not require additional tape. Remove and discard gloves.	
___	___	___	27. After securing the dressing, label it with date and time. Remove all remaining equipment; place the patient in a comfortable position, with side rails up as indicated and bed in the lowest position.	
___	___	___	28. Remove PPE, if used. Perform hand hygiene.	
___	___	___	29. Check all wound dressings at least every shift. More frequent checks may be needed if the wound is more complex or dressings become saturated quickly.	

Skill Checklists for Taylor's Clinical Nursing Skills. A Nursing Process Approach, 5th edition

Name ______________________ Date ______________________

Unit ______________________ Position ______________________

Instructor/Evaluator: ______________________ Position ______________________

SKILL 8-3
Performing Irrigation of a Wound

Excellent	Satisfactory	Needs Practice	**Goal:** The wound is cleaned without contamination or trauma; without damaging proliferative cells and newly formed tissues; and without causing the patient to experience pain or discomfort.	**Comments**
___	___	___	1. Review the patient's health record for prescribed wound care or the nursing care plan related to wound care. Gather necessary supplies.	
___	___	___	2. Perform hand hygiene and put on PPE, if indicated.	
___	___	___	3. Identify the patient.	
___	___	___	4. Assemble equipment on the overbed table or other surface within reach.	
___	___	___	5. Close the curtains around the bed and close the door to the room if possible. Explain what you are going to do and why you are going to do it to the patient.	
___	___	___	6. Assess the patient for possible need for nonpharmacologic pain-reducing interventions or analgesic medication before wound care and/or dressing change. Administer appropriate prescribed analgesic. Allow enough time for the analgesic to achieve its effectiveness before beginning the procedure.	
___	___	___	7. Place a waste receptacle or bag at a convenient location for use during the procedure.	
___	___	___	8. Adjust the bed to a comfortable working height, usually elbow height of the caregiver (VHACEOSH, 2016).	
___	___	___	9. Assist the patient to a comfortable position that provides easy access to the wound area. Position the patient so the irrigation solution will flow from the clean end of the wound toward the dirtier end or top to bottom. Use the bath blanket to cover any exposed area other than the wound. Place a waterproof pad under the wound site.	
___	___	___	10. Put on a gown, mask, and eye protection or face shield.	

SKILL 8-3

Performing Irrigation of a Wound *(Continued)*

Excellent	Satisfactory	Needs Practice		Comments
___	___	___	11. Check the position of drains, tubes, or other adjuncts before removing the dressing. Put on clean, disposable gloves and loosen the tape on the old dressings by removing in the direction of hair growth and the use of a push–pull method. Push–pull method: lift a corner of the dressing away from the skin, then gently push the skin away from the dressing/adhesive. Continue moving fingers of the opposite hand to support the skin as the product is removed (McNichol et al., 2013). Carefully lift the adhesive barrier from the surrounding skin to prevent medical adhesive–related skin injury (MARSI). Remove the sides/edges first, then the center. If there is resistance, use an adhesive remover (McNichol et al., 2013).	
___	___	___	12. Carefully remove the soiled dressings. If any part of the dressing sticks to the underlying skin, use small amounts of sterile saline to help loosen and remove it.	
___	___	___	13. After removing the dressing, note the presence, amount, type, color, and odor of any drainage on the dressings. Place soiled dressings in the appropriate waste receptacle.	
___	___	___	14. Assess the wound for appearance, stage, presence of eschar, granulation tissue, ***epithelialization***, undermining, tunneling, necrosis, ***sinus tract***, and drainage. Assess the appearance of the surrounding tissue. Measure the wound.	
___	___	___	15. Remove your gloves and put them in the receptacle. Perform hand hygiene.	
___	___	___	16. Set up a sterile field, if indicated, and wound cleaning and irrigation supplies. Pour warmed sterile irrigating solution into the sterile container. Put on the sterile gloves. Alternately, clean gloves (clean technique) may be used when cleaning a chronic wound or pressure injury.	
___	___	___	17. Position the sterile basin below the wound to collect the irrigation fluid.	
___	___	___	18. Fill the irrigation syringe with solution. ***Alternately, irrigation solution may be packaged in individual, single-use syringe; remove cap on syringe. Using your nondominant hand,*** gently apply pressure to the basin against the skin below the wound to form a seal with the skin.	
___	___	___	19. ***Direct a stream of solution into the wound. Keep the tip of the syringe at least 1 in above the upper edge of the wound. Flush all wound areas.***	

Excellent	Satisfactory	Needs Practice	SKILL 8-3 **Performing Irrigation of a Wound** *(Continued)*	Comments
___	___	___	20. Watch for the solution to flow smoothly and evenly. When the solution from the wound flows out clear, discontinue irrigation.	
___	___	___	21. Once the wound is cleaned, dry the surrounding skin using a gauze sponge.	
___	___	___	22. If a drain is in use at the wound location, clean around the drain. Refer to Skills 8-6, 8-7, 8-8, and 8-9.	
___	___	___	23. Remove gloves and place in a waste receptacle. Perform hand hygiene.	
___	___	___	24. Put on sterile gloves. Alternately, clean gloves (clean technique) may be used when cleaning a chronic wound or pressure injury. Apply a skin protectant or barrier to the healthy skin around the wound where the dressing adhesive or tape will be placed and where wound drainage may come in contact with skin.	
___	___	___	25. Apply any topical medications, foams, gels, and/or gauze to the wound as prescribed; ensure products stay confined to the wound and do not impact on intact surrounding tissue/skin.	
___	___	___	26. Gently place a layer of dry, sterile dressing or other prescribed cover dressing at the wound center and extend it at least 1 in beyond the wound in all directions. Alternately, follow the manufacturer's directions for application. Forceps may be used to apply the dressing.	
___	___	___	27. Apply tape, Montgomery straps, or roller gauze to secure the dressings, if needed. Alternately, many commercial wound products are self-adhesive and do not require additional tape. Remove and discard gloves.	
___	___	___	28. After securing the dressing, label it with date and time. Remove all remaining equipment; place the patient in a comfortable position, with side rails up as indicated and bed in the lowest position.	
___	___	___	29. Remove PPE, if used. Perform hand hygiene.	
___	___	___	30. Check all wound dressings at least every shift. More frequent checks may be needed if the wound is more complex or dressings become saturated quickly.	

Skill Checklists for Taylor's Clinical Nursing Skills. A Nursing Process Approach, 5th edition

Name ______________________ Date ______________________

Unit ______________________ Position ______________________

Instructor/Evaluator: ______________________ Position ______________________

SKILL 8-4

Collecting a Wound Culture

Goal: The culture is obtained without contamination, without exposing the patient to additional pathogens, and without causing discomfort for the patient; and the patient demonstrates an understanding of the reason for the wound culture.

Excellent	Satisfactory	Needs Practice		Comments
___	___	___	1. Review the patient's health record for prescribed orders for obtaining a wound culture. Gather necessary supplies. If possible, obtain the wound culture prior to the start of antimicrobial therapy.	
___	___	___	2. Perform hand hygiene and put on PPE, if indicated.	
___	___	___	3. Identify the patient.	
___	___	___	4. Assemble equipment on the overbed table or other surface within reach.	
___	___	___	5. Close the curtains around the bed and close the door to the room, if possible. Explain to the patient what you are going to do and why you are going to do it.	
___	___	___	6. Assess the patient for possible need for nonpharmacologic pain-reducing interventions or analgesic medication before obtaining the wound culture. Administer appropriate prescribed analgesic. Allow enough time for the analgesic to achieve its effectiveness before beginning the procedure.	
___	___	___	7. Place an appropriate waste receptacle within easy reach for use during the procedure.	
___	___	___	8. Adjust the bed to a comfortable working height, usually elbow height of the caregiver (VHACEOSH, 2016).	
___	___	___	9. Assist the patient to a comfortable position that provides easy access to the wound. If necessary, drape the patient with the bath blanket to expose only the wound area. Place a waterproof pad under the wound site. Check the culture label against the patient's identification bracelet.	
___	___	___	10. If there is a dressing in place on the wound, put on clean gloves and carefully remove the dressing. Refer to Skill 8-2. Note the presence, amount, type, color, and odor of any drainage on the dressings. Place soiled dressings in the appropriate waste receptacle.	
___	___	___	11. Remove gloves and perform hand hygiene.	
___	___	___	12. Assess and clean the wound, ***using a nonantimicrobial cleanser,*** as outlined in Skills 8-2 and 8-3.	

Excellent	Satisfactory	Needs Practice	SKILL 8-4 **Collecting a Wound Culture** *(Continued)*	Comments
___	___	___	13. Dry the surrounding skin with gauze dressings. Put on clean gloves.	
___	___	___	14. Twist the cap to loosen the swab on the Culturette tube, or open the separate swab(s) and remove the cap from the culture tube. ***Keep the swab and inside of the culture tube(s) sterile.***	
___	___	___	15. If contact with the wound is necessary to separate wound margins to permit insertion of the swab deep into the wound, put a sterile glove on one hand to manipulate the wound margins. Clean gloves may be appropriate for contact with pressure injuries and chronic wounds.	
___	___	___	16. ***Identify a 1 cm area of the wound that is free from necrotic tissue.*** Carefully insert the swab into this area of clean viable tissue. ***Press the swab to apply sufficient pressure to express fluid from the wound tissue and rotate the swab several times. Avoid touching the swab to intact skin at the wound edges.***	
___	___	___	17. Place the swab back in the culture tube. ***Do not touch the outside of the tube with the swab.*** Secure the cap. Some swab containers have an ampule of medium at the bottom of the tube. It might be necessary to crush this ampule to activate. Follow the manufacturer's instructions for use.	
___	___	___	18. Use another swab if collecting a specimen from another area of the wound or site and repeat the procedure.	
___	___	___	19. Remove gloves and discard them accordingly. Perform hand hygiene.	
___	___	___	20. Put on gloves. Place a dressing on the wound, as appropriate, based on prescribed orders and/or the nursing care plan. Refer to Skill 8-2. Remove gloves. Perform hand hygiene.	
___	___	___	21. After securing the dressing, label dressing with date and time. Remove all remaining equipment; place the patient in a comfortable position, with side rails up as indicated and bed in the lowest position.	
___	___	___	22. Label the specimen according to your institution's guidelines. Information included may include wound site, time the specimen was collected, any antimicrobials the patient is receiving, and the identity of the person who obtained the specimen (Huddleston Cross, 2014). Send or transport specimen to the laboratory in a biohazard bag immediately or within the optimal time from for transport as indicated by facility policy and guidelines.	
___	___	___	23. Remove PPE, if used. Perform hand hygiene.	

Skill Checklists for Taylor's Clinical Nursing Skills.
A Nursing Process Approach, 5th edition

Name ______________________ Date ______________________

Unit ______________________ Position ______________________

Instructor/Evaluator: ______________________ Position ______________________

SKILL 8-5

Applying Montgomery Straps

Goal: The Montgomery straps are applied and the patient's skin is free from irritation and injury.

Excellent	Satisfactory	Needs Practice		Comments
___	___	___	1. Review the patient's health record for prescribed wound care or the nursing care plan related to wound care. Gather necessary supplies.	
___	___	___	2. Perform hand hygiene and put on PPE, if indicated.	
___	___	___	3. Identify the patient.	
___	___	___	4. Assemble equipment on the overbed table or other surface within reach.	
___	___	___	5. Close the curtains around the bed and close the door to the room, if possible. Explain what you are going to do and why you are going to do it to the patient.	
___	___	___	6. Assess the patient for possible need for nonpharmacologic pain-reducing interventions or analgesic medication before wound care dressing change. Administer appropriate prescribed analgesic. Allow enough time for the analgesic to achieve its effectiveness before beginning the procedure.	
___	___	___	7. Place a waste receptacle at a convenient location for use during the procedure.	
___	___	___	8. Adjust the bed to a comfortable working height, usually elbow height of the caregiver (VHACEOSH, 2016).	
___	___	___	9. Assist the patient to a comfortable position that provides easy access to the wound area. Use a bath blanket to cover any exposed area other than the wound. Place a waterproof pad under the wound site.	
___	___	___	10. Perform wound care and a dressing change as ordered and outlined in Skills 8-2 and 8-3.	
___	___	___	11. Put on clean gloves. Clean the skin on either side of the wound with the gauze, moistened with normal saline. Dry the skin.	
___	___	___	12. ***Apply a skin protectant/barrier to the skin where the straps will be placed.***	
___	___	___	13. Cut the Montgomery strap to size, based on the size of the wound. Write the date and time of application on strap.	

Excellent	Satisfactory	Needs Practice	SKILL 8-5 **Applying Montgomery Straps** *(Continued)*	Comments
___	___	___	14. Cut the hydrocolloidal or nonhydrocolloidal skin barrier sheet to the size of the strap and apply to the patient's skin, near the dressing. Apply the sticky side of each strap to the skin barrier sheet, so the openings for the strings are at the edge of the dressing. Repeat for the other side.	
___	___	___	15. Tie the opposing ties together, over the dressing, like a shoelace. ***Do not secure too tightly.***	
___	___	___	16. Remove gloves. Perform hand hygiene. Label dressing with date and time. Remove all remaining equipment; place the patient in a comfortable position, with side rails up as indicated and the bed in the lowest position.	
___	___	___	17. If nondisposable scissors were used, put on gloves. Clean scissors with antimicrobial wipe.	
___	___	___	18. Remove gloves and additional PPE, if used. Perform hand hygiene.	
___	___	___	19. Check all wound dressings at least every shift. More frequent checks may be needed if the wound is more complex or dressings become saturated quickly.	
___	___	___	20. Replace the ties and straps whenever they are soiled, or every 2 to 3 days. Straps can be reapplied onto skin barrier. Skin barrier can remain in place up to 7 days. Use a silicone-based adhesive remover to help remove the skin barrier.	

Skill Checklists for Taylor's Clinical Nursing Skills. A Nursing Process Approach, 5th edition

Name ______________________ Date ______________________

Unit ______________________ Position ______________________

Instructor/Evaluator: ______________________ Position ______________________

SKILL 8-6

Caring for a Penrose Drain

Excellent	Satisfactory	Needs Practice	**Goal:** The Penrose drain remains patent and intact; the wound care is accomplished without contaminating the wound area, or causing trauma to the wound; and without causing the patient to experience pain or discomfort.	**Comments**
___	___	___	1. Review the patient's health record for prescribed wound care or the nursing care plan related to wound/drain care. Gather necessary supplies.	
___	___	___	2. Perform hand hygiene and put on PPE, if indicated.	
___	___	___	3. Identify the patient.	
___	___	___	4. Assemble equipment on the overbed table or other surface within reach.	
___	___	___	5. Close the curtains around the bed and close the door to the room, if possible. Explain what you are going to do and why you are going to do it to the patient.	
___	___	___	6. Assess the patient for possible need for nonpharmacologic pain-reducing interventions or analgesic medication before wound care dressing change. Administer appropriate prescribed analgesic. Allow enough time for the analgesic to achieve its effectiveness before beginning the procedure.	
___	___	___	7. Place a waste receptacle at a convenient location for use during the procedure.	
___	___	___	8. Adjust the bed to a comfortable working height, usually elbow height of the caregiver (VHACEOSH, 2016).	
___	___	___	9. Assist the patient to a comfortable position that provides easy access to the drain and/or wound area. Use a bath blanket to cover any exposed area other than the wound. Place a waterproof pad under the wound site.	
___	___	___	10. Put on clean, disposable gloves. Check the position of the drain or drains before removing the dressing. Loosen the tape on the old dressings by removing in the direction of hair growth and the use of a push–pull method. Push–pull method: lift a corner of the dressing away from the skin, then gently push the skin away from the dressing/adhesive. Continue moving fingers of the opposite hand to support the skin as the product is removed (McNichol et al., 2013). Carefully lift the adhesive from the surrounding skin to prevent medical adhesive–related skin injury (MARSI). Remove the sides/edges first, then the center. If there is resistance, use an adhesive remover (McNichol et al., 2013).	

Excellent	Satisfactory	Needs Practice	SKILL 8-6 **Caring for a Penrose Drain** *(Continued)*	Comments
___	___	___	11. Carefully remove the soiled dressings. If any part of the dressing sticks to the underlying skin, use small amounts of sterile saline to help loosen and remove it. Note the presence, amount, type, color, and odor of any drainage on the dressings. Place soiled dressings in the appropriate waste receptacle.	
___	___	___	12. Inspect the drain site for appearance and drainage. Assess if any pain is present.	
___	___	___	13. Remove gloves and perform hand hygiene.	
___	___	___	14. Using sterile technique, prepare a sterile work area and open the needed supplies.	
___	___	___	15. Open the sterile cleaning solution. Pour it into the basin. Add the gauze sponges.	
___	___	___	16. Put on sterile gloves.	
___	___	___	17. Cleanse the drain site with the cleaning solution. Use the forceps and the moistened gauze or cotton-tipped applicators. ***Start at the drain insertion site, moving in a circular motion toward the periphery. Use each gauze sponge or applicator only once.*** Discard and use new gauze if additional cleansing is needed.	
___	___	___	18. Dry the skin with a new gauze pad in the same manner. Apply skin protectant/barrier to the skin around the drain; extend out to include the area of skin that will be taped. Place a pre-split drain sponge under and around the drain. Closely observe the safety pin in the drain. If the pin or drain is crusted, replace the pin with a new sterile pin. ***Take care not to dislodge the drain.***	
___	___	___	19. Apply gauze pads over the drain. Apply surgical pad, ABD, or other cover dressing over the gauze.	
___	___	___	20. Apply tape, Montgomery straps, or roller gauze to secure the dressings. Remove and discard gloves. Perform hand hygiene.	
___	___	___	21. After securing the dressing, label dressing with date and time. Remove all remaining equipment; place the patient in a comfortable position, with side rails up as indicated and bed in the lowest position.	
___	___	___	22. Remove additional PPE, if used. Perform hand hygiene.	
___	___	___	23. Check all wound dressings at least every shift. More frequent checks may be needed if the wound is more complex or dressings become saturated quickly.	

Skill Checklists for Taylor's Clinical Nursing Skills. A Nursing Process Approach, 5th edition

Name ____________________ Date ____________________

Unit ____________________ Position ____________________

Instructor/Evaluator: ____________________ Position ____________________

SKILL 8-7

Caring for a T-Tube Drain

Excellent	Satisfactory	Needs Practice	**Goal:** The drain remains patent and intact; drain care is accomplished without contaminating the wound area and/or without causing trauma to the wound; and the patient does not experience pain or discomfort.	**Comments**
___	___	___	1. Review the patient's health record for prescribed wound care or the nursing care plan related to wound/drain care. Gather necessary supplies.	
___	___	___	2. Perform hand hygiene and put on PPE, if indicated.	
___	___	___	3. Identify the patient.	
___	___	___	4. Assemble equipment on the overbed table or other surface within reach.	
___	___	___	5. Close the curtains around the bed and close the door to the room, if possible. Explain what you are going to do and why you are going to do it to the patient.	
___	___	___	6. Assess the patient for possible need for nonpharmacologic pain-reducing interventions or analgesic medication before wound care dressing change. Administer appropriate prescribed analgesic. Allow enough time for the analgesic to achieve its effectiveness before beginning the procedure.	
___	___	___	7. Place a waste receptacle at a convenient location for use during the procedure.	
___	___	___	8. Adjust the bed to a comfortable working height, usually elbow height of the caregiver (VHACEOSH, 2016).	
___	___	___	9. Assist the patient to a comfortable position that provides easy access to the drain and/or wound area. Use a bath blanket to cover any exposed area other than the drain. Place a waterproof pad under the drain site.	
			Emptying Drainage	
___	___	___	10. Put on clean gloves; put on mask or face shield, as indicated.	
___	___	___	11. Using sterile technique, open a gauze pad, making a sterile field with the outer wrapper.	
___	___	___	12. Place the graduated collection container under the outlet valve of the drainage bag. ***Without touching the outlet, pull off the cap and empty the bag's contents completely into the container. Use the gauze to wipe the outlet, and replace the cap.***	
___	___	___	13. Carefully measure and note the characteristics of the drainage. Discard the drainage according to facility policy.	

SKILL 8-7

Caring for a T-Tube Drain *(Continued)*

Excellent	Satisfactory	Needs Practice		Comments
___	___	___	14. Remove gloves and perform hand hygiene.	
			Cleaning the Drain Site	
___	___	___	15. Put on clean, disposable gloves. Check the position of the drain before removing the dressing. Loosen the tape on the old dressings by removing in the direction of hair growth and the use of a push–pull method. Push–pull method: lift a corner of the dressing away from the skin, then gently push the skin away from the dressing/adhesive. Continue moving fingers of the opposite hand to support the skin as the product is removed (McNichol et al., 2013). Carefully lift the adhesive from the surrounding skin to prevent medical adhesive–related skin injury (MARSI). Remove the sides/edges first, then the center. If there is resistance, use an adhesive remover (McNichol et al., 2013).	
___	___	___	16. Carefully remove the soiled dressings. If any part of the dressing sticks to the underlying skin, use small amounts of sterile saline to help loosen and remove it. Note the presence, amount, type, color, and odor of any drainage on the dressings. Place soiled dressings in the appropriate waste receptacle.	
___	___	___	17. Inspect the drain site for appearance and drainage. Assess if any pain is present.	
___	___	___	18. Remove gloves and perform hand hygiene.	
___	___	___	19. Using sterile technique, prepare a sterile work area and open the needed supplies.	
___	___	___	20. Open the sterile cleaning solution. Pour it into the basin. Add the gauze sponges.	
___	___	___	21. Put on sterile gloves.	
___	___	___	22. Cleanse the drain site with the cleaning solution. Use the forceps and the moistened gauze or cotton-tipped applicators. ***Start at the drain insertion site, moving in a circular motion toward the periphery. Use each gauze sponge only once.*** Discard and use new gauze if additional cleansing is needed.	
___	___	___	23. Dry with new sterile gauze in the same manner. Apply skin protectant/barrier to the skin around the drain; extend out to include the area of skin that will be taped.	
___	___	___	24. Place a pre-split drain sponge under the drain. Apply gauze pads or other cover dressing, such as a transparent dressing, as indicated by facility policy, over the drain. Secure the dressings with tape, as needed. Remove and discard gloves. Perform hand hygiene.	

Excellent	Satisfactory	Needs Practice	SKILL 8-7 **Caring for a T-Tube Drain** *(Continued)*	**Comments**
____	____	____	25. Secure the drain tubing to the patient's skin using a tape or a commercial securement/stabilization device, allowing slack in the tubing to avoid excessive tension. ***Be careful not to kink the tubing and ensure the collection bag remains below the drain site.***	
____	____	____	26. Label the dressing with date and time. Remove all remaining equipment; place the patient in a comfortable position, with side rails up as indicated and bed in the lowest position.	
____	____	____	27. Remove additional PPE, if used. Perform hand hygiene.	
____	____	____	28. Check drain status at least every 4 hours. Check all wound dressings every shift. Perform more frequent checks if the wound is more complex or dressings become saturated quickly.	

Skill Checklists for Taylor's Clinical Nursing Skills. A Nursing Process Approach, 5th edition

Name ______________________ Date ______________________

Unit ______________________ Position ______________________

Instructor/Evaluator: ______________________ Position ______________________

SKILL 8-8

Caring for a Jackson–Pratt Drain

Excellent	Satisfactory	Needs Practice	**Goal:** The drain is patent and intact; drain care is accomplished without contaminating the wound area and/or without causing trauma to the wound; and the patient does not experience pain or discomfort.	**Comments**
___	___	___	1. Review the patient's health record for prescribed wound care or the nursing care plan related to wound/drain care. Gather necessary supplies.	
___	___	___	2. Perform hand hygiene and put on PPE, if indicated.	
___	___	___	3. Identify the patient.	
___	___	___	4. Assemble equipment on the overbed table or other surface within reach.	
___	___	___	5. Close the curtains around the bed and close the door to the room, if possible. Explain what you are going to do and why you are going to do it to the patient.	
___	___	___	6. Assess the patient for possible need for nonpharmacologic pain-reducing interventions or analgesic medication before wound care dressing change. Administer appropriate prescribed analgesic. Allow enough time for the analgesic to achieve its effectiveness before beginning the procedure.	
___	___	___	7. Place a waste receptacle at a convenient location for use during the procedure.	
___	___	___	8. Adjust the bed to a comfortable working height, usually elbow height of the caregiver (VHACEOSH, 2016).	
___	___	___	9. Assist the patient to a comfortable position that provides easy access to the drain and/or wound area. Use a bath blanket to cover any exposed area other than the drain. Place a waterproof pad under the drain site.	
___	___	___	10. Put on clean gloves; put on mask or face shield, as indicated.	
___	___	___	11. Using sterile technique, open a gauze pad, making a sterile field with the outer wrapper.	
___	___	___	12. Place the graduated collection container under the drain outlet. Without contaminating the outlet valve, pull off the cap. The chamber will expand completely as it draws in air. ***Empty the chamber's contents completely into the container. Use the gauze pad to wipe the outlet. Fully compress the chamber with one hand and replace the cap with your other hand.***	

Excellent	Satisfactory	Needs Practice	SKILL 8-8 **Caring for a Jackson–Pratt Drain** *(Continued)*	Comments
___	___	___	13. Check the patency of the equipment. Bulb should remain compressed. ***Check that the tubing is free from twists and kinks.***	
___	___	___	14. Secure the JP drain to the patient's gown below the wound with a safety pin, ***making sure that there is no tension on the tubing.***	
___	___	___	15. Carefully measure and record the character, color, and amount of the drainage. Discard the drainage according to facility policy. Remove gloves. Perform hand hygiene.	
___	___	___	16. Put on clean gloves. If the drain site has a dressing, remove the dressing (as outlined in Skill 8-7) and assess the site.	
___	___	___	17. Remove gloves and perform hand hygiene.	
___	___	___	18. Cleanse the drain site and redress as outlined in Skill 8-7.	
___	___	___	19. If the drain site is open to air, observe the sutures that secure the drain to the skin. Look for signs of pulling, tearing, swelling, or infection of the surrounding skin. Gently clean the sutures with the gauze pad moistened with normal saline. Dry with a new gauze pad. Apply skin protectant/barrier to the surrounding skin.	
___	___	___	20. Remove and discard gloves. Perform hand hygiene.	
___	___	___	21. Remove all remaining equipment; place the patient in a comfortable position, with side rails up as indicated and bed in the lowest position.	
___	___	___	22. Remove additional PPE, if used. Perform hand hygiene.	
___	___	___	23. Check drain status at least every 4 hours. Empty and reengage suction (compress device) when device is half to two thirds full. Check all wound dressings at least every shift. More frequent checks may be needed if the wound is more complex or dressings become saturated quickly.	

Skill Checklists for Taylor's Clinical Nursing Skills. A Nursing Process Approach, 5th edition

Name ______________________________ Date ______________

Unit ______________________________ Position ______________

Instructor/Evaluator: ______________________________ Position ______________

SKILL 8-9

Caring for a Hemovac Drain

Excellent	Satisfactory	Needs Practice	**Goal:** The drain is patent and intact; drain care is accomplished without contaminating the wound area and/or without causing trauma to the wound; and the patient does not experience pain or discomfort.	Comments
___	___	___	1. Review the patient's health record for prescribed wound care or the nursing care plan related to wound/drain care. Gather necessary supplies.	
___	___	___	2. Perform hand hygiene and put on PPE, if indicated.	
___	___	___	3. Identify the patient.	
___	___	___	4. Assemble equipment on the overbed table or other surface within reach.	
___	___	___	5. Close the curtains around the bed and close the door to the room, if possible. Explain what you are going to do and why you are going to do it to the patient.	
___	___	___	6. Assess the patient for possible need for nonpharmacologic pain-reducing interventions or analgesic medication before wound care dressing change. Administer appropriate prescribed analgesic. Allow enough time for analgesic to achieve its effectiveness before beginning the procedure.	
___	___	___	7. Place a waste receptacle at a convenient location for use during the procedure.	
___	___	___	8. Adjust the bed to a comfortable working height, usually elbow height of the caregiver (VHACEOSH, 2016).	
___	___	___	9. Assist the patient to a comfortable position that provides easy access to the drain and/or wound area. Use a bath blanket to cover any exposed area other than the drain. Place a waterproof pad under the drain site.	
___	___	___	10. Put on clean gloves; put on mask or face shield, as indicated.	
___	___	___	11. Using sterile technique, open a gauze pad, making a sterile field with the outer wrapper.	
___	___	___	12. Place the graduated collection container under the drain outlet. ***Without contaminating the outlet, pull off the cap.*** The chamber will expand completely as it draws in air. ***Empty the chamber's contents completely into the container. Use the gauze pad to wipe the outlet. Fully compress the chamber by pushing the top and bottom together with your hands. Keep the device tightly compressed while you apply the cap.***	

SKILL 8-9

Caring for a Hemovac Drain *(Continued)*

Excellent	Satisfactory	Needs Practice		Comments
___	___	___	13. Device should remain compressed. Check the patency of the equipment. ***Make sure the tubing is free from twists and kinks.***	
___	___	___	14. Secure the Hemovac drain to the patient's gown below the wound with a safety pin, ***making sure that there is no tension on the tubing.***	
___	___	___	15. Carefully measure and record the character, color, and amount of the drainage. Discard the drainage according to facility policy. Remove gloves. Perform hand hygiene.	
___	___	___	16. Put on clean gloves. If the drain site has a dressing, remove the dressing, assess and clean the site, and replace the dressing as outlined in Skill 8-7. Include cleaning of the sutures with the gauze pad moistened with normal saline. Dry sutures with gauze before applying new dressing.	
___	___	___	17. If the drain site is open to air, observe the sutures that secure the drain to the skin. Look for signs of pulling, tearing, swelling, or infection of the surrounding skin. Gently clean the sutures with the gauze pad moistened with normal saline. Dry with a new gauze pad. Apply skin protectant/barrier to the surrounding skin, if needed.	
___	___	___	18. Remove and discard gloves. Perform hand hygiene.	
___	___	___	19. Remove all remaining equipment; place the patient in a comfortable position, with side rails up as indicated and bed in the lowest position.	
___	___	___	20. Remove additional PPE, if used. Perform hand hygiene.	
___	___	___	21. Check drain status at least every 4 hours. Empty and reengage suction (compress device) when device is half to two thirds full. Check all wound dressings at least every shift. More frequent checks may be needed if the wound is more complex or dressings become saturated quickly.	

Skill Checklists for Taylor's Clinical Nursing Skills.
A Nursing Process Approach, 5th edition

Name ______________________ Date ______________________

Unit ______________________ Position ______________________

Instructor/Evaluator: ______________________ Position ______________________

SKILL 8-10

Applying Negative Pressure Wound Therapy

Excellent	Satisfactory	Needs Practice	**Goal:** The a is accomplished without contaminating the wound area, without causing trauma to the wound, without causing the patient to experience pain or discomfort, and with the device functioning correctly.	Comments
____	____	____	1. Review the patient's health record for prescribed application of NPWT therapy, including the ordered pressure setting for the device. Gather necessary supplies.	
____	____	____	2. Perform hand hygiene and put on PPE, if indicated.	
____	____	____	3. Identify the patient.	
____	____	____	4. Assemble equipment on the overbed table or other surface within reach.	
____	____	____	5. Close the curtains around the bed and close the door to the room, if possible. Explain what you are going to do and why you are going to do it to the patient.	
____	____	____	6. Assess the patient for possible need for nonpharmacologic pain-reducing interventions or analgesic medication before wound care dressing change. Administer appropriate prescribed analgesic. Allow enough time for the analgesic to achieve its effectiveness before beginning the procedure.	
____	____	____	7. Adjust the bed to a comfortable working height, usually elbow height of the caregiver (VHACEOSH, 2016).	
____	____	____	8. Assist the patient to a comfortable position that provides easy access to the wound area. Position the patient so the cleaning/irrigation solution will flow from the clean end of the wound toward the dirty end. Expose the area and drape the patient with a bath blanket, if needed. Put a waterproof pad under the wound area.	
____	____	____	9. Have the disposal bag or waste receptacle within easy reach for use during the procedure.	
____	____	____	10. Using sterile technique, prepare a sterile field and add all the sterile supplies needed for the procedure to the field. Pour warmed, sterile irrigating solution into the sterile container, as indicated.	
____	____	____	11. Put on a gown, mask, and eye protection.	

SKILL 8-10

Applying Negative Pressure Wound Therapy *(Continued)*

Excellent	Satisfactory	Needs Practice		Comments
___	___	___	12. If NPWT is currently in use, turn off the negative pressure unit. Put on clean, disposable gloves. Loosen the tape on the old dressings by removing in the direction of hair growth and the use of a push–pull method. Push–pull method: lift a corner of the dressing away from the skin, then gently push the skin away from the dressing/adhesive. Continue moving fingers of the opposite hand to support the skin as the product is removed (McNichol et al., 2013). Carefully lift the adhesive from the surrounding skin to prevent medical adhesive–related skin injury (MARSI). Remove the sides/edges first, then the center. If there is resistance, use an adhesive remover (McNichol et al., 2013).	
___	___	___	13. Carefully remove the soiled dressings. If any part of the dressing sticks to the underlying skin, use small amounts of sterile saline to help loosen and remove it.	
___	___	___	14. Note the presence, amount, type, color, and odor of any drainage on the dressings. ***Note the number of pieces of wound contact material removed from the wound. Compare with the documented number from the previous dressing change.***	
___	___	___	15. Discard the dressings in the receptacle. Remove your gloves and put them in the receptacle. Perform hand hygiene.	
___	___	___	16. Put on sterile gloves. Using sterile technique, clean or irrigate the wound, based on wound care plan and prescribed wound care.	
___	___	___	17. Clean the area around the wound with normal saline or prescribed skin cleanser. Dry the surrounding skin with a sterile gauze sponge.	
___	___	___	18. Assess the wound for appearance, stage, presence of eschar, granulation tissue, epithelialization, undermining, tunneling, necrosis, sinus tract, and drainage. Assess the appearance of the surrounding tissue. Measure the wound.	
___	___	___	19. Remove gloves and perform hand hygiene.	
___	___	___	20. Put on sterile gloves. ***Wipe intact skin around the wound with a skin protectant/barrier wipe and allow it to dry.***	
___	___	___	21. If the use of a wound contact layer (impregnated porous gauze or silicone adhesive contact layer) is indicated, use sterile scissors to cut the wound contact layer to fit the wound bed. Apply wound contact layer to the wound bed.	

SKILL 8-10

Applying Negative Pressure Wound Therapy *(Continued)*

Excellent	Satisfactory	Needs Practice		Comments
___	___	___	22. Fit the wound contact material to the shape of the wound.	
___	___	___	• If using foam wound contact material, use sterile scissors to cut the foam to the shape and measurement of the wound. ***Do not cut foam over the wound.*** More than one piece of foam may be necessary if the first piece is cut too small. Carefully place the foam in the wound. ***Ensure foam-to-foam contact if more than one piece is required.***	
___	___	___	• If using gauze wound filler, ***carefully place in wound to fill cavity.***	
___	___	___	• ***Note the number of pieces of wound filler placed in the wound.***	
___	___	___	• ***Do not under- or over-fill.***	
___	___	___	23. Trim and place the transparent adhesive drape to cover the wound contact material and an additional 3 to 5 cm border of intact periwound tissue. ***Avoid stretching the transparent adhesive drape tight over the wound.***	
___	___	___	24. Choose an appropriate site to apply the connector pad/tubing port. Pinch the transparent adhesive drape and cut a hole through it. Apply the connector pad/tubing port and connective tubing over the hole. Position tubing away from the periwound area and anchor (Schreiber, 2016).	
___	___	___	25. Remove the drainage collection canister from the package and insert into the negative pressure unit until it locks into place. Attach the connective tubing to the canister and check that the clamps on the tubing are open, if present.	
___	___	___	26. Remove gloves and discard. Perform hand hygiene. Turn on the power to the negative pressure unit. Select the prescribed therapy settings (suction and cycle type) and start the device.	
___	___	___	27. ***Assess the dressing to ensure seal integrity. The dressing should be collapsed, shrinking to the wound contact material and skin. Observe drainage in tubing.***	
___	___	___	28. Label dressing with date and time. Remove all remaining equipment; place the patient in a comfortable position, with side rails up as indicated and bed in the lowest position.	
___	___	___	29. Remove PPE, if used. Perform hand hygiene.	
___	___	___	30. Check all wound dressings at least every shift. More frequent checks may be needed if the wound is more complex or dressings become saturated quickly. Check negative pressure settings at least every shift. Assess the patient's tolerance of and response to the therapy at least every shift.	

Skill Checklists for Taylor's Clinical Nursing Skills. A Nursing Process Approach, 5th edition

Name ______________________ Date ______________________

Unit ______________________ Position ______________________

Instructor/Evaluator: ______________________ Position ______________________

SKILL 8-11

Removing Sutures

Excellent	Satisfactory	Needs Practice	**Goal:** The sutures are removed without contaminating the incisional area, without causing trauma to the wound, and without causing the patient to experience pain or discomfort.	Comments
___	___	___	1. Review the patient's health record for prescribed orders for suture removal. Gather necessary supplies.	
___	___	___	2. Perform hand hygiene and put on PPE, if indicated.	
___	___	___	3. Identify the patient.	
___	___	___	4. Assemble equipment on the overbed table or other surface within reach.	
___	___	___	5. Close the curtains around the bed and close the door to the room, if possible. Explain what you are going to do and why you are going to do it to the patient. Describe the sensation of suture removal as a pulling or slightly uncomfortable experience.	
___	___	___	6. Assess the patient for possible need for nonpharmacologic pain-reducing interventions or analgesic medication before beginning the procedure. Administer appropriate prescribed analgesic. Allow enough time for the analgesic to achieve its effectiveness before beginning the procedure.	
___	___	___	7. Place a waste receptacle at a convenient location for use during the procedure.	
___	___	___	8. Adjust the bed to a comfortable working height, usually elbow height of the caregiver (VHACEOSH, 2016).	
___	___	___	9. Assist the patient to a comfortable position that provides easy access to the incision area. Use a bath blanket to cover any exposed area other than the incision. Place a waterproof pad under the incision site.	
___	___	___	10. Put on clean gloves. Carefully and gently remove any dressings that may be in place.	
___	___	___	11. Clean the incision, according to prescribed wound care or facility policy and procedure. Assess the wound.	
___	___	___	12. Perform hand hygiene. Open the suture removal kit. Put on clean disposable gloves.	

Excellent	Satisfactory	Needs Practice	SKILL 8-11 **Removing Sutures** *(Continued)*	Comments
___	___	___	13. Using the forceps, grasp the knot of the first suture and gently lift the knot up off the skin.	
___	___	___	14. Using the scissors, cut one side of the suture below the knot, close to the skin. Grasp the knot with the forceps and pull the cut suture through the skin. ***Avoid pulling the visible portion of the suture through the underlying tissue.***	
___	___	___	15. Remove every other suture to be sure the wound edges are healed. If the wound edges remain approximated, remove the remaining sutures, as ordered. Dispose of sutures according to facility policy.	
___	___	___	16. If wound closure strips are to be used, apply skin protectant/barrier to skin around incision. ***Do not apply to incision.*** Apply adhesive closure strips. Take care to handle the strips by the paper backing.	
___	___	___	17. Reapply the dressing, based on the prescribed orders and facility policy.	
___	___	___	18. Remove and discard gloves. Perform hand hygiene.	
___	___	___	19. Remove all remaining equipment; place the patient in a comfortable position, with side rails up as indicated and bed in the lowest position.	
___	___	___	20. Remove additional PPE, if used. Perform hand hygiene.	
___	___	___	21. Assess all wounds every shift. More frequent checks may be needed if the wound is more complex.	

Skill Checklists for Taylor's Clinical Nursing Skills. A Nursing Process Approach, 5th edition

Name ____________________ Date ____________________

Unit ____________________ Position ____________________

Instructor/Evaluator: ____________________ Position ____________________

SKILL 8-12

Removing Surgical Staples

Goal: The staples are removed without contaminating the incisional area, without causing trauma to the wound, and without causing the patient to experience pain or discomfort.

Excellent	Satisfactory	Needs Practice		Comments
___	___	___	1. Review the patient's health record for prescribed order for staple removal. Gather necessary supplies.	
___	___	___	2. Perform hand hygiene and put on PPE, if indicated.	
___	___	___	3. Identify the patient.	
___	___	___	4. Assemble equipment on the overbed table or other surface within reach.	
___	___	___	5. Close the curtains around the bed and close the door to the room, if possible. Explain what you are going to do and why you are going to do it to the patient. Describe the sensation of staple removal as a pulling experience.	
___	___	___	6. Assess the patient for possible need for nonpharmacologic pain-reducing interventions or analgesic medication before beginning the procedure. Administer the appropriate prescribed analgesic. Allow enough time for the analgesic to achieve its effectiveness before beginning the procedure.	
___	___	___	7. Place a waste receptacle at a convenient location for use during the procedure.	
___	___	___	8. Adjust the bed to a comfortable working height, usually elbow height of the caregiver (VHACEOSH, 2016).	
___	___	___	9. Assist the patient to a comfortable position that provides easy access to the incision area. Use a bath blanket to cover any exposed area other than the incision. Place a waterproof pad under the incision site.	
___	___	___	10. Put on clean gloves. Carefully remove any dressings that may be in place.	
___	___	___	11. Clean the incision, according to prescribed wound care or facility policy and procedure.	
___	___	___	12. Perform hand hygiene. Open the staple remover kit. Put on clean disposable gloves.	
___	___	___	13. Grasp the staple remover. ***Position the staple remover under the staple to be removed. Firmly close the staple remover.*** The staple will bend in the middle and the edges will pull up out of the skin.	

Excellent	Satisfactory	Needs Practice	SKILL 8-12 **Removing Surgical Staples** *(Continued)*	Comments
___	___	___	14. Remove every other staple to be sure the wound edges are healed. If the wound edges remain approximated, remove the remaining staples, as ordered. Dispose of staples in the sharps container.	
___	___	___	15. If wound closure strips are to be used, apply skin protectant to the skin around the incision. ***Do not apply to the incision.*** Apply adhesive closure strips. Take care to handle the strips by the paper backing. (Refer to Skill 8-11, step 16).	
___	___	___	16. Reapply the dressing, based on the prescribed orders and facility policy.	
___	___	___	17. Remove and discard gloves. Perform hand hygiene.	
___	___	___	18. Remove all remaining equipment; place the patient in a comfortable position, with side rails up as indicated and bed in the lowest position.	
___	___	___	19. Remove additional PPE, if used. Perform hand hygiene.	
___	___	___	20. Assess all wounds every shift. More frequent checks may be needed if the wound is more complex.	

Skill Checklists for Taylor's Clinical Nursing Skills. A Nursing Process Approach, 5th edition

Name ______________________ Date ______________________

Unit ______________________ Position ______________________

Instructor/Evaluator: ______________________ Position ______________________

SKILL 8-13

Applying an External Heating Pad

Goal: Desired outcome depends on the patient's nursing diagnosis.

Excellent	Satisfactory	Needs Practice		Comments
___	___	___	1. Review the patient's health record for prescribed order for the application of heat therapy, including frequency, type of therapy, body area to be treated, and length of time for the application. Gather necessary supplies.	
___	___	___	2. Perform hand hygiene and put on PPE, if indicated.	
___	___	___	3. Identify the patient.	
___	___	___	4. Assemble equipment on the overbed table or other surface within reach.	
___	___	___	5. Close the curtains around the bed and close the door to the room if possible. Explain what you are going to do and why you are going to do it to the patient.	
___	___	___	6. Adjust the bed to a comfortable working height, usually elbow height of the caregiver (VHACEOSH, 2016).	
___	___	___	7. Assist the patient to a comfortable position that provides easy access to the area where the heat will be applied; use a bath blanket to cover any other exposed area.	
___	___	___	8. Assess the condition of the skin where the heat is to be applied.	
___	___	___	9. Check that the water in the electronic unit is at the appropriate level. Fill the unit two thirds full or to the fill mark, with distilled water, if necessary. Check the temperature setting on the unit to ensure it is within the safe range.	
___	___	___	10. Attach pad tubing to the electronic unit tubing.	
___	___	___	11. Plug in the unit and warm the pad before use. Apply the aquathermia pad to the prescribed area. Secure with gauze bandage or tape.	
___	___	___	12. Remove PPE, if used, and perform hand hygiene.	
___	___	___	13. ***Monitor the condition of the skin and the patient's response to the heat at frequent intervals, according to facility policy. Do not exceed the prescribed length of time for the application of heat.***	

Excellent	Satisfactory	Needs Practice	SKILL 8-13 **Applying an External Heating Pad** *(Continued)*	Comments
____	____	____	14. After the prescribed time for the treatment (up to 30 minutes), remove the aquathermia pad. ***Do not exceed the prescribed amount of time.*** Reassess the patient and area of application, noting the effect and presence of any adverse effects.	
____	____	____	15. Remove all remaining equipment; place the patient in a comfortable position, with side rails up as indicated and bed in the lowest position.	
____	____	____	16. Remove additional PPE, if used. Perform hand hygiene.	

Skill Checklists for Taylor's Clinical Nursing Skills. A Nursing Process Approach, 5th edition

Name ______________________ Date ______________________

Unit ______________________ Position ______________________

Instructor/Evaluator: ______________________ Position ______________________

SKILL 8-14

Applying a Warm Compress

Excellent	Satisfactory	Needs Practice	**Goal:** Desired outcome depends on the patient's nursing diagnosis and the rationale for application.	**Comments**
___	___	___	1. Review the patient's health record for prescribed order for the application of a moist warm compress, including the frequency and length of time for the application. Gather necessary supplies.	
___	___	___	2. Perform hand hygiene and put on PPE, if indicated.	
___	___	___	3. Identify the patient.	
___	___	___	4. Assemble equipment on the overbed table or other surface within reach.	
___	___	___	5. Assess the patient for possible need for nonpharmacologic pain-reducing interventions or analgesic medication before beginning the procedure. Administer appropriate analgesic, as ordered, and allow enough time for the analgesic to achieve its effectiveness before beginning the procedure.	
___	___	___	6. Close the curtains around the bed and close the door to the room, if possible. Explain what you are going to do and why you are going to do it to the patient.	
___	___	___	7. If using an electronic heating device with the compress, check that the water in the unit is at the appropriate level. Fill the unit two thirds full with distilled water, or to the fill mark, if necessary. Check the temperature setting on the unit to ensure it is within the safe range (refer to Skill 8-13).	
___	___	___	8. Assist the patient to a comfortable position that provides easy access to the area. Use a bath blanket to cover any exposed area other than the intended site. Place a waterproof pad under the site.	
___	___	___	9. Place a waste receptacle at a convenient location for use during the procedure.	
___	___	___	10. Pour the warmed solution into the container and drop the gauze for the compress into the solution. Alternately, if commercially packaged, prewarmed gauze is used, open packaging.	
___	___	___	11. Put on clean gloves. Assess the application site for inflammation, skin color, and ecchymosis.	

SKILL 8-14

Applying a Warm Compress *(Continued)*

Excellent	Satisfactory	Needs Practice		Comments
___	___	___	12. Retrieve the compress from the warmed solution, squeezing out any excess moisture. Alternately, remove pre-warmed gauze from open package. ***Apply the compress by gently and carefully molding it to the intended area. Ask the patient if the application feels too hot.***	
___	___	___	13. Cover the site with a clean dry bath towel; secure in place with a tape or roller gauze, if necessary.	
___	___	___	14. Place the aquathermia or heating device, if used, over the towel. Refer to Skill 8-13.	
___	___	___	15. Remove gloves and discard them appropriately. Perform hand hygiene and remove additional PPE, if used.	
___	___	___	16. ***Monitor the time the compress is in place to prevent burns and skin/tissue damage. Monitor the condition of the patient's skin and the patient's response at frequent intervals.***	
___	___	___	17. After the prescribed time for the treatment (up to 30 minutes), remove the external heating device (if used). ***Do not exceed the prescribed amount of time.*** Put on gloves.	
___	___	___	18. Carefully remove the compress while assessing the skin condition around the site and observing the patient's response to the heat application. Note any changes in the application area.	
___	___	___	19. Remove gloves. Perform hand hygiene.	
___	___	___	20. Place the patient in a comfortable position. Lower the bed. Dispose of any other supplies appropriately.	
___	___	___	21. Remove additional PPE, if used. Perform hand hygiene.	

Skill Checklists for Taylor's Clinical Nursing Skills.
A Nursing Process Approach, 5th edition

Name ________________________ Date ________________________

Unit ________________________ Position ________________________

Instructor/Evaluator: ________________________ Position ________________________

SKILL 8-15

Assisting With a Sitz Bath

Goal: The patient verbalizes an increase in comfort.

Excellent	Satisfactory	Needs Practice		Comments
___	___	___	1. Review the patient's health record for prescribed order for the application of a sitz bath, including the frequency and length of time for the application. Gather necessary supplies.	
___	___	___	2. Perform hand hygiene and put on PPE, if indicated.	
___	___	___	3. Identify the patient.	
___	___	___	4. Close the curtains around the bed and close the door to the room, if possible.	
___	___	___	5. Put on gloves. Assemble equipment either at the bedside if using a bedside commode or in the bathroom.	
___	___	___	6. Raise the lid of the toilet or commode. Place the bowl of the sitz bath, with drainage ports to the rear and infusion port in front, in the toilet. Fill the bowl of the sitz bath about halfway full with tepid to warm water (within a range of 105° to 109°F (40.5° to 43°C) (Taylor et al., 2019). ***Water temperature should not exceed 125°F*** (Burn Foundation, 2016).	
___	___	___	7. Clamp tubing on the bag. Fill the bag with same temperature water as mentioned above. Hang the bag above the patient's shoulder height on the IV pole.	
___	___	___	8. Assist the patient to sit on the toilet or commode. The patient should be able to sit in the basin or tub with the feet flat on the floor without any pressure on the sacrum or thighs. Wrap a blanket around the shoulders and provide extra draping, if needed. Insert tubing into the infusion port of the sitz bath. Slowly unclamp tubing and allow the sitz bath to fill.	
___	___	___	9. Clamp tubing once the sitz bath is full. Instruct the patient to open clamp when water in bowl becomes cool. ***Ensure that the call bell is within reach. Instruct the patient to call if he or she feels light-headed or dizzy or has any problems. Instruct the patient not to try standing without assistance.***	
___	___	___	10. Remove gloves and perform hand hygiene.	

Excellent	Satisfactory	Needs Practice	SKILL 8-15 **Assisting With a Sitz Bath** *(Continued)*	Comments
___	___	___	11. When the patient is finished (in about 15 to 20 minutes, or prescribed time), put on clean gloves. Assist the patient to stand and gently pat the perineal area dry. Remove gloves. Perform hand hygiene.	
___	___	___	12. Assist the patient to bed or chair. Ensure that the call bell is within reach.	
___	___	___	13. Put on gloves. Empty and disinfect sitz bath bowl according to facility policy.	
___	___	___	14. Remove gloves and any additional PPE, if used. Perform hand hygiene.	

Skill Checklists for Taylor's Clinical Nursing Skills. A Nursing Process Approach, 5th edition

Name ________________ Date ________________

Unit ________________ Position ________________

Instructor/Evaluator: ________________ Position ________________

SKILL 8-16

Applying Cold Therapy

Excellent	Satisfactory	Needs Practice	**Goal:** The desired outcome depends on the patient's nursing diagnosis.	**Comments**
___	___	___	1. Review the patient's health record for prescribed order or nursing care plan for the application of cold therapy, including frequency, type of therapy, body area to be treated, and length of time for the application. Gather necessary supplies.	
___	___	___	2. Perform hand hygiene and put on PPE, if indicated.	
___	___	___	3. Identify the patient. Determine if the patient has had any previous adverse reaction to hypothermia therapy.	
___	___	___	4. Assemble equipment on the overbed table or other surface within reach.	
___	___	___	5. Close the curtains around the bed and close the door to the room, if possible. Explain what you are going to do and why you are going to do it to the patient.	
___	___	___	6. Assess the condition of the skin where the cold is to be applied.	
___	___	___	7. Assist the patient to a comfortable position that provides easy access to the area to be treated. Expose the area and drape the patient with a bath blanket, if needed. Put the waterproof pad under the wound area, if necessary.	
___	___	___	8. Prepare device: Fill the bag, collar, or glove about three fourths full with ice. Remove any excess air from the device. Securely fasten the end of the bag or collar; tie the glove closed, checking for holes and leakage of water. Prepare commercially prepared ice pack, according to the manufacturer's directions, if appropriate.	
___	___	___	9. ***Cover the device with a towel or washcloth; commercially prepared devices may come with a cover.*** (If the device has a cloth exterior, this is not necessary.)	
___	___	___	10. Positioning the ice bag on the intended area and lightly secure in place, as needed.	
___	___	___	11. ***Remove the ice and assess the site for redness after 30 seconds. Ask the patient about the presence of burning sensations.***	
___	___	___	12. Replace the device snugly against the site if no problems are evident. Secure it in place with gauze wrap, ties, or tape.	

Excellent	Satisfactory	Needs Practice	SKILL 8-16 **Applying Cold Therapy** *(Continued)*	Comments
___	___	___	13. ***Monitor the time the compress is in place to prevent burns and skin/tissue damage. Monitor the condition of the patient's skin and the patient's response at frequent intervals.***	
___	___	___	14. After the prescribed time for the treatment (up to 30 minutes), remove the ice and dry the skin. ***Do not exceed the prescribed amount of time.***	
___	___	___	15. Remove PPE, if used. Perform hand hygiene.	
___	___	___	16. Place the patient in a comfortable position. Lower the bed. Dispose of any other supplies appropriately.	
___	___	___	17. Remove additional PPE, if used. Perform hand hygiene.	

Skill Checklists for Taylor's Clinical Nursing Skills. A Nursing Process Approach, 5th edition

Name ______________________ Date ______________

Unit ______________________ Position ______________

Instructor/Evaluator: ______________________ Position ______________

SKILL 9-1
Assisting a Patient With Turning in Bed

Excellent	Satisfactory	Needs Practice	**Goal:** The activity takes place without injury to patient or nurse.	**Comments**
___	___	___	1. Review the medical orders and nursing care plan for patient activity. Identify any movement limitations and the ability of the patient to assist with turning. ***Consult patient handling algorithm, if available, to plan appropriate approach to moving the patient.***	
___	___	___	2. Gather any positioning aids or supports, if necessary.	
___	___	___	3. Perform hand hygiene. Put on PPE, as indicated.	
___	___	___	4. Identify the patient. Explain the procedure to the patient.	
___	___	___	5. Close the curtains around the bed and close the door to the room, if possible. Position at least one nurse on either side of the bed. Place pillows, wedges, or any other support to be used for positioning within easy reach. Place the bed at an appropriate and comfortable working height, usually elbow height of the caregiver (VHACEOSH, 2016). Lower both side rails.	
___	___	___	6. If not already in place, position a friction-reducing sheet under the patient.	
___	___	___	7. Using the friction-reducing sheet, move the patient to the edge of the bed, opposite the side to which he or she will be turned. Raise the side rails.	
___	___	___	8. If the patient is able, have the patient grasp the side rail on the side of the bed toward which he or she is turning. Alternately, place the patient's arms across his or her chest and cross his or her far leg over the leg toward which they are turning.	
___	___	___	9. If available, activate the bed-turn mechanism to inflate the side of the bed behind the patient's back.	

SKILL 9-1

Assisting a Patient With Turning in Bed *(Continued)*

Excellent	Satisfactory	Needs Practice		Comments
___	___	___	10. The nurse on the side of the bed toward which the patient is turning should stand opposite the patient's center with his or her feet spread about shoulder width and with one foot ahead of the other. Tighten your gluteal and abdominal muscles and flex your knees. Use your leg muscles to do the pulling. The other nurse should position his or her hands on the patient's shoulder and hip, assisting to roll the patient to the side. Instruct the patient to pull on the bed rail at the same time. Use the friction-reducing sheet to gently pull the patient over on his or her side.	
___	___	___	11. Use a pillow or other support behind the patient's back. Pull the shoulder blade forward and out from under the patient.	
___	___	___	12. Make the patient comfortable and position in proper alignment, using pillows or other supports under the leg and arm, as needed. Readjust the pillow under the patient's head. Elevate the head of the bed as needed for comfort.	
___	___	___	13. Place the bed in the lowest position, with the side rails up, as indicated. Make sure the call bell and other necessary items are within easy reach.	
___	___	___	14. Clean transfer aids, per facility policy, if not indicated for single patient use. Remove gloves and other PPE, if used. Perform hand hygiene.	

Skill Checklists for Taylor's Clinical Nursing Skills. A Nursing Process Approach, 5th edition

Name ______________________ Date ______________

Unit ______________________ Position ______________

Instructor/Evaluator: ______________________ Position ______________

SKILL 9-2

Moving a Patient Up in Bed With the Assistance of Another Caregiver

Excellent	Satisfactory	Needs Practice	**Goal:** The patient is repositioned, remains free from injury, and maintains proper body alignment.	Comments
____	____	____	1. Review the medical record and nursing care plan for conditions that may influence the patient's ability to move or to be positioned. Assess for tubes, IV lines, incisions, or equipment that may alter the positioning procedure. Identify any movement limitations. ***Consult patient handling algorithm, if available, to plan appropriate approach to moving the patient.***	
____	____	____	2. Perform hand hygiene and put on PPE, if indicated.	
____	____	____	3. Identify the patient. Explain the procedure to the patient.	
____	____	____	4. Close the curtains around the bed and close the door to the room, if possible. Place the bed at an appropriate and comfortable working height, usually elbow height of the caregiver (VHACEOSH, 2016). Adjust the head of the bed to a flat position or as low as the patient can tolerate. Place the bed in slight Trendelenburg position, if the patient is able to tolerate it.	
____	____	____	5. Remove all pillows from under the patient. Leave one at the head of the bed, leaning upright against the headboard.	
____	____	____	6. Position at least one nurse on either side of the bed, and lower both side rails.	
____	____	____	7. If a friction-reducing sheet (or device) is not in place under the patient, place one under the patient's midsection.	
____	____	____	8. Ask the patient (if able) to bend his or her legs and put his or her feet flat on the bed to assist with the movement.	
____	____	____	9. Have the patient fold the arms across the chest. Have the patient (if able) lift the head with chin on chest.	
____	____	____	10. One nurse should be positioned on each side of the bed, at the patient's midsection, with feet spread shoulder width apart and one foot slightly in front of the other.	
____	____	____	11. If available on bed, engage mechanism to make the bed surface firmer for repositioning.	
____	____	____	12. Grasp the friction-reducing sheet securely, close to the patient's body.	

Excellent	Satisfactory	Needs Practice	SKILL 9-2 **Moving a Patient Up in Bed With the Assistance of Another Caregiver** *(Continued)*	Comments
___	___	___	13. Flex your knees and hips. Tighten your abdominal and gluteal muscles and keep your back straight.	
___	___	___	14. If possible, the patient can assist with the move by pushing with the legs. Shift your weight back and forth from your back leg to your front leg and count to three. On the count of three, move the patient up in bed. Repeat the process, if necessary, to get the patient to the right position.	
___	___	___	15. Assist the patient to a comfortable position and readjust the pillows and supports, as needed. Take bed out of Trendelenburg position and return bed surface to normal setting, if necessary. Raise the side rails. Place the bed in the lowest position. Make sure the call bell and other necessary items are within easy reach.	
___	___	___	16. Clean transfer aids, per facility policy, if not indicated for single patient use. Remove gloves or other PPE, if used. Perform hand hygiene.	

Skill Checklists for Taylor's Clinical Nursing Skills. A Nursing Process Approach, 5th edition

Name ______________________ Date ______________________

Unit ______________________ Position ______________________

Instructor/Evaluator: ______________________ Position ______________________

SKILL 9-3
Transferring a Patient From the Bed to a Stretcher

Goal: The patient is transferred without injury to patient or nurse.

Excellent	Satisfactory	Needs Practice	Step	Comments
___	___	___	1. Review the medical record and nursing care plan for any conditions that may influence the patient's ability to move or to be positioned. Assess for tubes, IV lines, incisions, or equipment that may alter the positioning procedure. Identify any movement limitations. ***Consult patient handling algorithm, if available, to plan appropriate approach to moving the patient.***	
___	___	___	2. Perform hand hygiene and put on PPE, if indicated.	
___	___	___	3. Identify the patient. Explain the procedure to the patient.	
___	___	___	4. Close the curtains around the bed and close the door to the room, if possible. Adjust the head of the bed to a flat position or as low as the patient can tolerate. Raise the bed to a height that is even with the transport stretcher (VHACEOSH, 2016). Lower the side rails, if in place.	
___	___	___	5. Place the bath blanket over the patient and remove the top covers from underneath.	
___	___	___	6. If a friction-reducing transfer sheet is not in place under the patient, place one under the patient's midsection. Have patient fold arms against chest and move chin to chest. Use the friction-reducing sheet to move the patient to the side of the bed where the stretcher will be placed. Alternately, place a lateral-assist device under the patient. Follow manufacturer's directions for use.	
___	___	___	7. Position the stretcher next (and parallel) to the bed. ***Lock the wheels on the stretcher and the bed.***	
___	___	___	8. Two nurses should stand on the stretcher side of the bed. A third nurse should stand on the side of the bed without the stretcher.	
___	___	___	9. Use the friction-reducing sheet to roll the patient away from the stretcher. Place the transfer board across the space between the stretcher and the bed, partially under the patient. Roll the patient onto his or her back, so that the patient is partially on the transfer board.	

Excellent	Satisfactory	Needs Practice	SKILL 9-3 **Transferring a Patient From the Bed to a Stretcher** *(Continued)*	Comments
___	___	___	10. The nurse on the side of the bed without the stretcher should grasp the friction-reducing sheet at the head and chest areas of the patient. The nurse on the stretcher side of the bed should grasp the friction-reducing sheet at the head and chest, and the other nurse on that side should grasp the friction-reducing sheet at the chest and leg areas of the patient.	
___	___	___	11. ***At a signal given by one of the nurses, have the nurses standing on the stretcher side of the bed pull the friction-reducing sheet. At the same time, the nurse (or nurses) on the other side push, transferring the patient's weight toward the transfer board, and pushing the patient from the bed to the stretcher.***	
___	___	___	12. Once the patient is transferred to the stretcher, remove the transfer board, and secure the patient until the side rails are raised. Raise the side rails. To ensure the patient's comfort, cover the patient with blanket and remove the bath blanket from underneath. Leave the friction-reducing sheet in place for the return transfer. Make sure the call bell and other necessary items are within easy reach.	
___	___	___	13. Clean transfer aids, per facility policy, if not indicated for single patient use. Remove gloves and any other PPE, if used. Perform hand hygiene.	

Skill Checklists for Taylor's Clinical Nursing Skills. A Nursing Process Approach, 5th edition

Name ______________________ Date ______________________

Unit ______________________ Position ______________________

Instructor/Evaluator: ______________________ Position ______________________

SKILL 9-4

Transferring a Patient From the Bed to a Chair

Excellent	Satisfactory	Needs Practice	**Goal:** The transfer is accomplished without injury to patient or nurse.	**Comments**
___	___	___	1. Review the medical record and nursing care plan for conditions that may influence the patient's ability to move or to be positioned. Assess for tubes, IV lines, incisions, or equipment that may alter the positioning procedure. Identify any movement limitations. ***Consult patient handling algorithm, if available, to plan appropriate approach to moving the patient.***	
___	___	___	2. Perform hand hygiene and put on PPE, as indicated.	
___	___	___	3. Identify the patient. Explain the procedure to the patient.	
___	___	___	4. If needed, move equipment to make room for the chair. Close the curtains around the bed and close the door to the room, if possible.	
___	___	___	5. Place the bed in the lowest position. Raise the head of the bed to a sitting position, or as high as the patient can tolerate.	
___	___	___	6. ***Make sure the bed brakes are locked. Put the chair next to the bed. If available, lock the brakes of the chair. If the chair does not have brakes, brace the chair against a secure object.***	
___	___	___	7. Encourage the patient to make use of a stand-assist aid, either freestanding or attached to the side of the bed, if available, to move to the side of the bed and to a side-lying position, facing the side of the bed on which the patient will sit.	
___	___	___	8. Lower the side rail, if necessary, and stand near the patient's hips. Stand with your legs shoulder width apart with one foot near the head of the bed, slightly in front of the other foot.	
___	___	___	9. Encourage the patient to make use of the stand-assist device. Assist the patient to sit up on the side of the bed; ask the patient to swing his or her legs over the side of the bed. At the same time, pivot on your back leg to lift the patient's trunk and shoulders. Keep your back straight; avoid twisting.	

Excellent	Satisfactory	Needs Practice	SKILL 9-4 **Transferring a Patient From the Bed to a Chair** *(Continued)*	Comments
___	___	___	10. ***Stand in front of the patient, and assess for any balance problems or complaints of dizziness. Allow the patient's legs to dangle a few minutes before continuing.***	
___	___	___	11. Assist the patient to put on a robe, as necessary and nonskid footwear.	
___	___	___	12. Wrap the gait belt around the patient's waist, based on assessed need and facility policy.	
___	___	___	13. Stand facing the patient. Spread your feet about shoulder width apart and flex your hips and knees.	
___	___	___	14. Ask the patient to slide his or her buttocks to the edge of the bed until the feet touch the floor. Position yourself as close as possible to the patient, with your foot positioned on the outside of the patient's foot. If a second staff person is assisting, have him or her assume a similar position. Grasp the gait belt.	
___	___	___	15. Encourage the patient to make use of the stand-assist device. If necessary, have second staff person grasp the gait belt on opposite side. Rock back and forth while counting to three. ***On the count of three, using the gait belt and your legs (not your back), assist the patient to a standing position.*** If indicated, brace your front knee against the patient's weak extremity as he or she stands. Assess the patient's balance and leg strength. If the patient is weak or unsteady, return the patient to bed.	
___	___	___	16. Pivot on your back foot and assist the patient to turn until the patient feels the chair against his or her legs.	
___	___	___	17. Ask the patient to use his or her arm to steady him- or herself on the arm of the chair while slowly lowering to a sitting position. Continue to brace the patient's knees with your knees and hold the gait belt. Flex your hips and knees when helping the patient sit in the chair.	
___	___	___	18. Assess the patient's alignment in the chair. Remove gait belt, if desired. Depending on patient comfort, it could be left in place to use when returning to bed. Cover with a blanket, if needed. Make sure call bell and other essential items are within easy reach.	
___	___	___	19. Clean transfer aids, per facility policy, if not indicated for single patient use. Remove gloves and any other PPE, if used. Perform hand hygiene.	

Skill Checklists for Taylor's Clinical Nursing Skills. A Nursing Process Approach, 5th edition

Name ______________________ Date ______________________

Unit ______________________ Position ______________________

Instructor/Evaluator: ______________________ Position ______________________

SKILL 9-5

Transferring a Patient Using a Powered Full-Body Sling Lift

Goal: The transfer is accomplished without injury to patient or nurse.

Excellent	Satisfactory	Needs Practice		Comments
___	___	___	1. Review the medical record and nursing care plan for conditions that may influence the patient's ability to move or to be positioned. Assess for tubes, IV lines, incisions, or equipment that may alter the positioning procedure. Identify any movement limitations. ***Consult patient handling algorithm, if available, to plan appropriate approach to moving the patient.***	
___	___	___	2. Perform hand hygiene and put on PPE, if indicated.	
___	___	___	3. Identify the patient. Explain the procedure to the patient.	
___	___	___	4. If needed, move the equipment to make room for the chair. Close the curtains around the bed and close the door to the room, if possible.	
___	___	___	5. Adjust the bed to a comfortable working height, usually elbow height of the caregiver (VHACEOSH, 2016). ***Lock the bed brakes.***	
___	___	___	6. Lower the side rail, if in use, on the side of the bed you are working. If the sling is for use with more than one patient, place a cover or pad on the sling. Place the sling evenly under the patient. Roll the patient to one side and place half of the sling with the sheet or pad on it under the patient from shoulders to mid-thigh. Raise the rail and move to the other side. Lower the rail, if necessary. Roll the patient to the other side and pull the sling under the patient. Raise the side rail.	
___	___	___	7. Bring the chair to the side of the bed. ***Lock the wheels, if present.***	
___	___	___	8. Lower the side rail on the chair side of the bed. Roll the base of the lift under the side of the bed nearest to the chair. ***Center the frame over the patient. Lock the wheels of the lift.***	
___	___	___	9. ***Using the base-adjustment lever, widen the stance of the base.***	
___	___	___	10. Lower the arms close enough to attach the sling to the frame.	

Excellent	Satisfactory	Needs Practice	SKILL 9-5 **Transferring a Patient Using a Powered Full-Body Sling Lift** *(Continued)*	Comments
____	____	____	11. Attach the straps on the sling to the hooks on the frame. Short straps attach behind the patient's back and long straps attach at the other end of the sling. Check the patient to make sure the straps are not pressing into the skin. Some lifts have straps or chains with hooks that attach to holes in the sling. Check the manufacturer's instructions for each lift.	
____	____	____	12. Check all equipment, lines, and drains attached to the patient so that they are not interfering with the device. Have the patient fold his or her arms across the chest.	
____	____	____	13. With a person standing on each side of the lift, tell the patient that he or she will be lifted from the bed. Support injured limbs as necessary. Engage the pump to raise the patient about 6 in above the bed.	
____	____	____	14. Unlock the wheels of the lift. ***Carefully wheel the patient straight back and away from the bed. Support the patient's limbs, as needed.***	
____	____	____	15. Position the patient over the chair with the base of the lift straddling the chair. Lock the wheels of the lift.	
____	____	____	16. Gently lower the patient to the chair until the hooks or straps are slightly loosened from the sling or frame. Guide the patient into the chair with your hands as the sling lowers.	
____	____	____	17. Disconnect the hooks or strap from the frame. Keep the sling in place under the patient.	
____	____	____	18. Adjust the patient's position, using pillows, if necessary. Check the patient's alignment in the chair. Cover the patient with a blanket, if necessary. Make sure call bell and other essential items are within easy reach. When it is time for the patient to return to bed, reattach the hooks or straps and reverse the steps.	
____	____	____	19. Clean transfer aids, per facility policy, if not indicated for single patient use. Remove gloves and any other PPE, if used. Perform hand hygiene.	

Skill Checklists for Taylor's Clinical Nursing Skills.
A Nursing Process Approach, 5th edition

Name ______________________ Date ______________________

Unit ______________________ Position ______________________

Instructor/Evaluator: ______________________ Position ______________________

SKILL 9-6

Providing Range-of-Motion Exercises

Goal: The patient completes the exercises and maintains or improves join mobility.

Excellent	Satisfactory	Needs Practice		Comments
___	___	___	1. Review the medical orders and nursing care plan for patient activity. Identify any movement limitations.	
___	___	___	2. Perform hand hygiene and put on PPE, if indicated.	
___	___	___	3. Identify the patient. Explain the procedure to the patient.	
___	___	___	4. Close the curtains around the bed and close the door to the room, if possible. Place the bed at an appropriate and comfortable working height, usually elbow height of the caregiver (VHACEOSH, 2016). Adjust the head of the bed to a flat position or as low as the patient can tolerate.	
___	___	___	5. Stand on the side of the bed where the joints are to be exercised. Lower side rail on that side, if in place. Uncover only the limb to be used during the exercise.	
___	___	___	6. Perform the exercises slowly and gently, providing support by holding the areas proximal and distal to the joint. Repeat each exercise two to five times, moving each joint in a smooth and rhythmic manner. ***Stop movement if the patient complains of pain or if you meet resistance.***	
___	___	___	7. While performing the exercises, begin at the head and move down one side of the body at a time. ***Encourage the patient to do as many of these exercises independently as possible.***	
___	___	___	8. Move the chin down to rest on the chest. Return the head to a normal upright position. Tilt the head as far as possible toward each shoulder.	
___	___	___	9. Move the head from side to side, bringing the chin toward each shoulder.	
___	___	___	10. Start with the arm at the patient's side and lift the arm forward to above the head. Return the arm to the starting position at the side of the body.	
___	___	___	11. With the arm back at the patient's side, move the arm laterally to an upright position above the head, and then return it to the original position. Move the arm across the body as far as possible.	

Excellent	Satisfactory	Needs Practice	SKILL 9-6 **Providing Range-of-Motion Exercises** *(Continued)*	Comments
___	___	___	12. Raise the arm at the side until the upper arm is in line with the shoulder. Bend the elbow at a 90-degree angle and move the forearm upward and downward, then return the arm to the side.	
___	___	___	13. Bend the elbow and move the lower arm and hand upward toward the shoulder. Return the lower arm and hand to the original position while straightening the elbow.	
___	___	___	14. Rotate the lower arm and hand so the palm is up. Rotate the lower arm and hand so the palm of the hand is down.	
___	___	___	15. Move the hand downward toward the inner aspect of the forearm. Return the hand to a neutral position even with the forearm. Then move the dorsal portion of the hand backward as far as possible.	
___	___	___	16. Bend the fingers to make a fist, and then straighten them out. Spread the fingers apart and return them back together. Touch the thumb to each finger on the hand.	
___	___	___	17. Extend the leg and lift it upward. Return the leg to the original position beside the other leg.	
___	___	___	18. Lift the leg laterally away from the patient's body. Return the leg back toward the other leg and try to extend it beyond the midline.	
___	___	___	19. Turn the foot and leg toward the opposite leg to rotate it internally. Turn the foot and leg outward away from the opposite leg to rotate it externally.	
___	___	___	20. Bend the leg and bring the heel toward the back of the leg. Return the leg to a straight position.	
___	___	___	21. At the ankle, move the foot up and back until the toes are upright. Move the foot with the toes pointing downward.	
___	___	___	22. Turn the sole of the foot toward the midline. Turn the sole of the foot outward.	
___	___	___	23. Curl the toes downward, and then straighten them out. Spread the toes apart and bring them together.	
___	___	___	24. Repeat these exercises on the other side of the body. Encourage the patient to do as many of these exercises independently as possible.	
___	___	___	25. When finished, make sure the patient is comfortable, with the side rails up and the bed in the lowest position. Place call bell and other essential items within reach.	
___	___	___	26. Remove gloves and any other PPE, if used. Perform hand hygiene.	

Skill Checklists for Taylor's Clinical Nursing Skills. A Nursing Process Approach, 5th edition

Name ______________________ Date ______________________

Unit ______________________ Position ______________________

Instructor/Evaluator: ______________________ Position ______________________

SKILL 9-7

Assisting a Patient With Ambulation

Goal: The patient ambulates safely, without falls or injury.

Excellent	Satisfactory	Needs Practice		Comments
____	____	____	1. Review the medical record and nursing care plan for conditions that may influence the patient's ability to move and ambulate. Assess for tubes, IV lines, incisions, or equipment that may alter the procedure for ambulation. Identify any movement limitations.	
____	____	____	2. Perform hand hygiene. Put on PPE, as indicated.	
____	____	____	3. Identify the patient. Explain the procedure to the patient. Ask the patient to report any feelings of dizziness, weakness, or shortness of breath while walking. Decide how far to walk.	
____	____	____	4. Place the bed in the lowest position.	
____	____	____	5. Encourage the patient to make use of a stand-assist aid, either freestanding or attached to the side of the bed, if available, to move to the side of the bed. Assist the patient to the side of the bed, if necessary.	
____	____	____	6. Have the patient sit on the side of the bed for several minutes and assess for dizziness or lightheadedness. Have the patient stay sitting until he or she feels secure.	
____	____	____	7. Assist the patient to put on footwear and a robe, if desired.	
____	____	____	8. Wrap the gait belt around the patient's waist, based on assessed need and facility policy.	
____	____	____	9. Encourage the patient to make use of the stand-assist device. Assist the patient to stand, using the gait belt, if necessary. Assess the patient's balance and leg strength. If the patient is weak or unsteady, return the patient to the bed or assist to a chair.	

Excellent	Satisfactory	Needs Practice	SKILL 9-7 **Assisting a Patient With Ambulation** *(Continued)*	Comments
____	____	____	10. If you are the only person assisting, position yourself to the side and slightly behind the patient. Support the patient by the waist or transfer belt.	
____	____	____	• When two caregivers assist, position yourself to the side and slightly behind the patient, supporting the patient by the waist or gait belt. Have the other caregiver carry or manage equipment or provide additional support from the other side.	
____	____	____	• Alternately, when two caregivers assist, stand at the patient's sides (one nurse on each side) with near hands grasping the gait belt and far hands holding the patient's lower arm or hand.	
____	____	____	11. Take several steps forward with the patient. Continue to assess the patient's strength and balance. Remind the patient to stand erect.	
____	____	____	12. Continue with ambulation for the planned distance and time. Return the patient to the bed or chair based on the patient's tolerance and condition. Remove gait belt.	
____	____	____	13. Ensure the patient is comfortable, with the side rails up and the bed in the lowest position, as necessary. Place call bell and other essential items within reach.	
____	____	____	14. Clean transfer aids per facility policy, if not indicated for single patient use. Remove gloves and any other PPE, if used. Perform hand hygiene.	

Skill Checklists for Taylor's Clinical Nursing Skills. A Nursing Process Approach, 5th edition

Name ______________________ Date ______________________

Unit ______________________ Position ______________________

Instructor/Evaluator: ______________________ Position ______________________

SKILL 9-8

Assisting a Patient With Ambulation Using a Walker

Goal: The patient ambulates safely with the walker and is free from falls or injury.

Excellent	Satisfactory	Needs Practice		Comments
___	___	___	1. Review the medical record and nursing care plan for conditions that may influence the patient's ability to move and ambulate, and for specific instructions for ambulation, such as distance. Assess for tubes, IV lines, incisions, or equipment that may alter the procedure for ambulation. Assess the patient's knowledge and previous experience regarding the use of a walker. Identify any movement limitations.	
___	___	___	2. Perform hand hygiene. Put on PPE, if indicated.	
___	___	___	3. Identify the patient. Explain the procedure to the patient. Tell the patient to report any feelings of dizziness, weakness, or shortness of breath while walking. Decide how far to walk.	
___	___	___	4. Place the bed in the lowest position, if the patient is in bed.	
___	___	___	5. Encourage the patient to make use of a stand-assist aid, either freestanding or attached to the side of the bed, if available, to move to the side of the bed.	
___	___	___	6. Assist the patient to the side of the bed, if necessary. Have the patient sit on the side of the bed. Assess for dizziness or lightheadedness. Have the patient stay seated until he or she feels secure.	
___	___	___	7. Assist the patient to put on footwear and a robe, if desired.	
___	___	___	8. Wrap the gait belt around the patient's waist, based on assessed need and facility policy.	
___	___	___	9. Place the walker directly in front of the patient. Ask the patient to push him- or herself off the bed or chair; make use of the stand-assist device, or assist the patient to stand. Once the patient is standing, have him or her hold the walker's handgrips firmly and equally. Stand slightly behind the patient, on one side.	
___	___	___	10. Have the patient move the walker forward 6 to 8 in and set it down, making sure all four feet of the walker stay on the floor. Then, tell the patient to step forward with either foot into the walker, supporting him- or herself on his or her arms. Follow through with the other leg.	

Excellent	Satisfactory	Needs Practice	SKILL 9-8 **Assisting a Patient With Ambulation Using a Walker** *(Continued)*	Comments
___	___	___	11. Move the walker forward again, and continue the same pattern. Continue with ambulation for the planned distance and time. Return the patient to the bed or chair based on the patient's tolerance and condition, ensuring that the patient is comfortable. Remove gait belt.	
___	___	___	12. Ensure the patient is comfortable, with the side rails up and the bed in the lowest position, as necessary. Place call bell and other essential items within reach.	
___	___	___	13. Clean transfer aids per facility policy, if not indicated for single patient use. Remove gloves and any other PPE, if used. Perform hand hygiene.	

Skill Checklists for Taylor's Clinical Nursing Skills. A Nursing Process Approach, 5th edition

Name ______________________ Date ______________

Unit ______________________ Position ______________

Instructor/Evaluator: ______________________ Position ______________

SKILL 9-9

Assisting a Patient With Ambulation Using Crutches

Goal: The patient ambulates safely without experiencing falls or injury and the patient demonstrates proper crutch-walking technique.

Excellent	Satisfactory	Needs Practice		Comments
___	___	___	1. Review the medical record and nursing care plan for conditions that may influence the patient's ability to move and ambulate. Assess for tubes, IV lines, incisions, or equipment that may alter the procedure for ambulation. Assess the patient's knowledge and previous experience regarding the use of crutches. Determine that the appropriate size crutch has been obtained.	
___	___	___	2. Perform hand hygiene. Put on PPE, if indicated.	
___	___	___	3. Identify the patient. Explain the procedure to the patient. Tell the patient to report any feelings of dizziness, weakness, or shortness of breath while walking. Decide how far to walk.	
___	___	___	4. Place the bed in the lowest position, if the patient is in bed.	
___	___	___	5. Encourage the patient to make use of a stand-assist aid, either freestanding or attached to the side of the bed, if available, to move to the side of the bed.	
___	___	___	6. Assist the patient to the side of the bed, if necessary. Have the patient sit on the side of the bed. Assess for dizziness or lightheadedness. Have the patient stay seated until he or she feels secure.	
___	___	___	7. Assist the patient to put on footwear and a robe, if desired.	
___	___	___	8. Wrap the gait belt around the patient's waist, based on assessed need and facility policy.	
___	___	___	9. Assist the patient to stand erect, face forward in the tripod position. This means the patient holds the crutches 12 in in front of, and 12 in to the side of, each foot.	
___	___	___	10. For the four-point gait:	
___	___	___	a. Have the patient move the right crutch forward 12 in and then move the left foot forward to the level of the right crutch.	
___	___	___	b. Then have the patient move the left crutch forward 12 in and then move the right foot forward to the level of the left crutch.	

Excellent	Satisfactory	Needs Practice	SKILL 9-9 **Assisting a Patient With Ambulation Using Crutches** *(Continued)*	Comments
___	___	___	11. For the three-point gait:	
___	___	___	a. Have the patient move the affected leg and both crutches forward about 12 in.	
___	___	___	b. Have the patient move the stronger leg forward to the level of the crutches.	
___	___	___	12. For the two-point gait:	
___	___	___	a. Have the patient move the left crutch and the right foot forward about 12 in at the same time.	
___	___	___	b. Have the patient move the right crutch and left leg forward to the level of the left crutch at the same time.	
___	___	___	13. For the swing-to gait:	
___	___	___	a. Have the patient move both crutches forward about 12 in.	
___	___	___	b. Have the patient lift the legs and swing them to the crutches, supporting his or her body weight on the crutches.	
___	___	___	14. Continue with ambulation for the planned distance and time. Return the patient to the bed or chair based on the patient's tolerance and condition. Remove gait belt.	
___	___	___	15. Ensure the patient is comfortable, with the side rails up and the bed in the lowest position, as necessary. Place call bell and other essential items within reach.	
___	___	___	16. Clean transfer aids per facility policy, if not indicated for single patient use. Remove gloves and any other PPE, if used. Perform hand hygiene.	

Skill Checklists for Taylor's Clinical Nursing Skills. A Nursing Process Approach, 5th edition

Name ______________________ Date ______________________

Unit ______________________ Position ______________________

Instructor/Evaluator: ______________________ Position ______________________

SKILL 9-10

Assisting a Patient With Ambulation Using a Cane

Excellent	Satisfactory	Needs Practice	**Goal:** The patient ambulates safely without falls or injury.	**Comments**
____	____	____	1. Review the medical record and nursing care plan for conditions that may influence the patient's ability to move and ambulate. Assess for tubes, IV lines, incisions, or equipment that may alter the procedure for ambulation.	
____	____	____	2. Perform hand hygiene. Put on PPE, as indicated.	
____	____	____	3. Identify the patient. Explain the procedure to the patient. Tell the patient to report any feelings of dizziness, weakness, or shortness of breath while walking. Decide how far to walk.	
____	____	____	4. Place the bed in the lowest position, if the patient is in bed.	
____	____	____	5. Encourage the patient to make use of a stand-assist aid, either freestanding or attached to the side of the bed, if available, to move to the side of the bed.	
____	____	____	6. Assist the patient to the side of the bed, if necessary. Have the patient sit on the side of the bed. Assess for dizziness or lightheadedness. Have the patient stay seated until he or she feels secure.	
____	____	____	7. Assist the patient to put on footwear and a robe, if desired.	
____	____	____	8. Wrap the gait belt around the patient's waist, based on assessed need and facility policy.	
____	____	____	9. Encourage the patient to make use of the stand-assist device to stand with weight evenly distributed between the feet and the cane.	
____	____	____	10. Have the patient hold the cane on his or her stronger side, close to the body, while the nurse stands to the side and slightly behind the patient.	
____	____	____	11. Tell the patient to advance the cane 4 to 12 in (10 to 30 cm) and then, while supporting his or her weight on the stronger leg and the cane, advance the weaker foot forward, parallel with the cane.	
____	____	____	12. While supporting his or her weight on the weaker leg and the cane, have the patient advance the stronger leg forward to finish the step.	
____	____	____	13. Continue with ambulation for the planned distance and time. Return the patient to the bed or chair based on the patient's tolerance and condition. Remove gait belt.	

Excellent	Satisfactory	Needs Practice	SKILL 9-10 **Assisting a Patient With Ambulation Using a Cane** *(Continued)*	Comments
___	___	___	14. Ensure the patient is comfortable, with the side rails up and the bed in the lowest position, as necessary. Place call bell and other essential items within reach.	
___	___	___	15. Clean transfer aids per facility policy, if not indicated for single patient use. Remove gloves and any other PPE, if used. Perform hand hygiene.	

Skill Checklists for Taylor's Clinical Nursing Skills. A Nursing Process Approach, 5th edition

Name ______________________ Date ______________________

Unit ______________________ Position ______________________

Instructor/Evaluator: ______________________ Position ______________________

SKILL 9-11

Applying and Removing Graduated Compression Stockings

Excellent	Satisfactory	Needs Practice	**Goal:** The stockings are applied and removed with minimal discomfort to the patient.	Comments
___	___	___	1. Review the medical record and medical orders to determine the need for graduated compression stockings.	
___	___	___	2. Perform hand hygiene. Put on PPE, as indicated.	
___	___	___	3. Identify the patient. Explain what you are going to do and the rationale for use of elastic stockings.	
___	___	___	4. Close the curtains around the bed and close the door to the room, if possible.	
___	___	___	5. Adjust the bed to a comfortable working height, usually elbow height of the caregiver (VHACEOSH, 2016).	
___	___	___	6. Assist patient to supine position. If patient has been sitting or walking, have him or her lie down with legs and feet well elevated for at least 15 minutes before applying stockings.	
___	___	___	7. Expose legs one at a time. Wash and dry legs, if necessary. Powder the leg lightly unless patient has a respiratory problem, dry skin, or sensitivity to the powder. If the skin is dry, a lotion may be used. Powders and lotions are not recommended by some manufacturers; check the package material for manufacturer specifications.	
___	___	___	8. Stand at the foot of the bed. Place hand inside stocking and grasp heel area securely. Turn stocking inside-out to the heel area, leaving the foot inside the stocking leg.	
___	___	___	9. With the heel pocket down, ease the stocking foot over the foot and heel. Check that the patient's heel is centered in heel pocket of stocking.	
___	___	___	10. Using your fingers and thumbs, carefully grasp edge of stocking and pull it up smoothly over ankle and calf, toward the knee. Make sure it is distributed evenly.	
___	___	___	11. Pull forward slightly on toe section. If the stocking has a toe window, make sure it is properly positioned. Adjust if necessary to ensure material is smooth.	
___	___	___	12. If the stockings are knee-length, make sure each stocking top is 1 to 2 in below the patella. Make sure the stocking does not roll down.	

Excellent	Satisfactory	Needs Practice	SKILL 9-11 **Applying and Removing Graduated Compression Stockings** *(Continued)*	Comments
____	____	____	13. If applying thigh-length stocking, continue the application. Flex the patient's leg. Stretch the stocking over the knee.	
____	____	____	14. Pull the stocking over the thigh until the top is 1 to 3 in below the gluteal fold. Adjust the stocking, as necessary, to distribute the fabric evenly. Make sure the stocking does not roll down.	
____	____	____	15. Remove equipment and return patient to a position of comfort. Remove gloves. Raise side rail and lower bed. Place call bell and other essential items within reach.	
____	____	____	16. Remove any other PPE, if used. Perform hand hygiene.	
			Removing Stockings	
____	____	____	17. To remove stocking, grasp top of stocking with your thumb and fingers and smoothly pull stocking off inside-out to heel. Support foot and ease stocking over it.	

Skill Checklists for Taylor's Clinical Nursing Skills. A Nursing Process Approach, 5th edition

Name ______________________ Date ______________________

Unit ______________________ Position ______________________

Instructor/Evaluator: ______________________ Position ______________________

SKILL 9-12

Applying Pneumatic Compression Devices

Goal: The patient maintains adequate circulation in extremities and is free from symptoms of neurovascular compromise and deep vein thrombosis.

Excellent	Satisfactory	Needs Practice	Step	Comments
____	____	____	1. Review the medical record and nursing care plan to determine the need for a pneumatic compression device (PCD) and for conditions that may contraindicate its use.	
____	____	____	2. Perform hand hygiene. Put on PPE, as indicated.	
____	____	____	3. Identify the patient. Explain the procedure to the patient.	
____	____	____	4. Close the curtains around the bed and close the door to the room, if possible. Place the bed at an appropriate and comfortable working height, usually elbow height of the caregiver (VHACEOSH, 2016).	
____	____	____	5. Hang the compression pump on the foot of the bed and plug it into an electrical outlet. Attach the connecting tubing to the pump.	
____	____	____	6. Remove the compression sleeves from the package and unfold them. Lay the unfolded sleeves on the bed with the cotton lining facing up. ***Note the markings indicating the correct placement for the ankle and popliteal areas.***	
____	____	____	7. Apply graduated compression stockings, if ordered. Place a sleeve under the patient's leg with the tubing toward the heel. Each one fits either leg. ***For total leg sleeves, place the behind-the-knee opening at the popliteal space to prevent pressure there. For knee-high sleeves, make sure the back of the ankle is over the ankle marking.***	
____	____	____	8. Wrap the sleeve snugly around the patient's leg so that two fingers fit between the leg and the sleeve. Secure the sleeve with the Velcro fasteners. Repeat for the second leg, if bilateral therapy is ordered. Connect each sleeve to the tubing, following manufacturer's recommendations.	
____	____	____	9. Set the pump to the prescribed maximal pressure (usually 35 to 55 mm Hg). Make sure the tubing is free from kinks. Check that the patient can move about without interrupting the airflow. Turn on the pump. Initiate cooling setting, if available.	
____	____	____	10. ***Observe the patient and the device during the first cycle. Check the audible alarms. Check the sleeves and pump at least once per shift or per facility policy.***	

Excellent	Satisfactory	Needs Practice	SKILL 9-12 **Applying Pneumatic Compression Devices** *(Continued)*	Comments
____	____	____	11. Place the bed in the lowest position. Make sure the call bell and other essential items are within easy reach.	
____	____	____	12. Remove PPE, if used. Perform hand hygiene.	
____	____	____	13. Assess the extremities for peripheral pulses, edema, changes in sensation, and movement. Remove the sleeves and assess for document skin integrity every 8 hours.	

Skill Checklists for Taylor's Clinical Nursing Skills. A Nursing Process Approach, 5th edition

Name ______________________ Date ______________

Unit ______________________ Position ______________

Instructor/Evaluator: ______________________ Position ______________

SKILL 9-13

Applying a Continuous Passive Motion Device

Goal: The patient experiences increased joint mobility and does not exhibit atrophy or contractures.

Excellent	Satisfactory	Needs Practice		Comments
___	___	___	1. Review the medical record and nursing care plan for the appropriate degrees of flexion and extension, the cycle rate, and the length of time the CPM is to be used.	
___	___	___	2. Obtain equipment. Apply the soft goods to the CPM device.	
___	___	___	3. Perform hand hygiene. Put on PPE, as indicated.	
___	___	___	4. Identify the patient. Explain the procedure to the patient.	
___	___	___	5. Close the curtains around the bed and close the door to the room, if possible. Place the bed at an appropriate and comfortable working height, usually elbow height of the caregiver (VHACEOSH, 2016).	
___	___	___	6. Using the tape measure, determine the distance between the gluteal crease and the popliteal space.	
___	___	___	7. Measure the leg from the knee to 14 in beyond the bottom of the foot.	
___	___	___	8. Position the patient in the middle of the bed. Make sure the affected extremity is in a slightly abducted position.	
___	___	___	9. Support the affected extremity and elevate it, placing it in the padded CPM device.	
___	___	___	10. ***Make sure the knee is at the hinged joint of the CPM device.***	
___	___	___	11. ***Adjust the footplate to maintain the patient's foot in a neutral position. Assess the patient's position to make sure the leg is not internally or externally rotated.***	
___	___	___	12. Apply the restraining straps under the CPM device and around the leg. ***Check that two fingers fit between the strap and the leg.***	
___	___	___	13. Explain the use of the STOP/GO button to the patient. Set the controls to the prescribed levels of flexion and extension and cycles per minute. Turn on the power to the CPM.	
___	___	___	14. Set the device to ON and start the therapy by pressing the GO button. Observe the patient and the device during the first cycle. Determine the angle of flexion when the device reaches its greatest height using the goniometer. Compare with prescribed degree.	

Excellent	Satisfactory	Needs Practice	SKILL 9-13 **Applying a Continuous Passive Motion Device** *(Continued)*	Comments
____	____	____	15. Place the bed in the lowest position, with the side rails up. Make sure the call bell and other essential items are within easy reach.	
____	____	____	16. Remove PPE, if used. Perform hand hygiene.	
____	____	____	17. Check the patient's level of comfort and perform skin and neurovascular assessments at least every 4 hours or per facility policy.	

Skill Checklists for Taylor's Clinical Nursing Skills. A Nursing Process Approach, 5th edition

Name ______________________ Date ______________

Unit ______________________ Position ______________

Instructor/Evaluator: ______________________ Position ______________

SKILL 9-14

Applying a Sling

Goal: The arm is immobilized in proper alignment.

Excellent	Satisfactory	Needs Practice		Comments
___	___	___	1. Review the medical record and nursing care plan to determine the need for the use of a sling.	
___	___	___	2. Perform hand hygiene. Put on PPE, as indicated.	
___	___	___	3. Identify the patient. Explain the procedure to the patient.	
___	___	___	4. Close the curtains around the bed and close the door to the room, if possible. Place the bed at an appropriate and comfortable working height, usually elbow height of the caregiver (VHACEOSH, 2016).	
___	___	___	5. Perform a pain assessment. If the patient reports pain, administer the prescribed medication in sufficient time to allow for the full effect of the analgesic.	
___	___	___	6. Assist the patient to a sitting position. Place the patient's forearm across the chest with the elbow flexed and the palm against the chest. Measure the sleeve length, if indicated.	
___	___	___	7. Enclose the arm in the sling, making sure the elbow fits into the corner of the fabric. Run the strap up the patient's back and across the shoulder opposite the injury, then down the chest to the fastener on the end of the sling.	
___	___	___	8. Place the ABD pad under the strap, between the strap and the patient's neck. ***Ensure that the sling and forearm are slightly elevated and at a right angle to the body.***	
___	___	___	9. Place the bed in the lowest position, with the side rails up. Make sure the call bell and other essential items are within easy reach.	
___	___	___	10. Remove PPE, if used. Perform hand hygiene.	
___	___	___	11. Check the patient's level of comfort, pain, arm positioning, and neurovascular status of the affected limb every 4 hours or according to facility policy. Assess the axillary and cervical skin frequently for irritation or breakdown.	

Skill Checklists for Taylor's Clinical Nursing Skills.
A Nursing Process Approach, 5th edition

Name ______________________________ Date ______________

Unit ______________________________ Position ______________

Instructor/Evaluator: ______________________________ Position ______________

SKILL 9-15

Applying a Figure-Eight Bandage

Goal: The bandage is applied correctly without injury or complications.

Excellent	Satisfactory	Needs Practice		Comments
___	___	___	1. Review the medical record and nursing care plan to determine the need for a figure-eight bandage.	
___	___	___	2. Perform hand hygiene. Put on PPE, as indicated.	
___	___	___	3. Identify the patient. Explain the procedure to the patient.	
___	___	___	4. Close the curtains around the bed and close the door to the room, if possible. Place the bed at an appropriate and comfortable working height, usually elbow height of the caregiver (VHACEOSH, 2016).	
___	___	___	5. Assist the patient to a comfortable position, with the affected body part in a normal-functioning position.	
___	___	___	6. Hold the bandage roll with the roll facing upward in one hand, while holding the free end of the roll in the other hand. Make sure to hold the bandage roll so it is close to the affected body part.	
___	___	___	7. Wrap the bandage around the limb twice, below the joint, to anchor it.	
___	___	___	8. Use alternating ascending and descending turns to form a figure eight. Overlap each turn of the bandage by one half to two thirds the width of the strip.	
___	___	___	9. Unroll the bandage as you wrap, not before wrapping.	
___	___	___	10. ***Wrap firmly, but not tightly. Assess the patient's comfort as you wrap. If the patient reports tingling, itching, numbness, or pain, loosen the bandage.***	
___	___	___	11. After the area is covered, wrap the bandage around the limb twice, above the joint, to anchor it. Secure the end of the bandage with tape, pins, or self-closures. Avoid metal clips.	
___	___	___	12. Place the bed in the lowest position, with the side rails up. Make sure the call bell and other necessary items are within easy reach.	
___	___	___	13. Remove PPE, if used. Perform hand hygiene.	
___	___	___	14. Elevate the wrapped extremity for 15 to 30 minutes after application of the bandage.	
___	___	___	15. Assess the distal circulation after the bandage is in place.	

Excellent	Satisfactory	Needs Practice	SKILL 9-15 **Applying a Figure-Eight Bandage** *(Continued)*	Comments
___	___	___	16. Lift the distal end of the bandage and assess the skin for color, temperature, and integrity. Assess for pain and perform a neurovascular assessment of the affected extremity after applying the bandage and at least every 4 hours thereafter, or per facility policy.	

Skill Checklists for Taylor's Clinical Nursing Skills. A Nursing Process Approach, 5th edition

Name ______________________ Date ______________________

Unit ______________________ Position ______________________

Instructor/Evaluator: ______________________ Position ______________________

SKILL 9-16

Assisting With Cast Application

Excellent	Satisfactory	Needs Practice	**Goal:** The cast is applied without interfering with neurovascular function.	**Comments**
___	___	___	1. Review the medical record and medical orders to determine the need for the cast.	
___	___	___	2. Perform hand hygiene. Put on gloves and/or other PPE, as indicated.	
___	___	___	3. Identify the patient. Explain the procedure to the patient and verify area to be casted.	
___	___	___	4. Perform a pain assessment and assess for muscle spasm. Administer prescribed medications in sufficient time to allow for the full effect of the analgesic and/or muscle relaxant.	
___	___	___	5. Close the curtains around the bed and close the door to the room, if possible. Place the bed at an appropriate and comfortable working height, usually elbow height of the caregiver (VHACEOSH, 2016).	
___	___	___	6. Position the patient, as needed, depending on the type of cast being applied and the location of the injury. Support the extremity or body part to be casted. Remove any rings or other jewelry from area to be casted.	
___	___	___	7. Drape the patient with the waterproof pads.	
___	___	___	8. Cleanse and dry the affected body part.	
___	___	___	9. Position and maintain the affected body part in the position indicated by the physician or advanced practice professional as the stockinette, sheet wadding, and padding are applied. The stockinette should extend beyond the ends of the cast. As the wadding is applied, check for wrinkles.	
___	___	___	10. Continue to position and maintain the affected body part in the position indicated by the physician or advanced practice professional as the casting material is applied. Assist with finishing by folding the stockinette or other padding down over the outer edge of the cast.	
___	___	___	11. ***Support the cast during hardening.*** Handle hardening plaster casts with the palms of hands, not fingers. Support the cast on a firm, smooth surface. Do not rest it on a hard surface or sharp edges. Avoid placing pressure on the cast.	

Excellent	Satisfactory	Needs Practice	SKILL 9-16 **Assisting With Cast Application** *(Continued)*	Comments
___	___	___	12. ***Elevate the injured limb at heart level with pillow or bath blankets, as ordered, making sure pressure is evenly distributed under the cast.***	
___	___	___	13. Place the bed in the lowest position, with the side rails up. Make sure the call bell and other essential items are within easy reach.	
___	___	___	14. Remove gloves and any other PPE, if used. Perform hand hygiene.	
___	___	___	15. Obtain x-rays, as ordered.	
___	___	___	16. Instruct the patient to report pain, odor, drainage, changes in sensation, abnormal sensation, or the inability to move fingers or toes of the affected extremity.	
___	___	___	17. Leave the cast uncovered and exposed to the air. Reposition the patient every 2 hours. Depending on facility policy, a fan may be used to dry the cast.	

Skill Checklists for Taylor's Clinical Nursing Skills. A Nursing Process Approach, 5th edition

Name ______________________ Date ______________________

Unit ______________________ Position ______________________

Instructor/Evaluator: ______________________ Position ______________________

SKILL 9-17

Caring for a Cast

Excellent	Satisfactory	Needs Practice	**Goal:** The cast remains intact, and the patient does not experience neurovascular compromise.	Comments
___	___	___	1. Review the medical record and the nursing care plan to determine the need for cast care and care for the affected body part.	
___	___	___	2. Perform hand hygiene. Put on PPE, as indicated.	
___	___	___	3. Identify the patient. Explain the procedure to the patient.	
___	___	___	4. Close the curtains around the bed and close the door to the room, if possible. Place the bed at an appropriate and comfortable working height, usually elbow height of the caregiver (VHACEOSH, 2016).	
___	___	___	5. If a plaster cast was applied, handle the casted extremity or body area with the palms of your hands for the first 24 to 36 hours, until the cast is fully dry.	
___	___	___	6. If the cast is on an extremity, elevate the affected area on pillows covered with waterproof pads. ***Maintain the normal curvatures and angles of the cast.***	
___	___	___	7. Keep cast (plaster) uncovered until fully dry.	
___	___	___	8. Assess the condition of the cast. Be alert for cracks, dents, or the presence of drainage from the cast. Perform skin assessment, particularly around edges of the cast, and neurovascular assessment according to facility policy, as often as every 1 to 2 hours. ***Check for pain, edema, inability to move body parts distal to the cast, pallor, pulses, and abnormal sensations. If the cast is on an extremity, compare it with the noncasted extremity.***	
___	___	___	9. If breakthrough bleeding or drainage is noted on the cast, mark the area on the cast, according to facility policy. Indicate the date and time next to the area. Follow medical orders or facility policy regarding the amount of drainage that needs to be reported to the primary care provider.	
___	___	___	10. Assess for signs of infection. Monitor the patient's temperature. Assess for a foul odor from the cast, increased pain, or extreme warmth over an area of the cast.	
___	___	___	11. Reposition the patient every 2 hours. Provide back and skin care frequently. Encourage range-of-motion exercise for unaffected joints. Encourage the patient to cough and breathe deeply.	

SKILL 9-17

Caring for a Cast *(Continued)*

Excellent	Satisfactory	Needs Practice		Comments
___	___	___	12. Instruct the patient to report pain, odor, drainage, changes in sensation, abnormal sensation, or the inability to move fingers or toes of the affected extremity.	
___	___	___	13. Place the bed in the lowest position, with the side rails up. Make sure the call bell and other essential items are within easy reach.	
___	___	___	14. Remove PPE, if used. Perform hand hygiene.	

Skill Checklists for Taylor's Clinical Nursing Skills.
A Nursing Process Approach, 5th edition

Name ______________________ Date ______________________

Unit ______________________ Position ______________________

Instructor/Evaluator: ______________________ Position ______________________

SKILL 9-18

Applying Skin Traction and Caring for a Patient in Skin Traction

Excellent	Satisfactory	Needs Practice	**Goal:** The traction is maintained with the appropriate counterbalance and the patient maintains proper body alignment.	Comments
____	____	____	1. Review the medical record and the nursing care plan to determine the type of traction being used and care for the affected body part.	
____	____	____	2. Perform hand hygiene. Put on PPE, as indicated.	
____	____	____	3. Identify the patient. Explain the procedure to the patient, emphasizing the importance of maintaining counterbalance, alignment, and position.	
____	____	____	4. Perform a pain assessment and assess for muscle spasm. Administer prescribed medications in sufficient time to allow for the full effect of the analgesic and/or muscle relaxant.	
____	____	____	5. Close the curtains around the bed and close the door to the room, if possible. Place the bed at an appropriate and comfortable working height, usually elbow height of the caregiver (VHACEOSH, 2016).	
			Applying Skin Traction	
____	____	____	6. Ensure the traction apparatus is attached securely to the bed. Assess the traction setup.	
____	____	____	7. Check that the ropes move freely through the pulleys. Check that all knots are tight and are positioned away from the pulleys. Pulleys should be free from the linens.	
____	____	____	8. Place the patient in a supine position with the foot of the bed elevated slightly. The patient's head should be near the head of the bed and in alignment.	
____	____	____	9. Cleanse the affected area. Place the compression stocking on the affected limb, as appropriate.	
____	____	____	10. Place the traction boot over the patient's leg. Be sure the patient's heel is in the heel of the boot. Secure the boot with the straps.	
____	____	____	11. Attach the traction cord to the boot footplate. Pass the rope over the pulley fastened at the end of the bed. Attach the weight to the hook on the rope, usually 5 to 10 lb for an adult. Gently let go of the weight. ***The weight should hang freely, not touching the bed or the floor.***	
____	____	____	12. ***Check the patient's alignment with the traction.***	

Excellent	Satisfactory	Needs Practice	SKILL 9-18 **Applying Skin Traction and Caring for a Patient in Skin Traction** *(Continued)*	Comments
___	___	___	13. ***Check the boot for placement and alignment. Make sure the line of pull is parallel to the bed and not angled downward.***	
___	___	___	14. Place the bed in the lowest position that still allows the weight to hang freely. Make sure the call bell and other essential items are within easy reach.	
___	___	___	15. Remove PPE, if used. Perform hand hygiene.	
			Caring for a Patient With Skin Traction	
___	___	___	16. Perform a skin-traction assessment per facility policy. This assessment includes checking the traction equipment, examining the affected body part, maintaining proper body alignment, and performing skin and neurovascular assessments.	
___	___	___	17. Remove the straps every 4 hours per the health care provider's order or facility policy. Check bony prominences for skin breakdown, abrasions, and pressure areas. Remove the boot, per medical order or facility policy, every 8 hours. Put on gloves and wash, rinse, and thoroughly dry the skin.	
___	___	___	18. Assess the extremity distal to the traction for edema, and assess peripheral pulses. Assess the temperature, color, and capillary refill, and compare with the unaffected limb. Check for pain, inability to move body parts distal to the traction, pallor, and abnormal sensations. Assess for indicators of deep vein thrombosis, including calf tenderness and swelling.	
___	___	___	19. Replace the traction; remove gloves and dispose of them appropriately.	
___	___	___	20. Check the boot for placement and alignment. ***Make sure the line of pull is parallel to the bed and not angled downward.***	
___	___	___	21. ***Ensure the patient is positioned in the center of the bed, with the affected leg aligned with the trunk of the patient's body. Check overall alignment of the patient's body.***	
___	___	___	22. Examine the weights and pulley system. ***Weights should hang freely, off the floor and bed. Knots should be secure. Ropes should move freely through the pulleys. The pulleys should not be constrained by knots.***	
___	___	___	23. Keep the bedsheets wrinkle free.	
___	___	___	24. Perform range-of-motion exercises on all unaffected joint areas, unless contraindicated. Encourage the patient to cough and deep breathe every 2 hours.	
___	___	___	25. Raise the side rails. Place the bed in the lowest position that still allows the weight to hang freely. Make sure the call bell and other essential items are within easy reach.	
___	___	___	26. Remove PPE, if used. Perform hand hygiene.	

*Skill Checklists for Taylor's Clinical Nursing Skills.
A Nursing Process Approach, 5th edition*

Name ______________________ Date ______________________

Unit ______________________ Position ______________________

Instructor/Evaluator: ______________________ Position ______________________

SKILL 9-19

Caring for a Patient in Skeletal Traction

Excellent	Satisfactory	Needs Practice	**Goal:** The traction is maintained appropriately and the patient maintains proper body alignment.	**Comments**
___	___	___	1. Review the medical record and the nursing care plan to determine the type of traction being used and the prescribed care.	
___	___	___	2. Perform hand hygiene. Put on PPE, as indicated.	
___	___	___	3. Identify the patient. Explain the procedure to the patient, emphasizing the importance of maintaining counterbalance, alignment, and position.	
___	___	___	4. Perform a pain assessment and assess for muscle spasm. Administer prescribed medications in sufficient time to allow for the full effect of the analgesic and/or muscle relaxant.	
___	___	___	5. Close the curtains around the bed and close the door to the room, if possible. Place the bed at an appropriate and comfortable working height, usually elbow height of the caregiver (VHACEOSH, 2016).	
___	___	___	6. Ensure the traction apparatus is attached securely to the bed. Assess the traction setup, including application of the ordered amount of weight. ***Be sure that the weights hang freely, not touching the bed or the floor.***	
___	___	___	7. ***Check that the ropes move freely through the pulleys. Check that all knots are tight and are positioned away from the pulleys. Pulleys should be free from the linens.***	
___	___	___	8. Check the alignment of the patient's body, as prescribed.	
___	___	___	9. Perform a skin assessment. Pay attention to pressure points, including the ischial tuberosity, popliteal space, Achilles tendon, sacrum, and heel.	
___	___	___	10. Perform a neurovascular assessment. Assess the extremity distal to the traction for edema and peripheral pulses. Assess the temperature and color and compare with the unaffected limb. Check for pain, inability to move body parts distal to the traction, pallor, and abnormal sensations. Assess for indicators of deep vein thrombosis, including calf tenderness, and swelling.	
___	___	___	11. Assess the site at and around the pins for redness, edema, and odor. Assess for skin tenting, prolonged or purulent drainage, elevated body temperature, elevated pin-site temperature, and bowing or bending of the pins.	

SKILL 9-19

Caring for a Patient in Skeletal Traction *(Continued)*

Excellent	Satisfactory	Needs Practice		Comments
___	___	___	12. Provide pin-site care.	
___	___	___	a. Using sterile technique, open the applicator package and pour the cleansing agent into the sterile container.	
___	___	___	b. Put on the sterile gloves.	
___	___	___	c. Place the applicators into the solution.	
___	___	___	d. ***Clean the pin site, starting at the insertion area and working outward, away from the pin site.***	
___	___	___	e. ***Use each applicator once. Use a new applicator for each pin site.*** Gently remove crusts or scabs appearing at the pin site if they can be removed easily; leave in place if there is difficulty during removal.	
___	___	___	13. Depending on medical order and facility policy, apply the antimicrobial ointment to pin sites and apply a dressing. Remove gloves and dispose of them appropriately.	
___	___	___	14. Perform ROM exercises on all joint areas, unless contraindicated. Encourage the patient to cough and deep breathe every 2 hours.	
___	___	___	15. Place the bed in the lowest position that still allows the weight to hang freely. Make sure the call bell and other essential items are within easy reach.	
___	___	___	16. Remove PPE, if used. Perform hand hygiene.	

Skill Checklists for Taylor's Clinical Nursing Skills. A Nursing Process Approach, 5th edition

Name ______________________ Date ______________________

Unit ______________________ Position ______________________

Instructor/Evaluator: ______________________ Position ______________________

SKILL 9-20

Caring for a Patient With an External Fixation Device

Goal: The patient shows no evidence of complication, such as infection, contractures, venous stasis, thrombus formation, or skin breakdown.

Excellent	Satisfactory	Needs Practice		Comments
___	___	___	1. Review the medical record and the nursing care plan to determine the type of device being used and prescribed care.	
___	___	___	2. Perform hand hygiene. Put on PPE, as indicated.	
___	___	___	3. Identify the patient. Explain the procedure to the patient. Assure the patient that there will be little pain after the fixation device is in place. Reinforce that the patient will be able to adjust to the device and will be able to move about with the device, allowing him or her to resume normal activities more quickly.	
___	___	___	4. ***After the fixation device is in place, apply ice to the surgical site, as ordered or per facility policy. Elevate the affected body part, if appropriate.***	
___	___	___	5. Perform a pain assessment and assess for muscle spasm. Administer prescribed medications in sufficient time to allow for the full effect of the analgesic and/or muscle relaxant.	
___	___	___	6. Administer analgesics, as ordered, before exercising or mobilizing the affected body part.	
___	___	___	7. Perform neurovascular assessments, per facility policy or medical order, usually every 2 to 4 hours for 24 hours, then every 4 to 8 hours. Assess the affected body part for color, motion, sensation, edema, capillary refill, and pulses. If appropriate, compare with the unaffected side. Assess for pain not relieved by analgesics, and for burning, tingling, and numbness.	
___	___	___	8. Close the curtains around the bed and close the door to the room, if possible. Place the bed at an appropriate and comfortable working height, usually elbow height of the caregiver (VHACEOSH, 2016).	
___	___	___	9. Assess the pin site for redness, tenting of the skin, prolonged or purulent drainage, swelling, and bowing, bending, or loosening of the pins. Monitor body temperature.	

Excellent	Satisfactory	Needs Practice	SKILL 9-20 **Caring for a Patient With an External Fixation Device** *(Continued)*	Comments
___	___	___	10. Perform pin-site care.	
___	___	___	a. Using sterile technique, open the applicator package and pour the cleansing agent into the sterile container.	
___	___	___	b. Put on the sterile gloves.	
___	___	___	c. Place the applicators into the solution.	
___	___	___	d. Clean the pin site starting at the insertion area and working outward, away from the pin site.	
___	___	___	e. ***Use each applicator once. Use a new applicator for each pin site.*** Gently remove crusts or scabs appearing at the pin site if they can be removed easily; leave in place if there is difficulty during removal.	
___	___	___	11. Depending on medical order and facility policy, apply the antimicrobial ointment to pin sites and apply a dressing. Remove gloves and dispose of them appropriately.	
___	___	___	12. Perform ROM exercises on all joint areas, unless contraindicated. Encourage the patient to cough and deep breathe every 2 hours.	
___	___	___	13. Place the bed in the lowest position that still allows the weight to hang freely, with the side rails up. Make sure the call bell and other essential items are within easy reach.	
___	___	___	14. Remove PPE, if used. Perform hand hygiene.	

Skill Checklists for Taylor's Clinical Nursing Skills. A Nursing Process Approach, 5th edition

Name ______________________ Date ______________________

Unit ______________________ Position ______________________

Instructor/Evaluator: ______________________ Position ______________________

SKILL 10-1

Promoting Patient Comfort

Excellent	Satisfactory	Needs Practice	**Goal**: The patient experiences relief from discomfort and/or pain without adverse effect.	Comments
___	___	___	1. Perform hand hygiene and put on PPE, if indicated.	
___	___	___	2. Identify the patient.	
___	___	___	3. Discuss pain with the patient, acknowledging that the patient's pain exists. Explain how pain medications and other pain management therapies work together to provide pain relief. Allow the patient to help choose interventions for pain relief. Discuss the patient's expectations for comfort and pain relief.	
___	___	___	4. Assess the patient's pain using an appropriate assessment tool and measurement scale.	
___	___	___	5. Provide pharmacologic interventions, if indicated and ordered.	
___	___	___	6. Adjust the patient's environment to promote comfort.	
___	___	___	a. Adjust and maintain the room temperature per the patient's preference.	
___	___	___	b. Reduce harsh lighting, but provide adequate lighting per the patient's preference.	
___	___	___	c. Reduce harsh and unnecessary noise. Avoid having conversations immediately outside the patient's room.	
___	___	___	d. Close the room door and/or curtain whenever possible.	
___	___	___	e. Provide good ventilation in the patient's room. Reduce unpleasant odors by promptly emptying bedpans, urinals, and emesis basins after use. Remove trash and laundry promptly.	
___	___	___	7. Prevent unnecessary interruptions and coordinate patient activities to group activities together. Allow for and plan rest periods without disturbance.	
___	___	___	8. Assist the patient to change position frequently. Assist the patient to a comfortable position, maintaining good alignment and supporting extremities, as needed. Raise the head of the bed, as appropriate.	
___	___	___	9. Provide oral hygiene as often as necessary (e.g., every 1 to 2 hours) to keep the mouth and mucous membranes clean and moist. This is especially important for patients who cannot drink or are not permitted fluids by mouth.	

SKILL 10-1
Promoting Patient Comfort *(Continued)*

Excellent	Satisfactory	Needs Practice		Comments
___	___	___	10. Ensure the availability of appropriate fluids for drinking, unless contraindicated. Make sure the patient's water pitcher is filled and within reach. Have other fluids of the patient's choice available.	
___	___	___	11. Remove physical situations that might cause discomfort.	
___	___	___	a. Change soiled and/or wet dressings; replace soiled and/or wet bed linens.	
___	___	___	b. Smooth wrinkles in bed linens.	
___	___	___	c. Ensure patient is not lying or sitting on tubes, tubing, wires, or other equipment.	
___	___	___	12. Assist the patient, as necessary, with ambulation, and active or passive range-of-motion exercises (ROM), as appropriate.	
___	___	___	13. Assess the patient's spiritual needs related to the pain experience. Ask the patient if he or she would like a spiritual counselor to visit.	
___	___	___	14. Consider the use of distraction. Distraction requires the patient to focus on something other than the pain.	
___	___	___	a. Have the patient recall a pleasant experience or focus attention on an enjoyable experience.	
___	___	___	b. Offer age or developmentally appropriate games, toys, books, audiobooks, access to television, and/or videos, or other items of interest to the patient.	
___	___	___	c. Encourage the patient to hold or stroke a loved person, pet, or toy.	
___	___	___	d. Offer access to music the patient prefers. Turn on the music when pain begins, or before anticipated painful stimuli. The patient can close his or her eyes and concentrate on listening. Raising or lowering the volume as pain increases or decreases can be helpful.	
___	___	___	15. Consider the use of guided imagery.	
___	___	___	a. Help the patient to identify a scene or experience that the patient describes as happy, pleasant, or peaceful.	
___	___	___	b. Encourage the patient to begin with several minutes of focused breathing, relaxation, or meditation (refer to specific information in steps 16 and 17).	
___	___	___	c. Help the patient concentrate on the peaceful, pleasant image.	
___	___	___	d. If indicated, read a description of the identified scene or experience, using a soothing, soft voice.	
___	___	___	e. Encourage the patient to concentrate on the details of the image, such as its sight, sounds, smells, tastes, and touch.	

SKILL 10-1

Promoting Patient Comfort *(Continued)*

Excellent	Satisfactory	Needs Practice		Comments
___	___	___	16. Consider the use of relaxation activities, such as deep breathing.	
___	___	___	a. Have the patient sit or recline comfortably and place hands on stomach. Close the eyes.	
___	___	___	b. Ask the patient to mentally count to maintain a comfortable rate and rhythm. Have the patient inhale slowly and deeply while letting the abdomen expand as much as possible. Have the patient hold his or her breath for a few seconds.	
___	___	___	c. Tell the patient to exhale slowly through the mouth, blowing through puckered lips. Have the patient continue to count to maintain comfortable rate and rhythm, concentrating on the rise and fall of the abdomen.	
___	___	___	d. When the patient's abdomen feels empty, have the patient begin again with a deep inhalation.	
___	___	___	e. Encourage patient to practice at least twice a day, for 10 minutes, and then use the technique, as needed, to assist with pain management.	
___	___	___	17. Consider the use of relaxation activities, such as progressive muscle relaxation.	
___	___	___	a. Assist the patient to a comfortable position.	
___	___	___	b. Direct the patient to focus on a particular muscle group. Start with the muscles of the jaw, then repeat with the muscles of the neck, shoulder, upper and lower arm, hand, abdomen, buttocks, thigh, lower leg, and foot.	
___	___	___	c. Ask the patient to tighten the muscle group and note the sensation that the tightened muscles produce. After 5 to 7 seconds, tell the patient to relax the muscles all at once and concentrate on the sensation of the relaxed state, noting the difference in feeling in the muscles when contracted and relaxed.	
___	___	___	d. Have the patient continue to tighten–hold–relax each muscle group until the entire body has been covered.	
___	___	___	e. Encourage the patient to practice at least twice a day, for 10 minutes, and then use the technique, as needed, to assist with pain management.	

Excellent	Satisfactory	Needs Practice	SKILL 10-1 **Promoting Patient Comfort** *(Continued)*	**Comments**
___	___	___	18. Consider the use of cutaneous stimulation, such as the intermittent application of heat or cold, or both.	
___	___	___	19. Consider the use of cutaneous stimulation, such as massage.	
___	___	___	20. Discuss consideration of consultation with a nurse trained in Healing Touch (HT) with the patient.	
___	___	___	21. Discuss the potential for use of cutaneous stimulation, such as TENS, with the patient and health care provider.	
___	___	___	22. Remove equipment and return patient to a position of comfort. Remove gloves, if used. Raise side rail and lower bed.	
___	___	___	23. Remove additional PPE, if used. Perform hand hygiene.	
___	___	___	24. Evaluate the patient's response to interventions. Reassess level of discomfort or pain using original assessment tools. Reassess and alter care plan, as appropriate.	

Skill Checklists for Taylor's Clinical Nursing Skills. A Nursing Process Approach, 5th edition

Name ______________________ Date ______________

Unit ______________________ Position ______________

Instructor/Evaluator: ______________________ Position ______________

SKILL 10-2
Giving a Back Massage

Goal: The patient reports increased comfort and/or decreased pain, and the patient is relaxed.

Excellent	Satisfactory	Needs Practice		Comments
___	___	___	1. Perform hand hygiene and put on PPE, if indicated.	
___	___	___	2. Identify the patient.	
___	___	___	3. Offer a back massage to the patient and explain the procedure.	
___	___	___	4. Put on gloves, if indicated.	
___	___	___	5. Close the room door and/or the curtain around the bed. Turn down the lights, if possible, and adjust the room temperature for patient comfort (Westman & Blaisdell, 2016).	
___	___	___	6. Assess the patient's pain using an appropriate assessment tool and measurement scale. Ask the patient if he or she has any aversion to touch (Westman & Blaisdell, 2016).	
___	___	___	7. Raise the bed to a comfortable working position, usually elbow height of the caregiver (VHA Center for Engineering & Occupational Safety and Health [CEOSH], 2016), and lower the side rail.	
___	___	___	8. Assist the patient to a comfortable position, preferably the prone or side-lying position. Remove the covers and move the patient's gown just enough to expose the patient's back from the shoulders to sacral area. Drape the patient, as needed, with the bath blanket.	
___	___	___	9. Warm the lubricant or lotion in the palm of your hand, or place the container in small basin of warm water. During massage, observe the patient's skin for reddened areas or injury. ***Avoid areas of injury, such as wounds, burns, and pressure ulcers and areas with rashes, tubes, and IV lines*** (Westman & Blaisdell, 2016).	
___	___	___	10. Using light, gliding strokes (*effleurage*), apply lotion to patient's shoulders, back, and sacral area.	
___	___	___	11. Place your hands beside each other at the base of the patient's spine and stroke upward to the shoulders and back downward to the buttocks in slow, continuous strokes. Continue for several minutes.	

SKILL 10-2

Giving a Back Massage *(Continued)*

Excellent	Satisfactory	Needs Practice		Comments
___	___	___	12. Massage the patient's shoulders, entire back, areas over iliac crests, and sacrum with circular, stroking motions, keeping hands in contact with the patient's skin. Continue for several minutes, applying additional lotion, as necessary.	
___	___	___	13. Knead the patient's back by gently alternating grasping and compression motions (*pétrissage*).	
___	___	___	14. Complete the massage with additional long, stroking movements that eventually become lighter in pressure.	
___	___	___	15. If excess lotion remains, use the towel to pat the patient dry.	
___	___	___	16. Remove gloves, if worn. Reposition patient's gown and covers. Raise side rail and lower bed. Assist patient to a position of comfort.	
___	___	___	17. Remove additional PPE, if used. Perform hand hygiene.	
___	___	___	18. Evaluate the patient's response to this intervention. Reassess level of discomfort or pain using original assessment tools. Reassess and alter care plan, as appropriate.	

Skill Checklists for Taylor's Clinical Nursing Skills.
A Nursing Process Approach, 5th edition

Name ______________________ Date ______________________

Unit ______________________ Position ______________________

Instructor/Evaluator: ______________________ Position ______________________

SKILL 10-3

Applying and Caring for a Patient Using a TENS Unit

Goal: The patient verbalizes decreased discomfort and pain, without experiencing any injury or skin irritation or breakdown.

Excellent	Satisfactory	Needs Practice		Comments
___	___	___	1. Perform hand hygiene and put on PPE, if indicated.	
___	___	___	2. Identify the patient.	
___	___	___	3. Show the patient the TENS device, and explain its function and the reason for its use.	
___	___	___	4. Assess the patient's pain using an appropriate assessment tool and measurement scale.	
___	___	___	5. Inspect the area where the electrodes are to be placed. Clean the patient's skin using the disposable cleansing wipe or skin cleanser and water. Dry the area thoroughly.	
___	___	___	6. Remove the adhesive backing from the self-adhering electrodes and apply them to the specified location.	
___	___	___	7. ***Check the placement of the electrodes; leave at least a 2-in (5-cm) space between them.***	
___	___	___	8. ***Check the controls on the TENS unit to make sure that they are off.*** Connect the wires to the electrodes (if not already attached) and plug them into the unit.	
___	___	___	9. Turn on the unit and adjust the intensity setting to the lowest intensity and determine if the patient can feel a tingling, burning, or buzzing sensation. Then adjust the intensity to the prescribed amount or the setting most comfortable for the patient. Secure the unit to the patient.	
___	___	___	10. Set the pulse width (duration of the each pulsation) as indicated or recommended.	
___	___	___	11. Assess the patient's pain level during therapy.	
___	___	___	a. If intermittent use is ordered, turn the unit off after the specified duration of treatment and remove the electrodes. Clean the patient's skin at the electrode sites.	
___	___	___	b. If continuous therapy is ordered, periodically remove the electrodes from the skin (after turning off the unit) to inspect the area and clean the skin, according to facility policy. Reapply the electrodes and continue therapy. Change the electrodes according to manufacturer's directions.	

Excellent	Satisfactory	Needs Practice	SKILL 10-3 **Applying and Caring for a Patient Using a TENS Unit** *(Continued)*	**Comments**
___	___	___	12. When therapy is discontinued, turn off the unit and remove the electrodes. Clean the patient's skin. Clean the unit and replace the batteries.	
___	___	___	13. Remove PPE, if used. Perform hand hygiene.	

Skill Checklists for Taylor's Clinical Nursing Skills. A Nursing Process Approach, 5th edition

Name ______________________ Date ______________________

Unit ______________________ Position ______________________

Instructor/Evaluator: ______________________ Position ______________________

SKILL 10-4

Caring for a Patient Receiving Patient-Controlled Analgesia

Goal: The patient reports increased comfort and/or decreased pain, without adverse effects, oversedation, or respiratory depression.

Excellent	Satisfactory	Needs Practice		Comments
___	___	___	1. Gather equipment. Check the medication order against the original order in the health care record, according to facility policy. Clarify any inconsistencies. Check the patient's health record for allergies.	
___	___	___	2. Know the actions, special nursing considerations, safe dose ranges, purpose of administration, and adverse effects of the medications to be administered. Consider the appropriateness of the medication for this patient.	
___	___	___	3. Prepare the medication syringe or other reservoir for administration, based on facility policy.	
___	___	___	4. Perform hand hygiene and put on PPE, if indicated.	
___	___	___	5. Identify the patient.	
___	___	___	6. Show the patient the device, and explain its function and the reason for use. Explain the purpose and action of the medication to the patient.	
___	___	___	7. Plug the PCA device into the electrical outlet, if necessary. Check status of battery power, if appropriate.	
___	___	___	8. Close the door to the room or pull the bedside curtain.	
___	___	___	9. Complete necessary assessments before administering medication. Check allergy bracelet or ask patient about allergies. Assess the patient's pain using an appropriate assessment tool and measurement scale.	
___	___	___	10. ***Check the label on the prefilled drug syringe or reservoir with the medication record and patient identification.*** Obtain verification of information from a second nurse, according to facility policy.	
___	___	___	11. Scan the patient's barcode on the identification band, if required.	
___	___	___	12. Connect tubing to prefilled syringe or other reservoir and place into the PCA device. ***Prime the tubing.*** Attach label to tubing, based on facility policy.	

Excellent	Satisfactory	Needs Practice	SKILL 10-4 **Caring for a Patient Receiving Patient-Controlled Analgesia** *(Continued)*	Comments
___	___	___	13. Set the PCA device to administer the loading dose, if ordered, and then program the device based on the prescriber's order for medication dosage, dose interval, and lockout interval. Obtain verification of information from a second nurse, according to facility policy.	
___	___	___	14. Put on gloves. Depending on facility policy, remove the passive disinfection cap from the connection port on the IV infusion tubing or other access site, based on route of administration. Alternately, use an antimicrobial swab to clean the connection port. Connect the PCA tubing to the patient's IV infusion line or appropriate access site, based on the specific site used. Secure the site per facility policy and procedure. Remove gloves. Initiate the therapy by activating the appropriate button on the pump. Lock the PCA device, per facility policy.	
___	___	___	15. Ensure the patient control (dosing button) is within the patient's reach. Attach the warning sign to the PCA control cord and/or PCA infusion device, per facility policy. Reinforce the steps for use with the patient and the need to press the button each time he or she needs relief from pain.	
___	___	___	16. Assess the patient's response to the medication: Assess the patient's pain at least every 4 hours or more often, as needed, based on patient's individual risk factors. Monitor vital signs, especially respiratory status, including respiratory rate, depth, and quality and oxygen saturation every 2 to 4 hours or more often, as needed, based on patient's individual risk factors and situation.	
___	___	___	17. Assess the patient's response to the medication: Assess the patient's sedation score and end-tidal carbon dioxide level (capnography) at least every 4 hours or more often, as needed, based on patient's individual risk factors.	
___	___	___	18. Assess the infusion site periodically, according to facility policy and nursing judgment. Assess the patient's use of the medication, noting number of attempts and number of doses delivered. Replace the drug syringe when it is empty.	
___	___	___	19. Make sure the patient control (dosing button) is within the patient's reach.	
___	___	___	20. Remove gloves and additional PPE, if used. Perform hand hygiene.	

Skill Checklists for Taylor's Clinical Nursing Skills.
A Nursing Process Approach, 5th edition

Name ____________________ Date ____________________

Unit ____________________ Position ____________________

Instructor/Evaluator: ____________________ Position ____________________

Excellent	Satisfactory	Needs Practice	SKILL 10-5 **Caring for a Patient Receiving Epidural Analgesia** **Goal:** The patient reports increased comfort and/or decreased pain, without adverse effects, oversedation, or respiratory depression.	**Comments**
___	___	___	1. Gather equipment. Check the medication order against the original order in the health care record, according to facility policy. Clarify any inconsistencies. Check the patient's health record for allergies.	
___	___	___	2. Know the actions, special nursing considerations, safe dose ranges, purpose of administration, and adverse effects of the medications to be administered. Consider the appropriateness of the medication for this patient.	
___	___	___	3. Prepare the medication syringe or other reservoir for administration, based on facility policy.	
___	___	___	4. Perform hand hygiene and put on PPE, if indicated.	
___	___	___	5. Identify the patient.	
___	___	___	6. Show the patient the device, and explain the function of the device and the reason for its use. Explain the purpose and action of the medication to the patient.	
___	___	___	7. Close the door to the room or pull the bedside curtain.	
___	___	___	8. Complete necessary assessments before administering the medication. Check allergy bracelet or ask the patient about allergies. Assess the patient's pain using an appropriate assessment tool and measurement scale. Put on gloves.	
___	___	___	9. ***Have an ampule of 0.4-mg naloxone and a syringe at the bedside, according to facility policy.***	
___	___	___	10. After the catheter has been inserted and the infusion initiated by the anesthesiologist or radiologist, ***identify the patient. Compare the label on the medication container and rate of infusion with the eMAR/MAR.*** Obtain verification of information from a second nurse, according to facility policy. If using a barcode administration system, scan the barcode on the medication label, if required.	
___	___	___	11. Tape all connection sites. ***Label the bag, tubing, and pump apparatus "For Epidural Infusion Only." Do not administer any other opioid or adjuvant drugs without the approval of the clinician responsible for the epidural injection.***	

Excellent	Satisfactory	Needs Practice	SKILL 10-5 **Caring for a Patient Receiving Epidural Analgesia** *(Continued)*	Comments
___	___	___	12. Assess the catheter exit site and apply a transparent dressing over the catheter insertion site, if not already in place. Secure the catheter and tubing, based on facility policy. Remove gloves and additional PPE, if used. Perform hand hygiene.	
___	___	___	13. Refer to Skill 10-4 for additional considerations if the epidural analgesia is being administered as PCA.	
___	___	___	14. Monitor the infusion rate according to facility policy. Assess and record the patient's vital signs, sedation level (in Skill 10-4), and respiratory status, including the patient's oxygen saturation, continuously for the first 20 minutes after initiation, then at least every hour for the first 12 hours, every 2 hours up to 24 hours, then at 4-hour intervals (or according to facility policy) (Sawhney, 2012). ***Notify the health care provider if the sedation rating is 3 or 4, the respiratory depth decreases, or the respiratory rate falls below 10 breaths/min.*** Refer to Skill 10-4. Monitor end-tidal carbon dioxide level (capnography) for patients at high risk of respiratory depression (Schreiber, 2015).	
___	___	___	15. Keep the head of bed elevated 30 degrees unless contraindicated.	
___	___	___	16. Assess the patient's level of pain and the effectiveness of pain relief.	
___	___	___	17. Monitor the patient's blood pressure and pulse.	
___	___	___	18. Monitor urinary output and assess for bladder distention.	
___	___	___	19. Assess motor strength and sensation every 4 hours or as specified by facility policy.	
___	___	___	20. Monitor for adverse effects (pruritus, nausea, decreased gastric motility, headache, and vomiting) (Schreiber, 2015).	
___	___	___	21. Assess for signs of infection at the insertion site.	
___	___	___	22. Assess the catheter-site dressing for drainage, based on facility policy. Notify the anesthesia provider or pain management team immediately of any abnormalities. Change the dressing over the catheter exit site per facility policy using aseptic technique. Change the infusion tubing as specified by facility policy.	

Skill Checklists for Taylor's Clinical Nursing Skills.
A Nursing Process Approach, 5th edition

Name ______________________ Date ______________________

Unit ______________________ Position ______________________

Instructor/Evaluator: ______________________ Position ______________________

SKILL 10-6

Caring for a Patient Receiving Continuous Wound Perfusion Pain Management

Excellent	Satisfactory	Needs Practice	**Goal:** The patient reports increased comfort and/or decreased pain, without adverse effects.	**Comments**
___	___	___	1. Check the medication order against the original health care provider's order, according to facility policy. Clarify any inconsistencies. Check the patient's health record for allergies.	
___	___	___	2. Know the actions, special nursing considerations, safe dose ranges, purpose of administration, and adverse effects of the medications to be administered. Consider the appropriateness of the medication for this patient.	
___	___	___	3. Perform hand hygiene and put on PPE, if indicated.	
___	___	___	4. Identify the patient.	
___	___	___	5. Close the door to the room or pull the bedside curtain.	
___	___	___	6. Assess the patient's pain. Administer postoperative analgesic, as ordered.	
___	___	___	7. Check the medication label attached to the pain management system balloon. Compare it with the health care provider's order and eMAR or MAR, per facility policy. Assess the patient for perioral numbness or tingling, numbness or tingling of fingers or toes, blurred vision, ringing in the ears, metallic taste in the mouth, confusion, seizures, drowsiness, nausea and/or vomiting. Assess the patient's vital signs.	
___	___	___	8. Put on gloves. Assess the wound perfusion system. Inspect tubing for kinks; check that the white tubing clamps are open. If tubing appears crimped, massage area on tubing to facilitate flow. Check filter in tubing, which should be unrestricted and free from tape.	
___	___	___	9. Check the flow restrictor to ensure it is in contact with the patient's skin. Tape in place, as necessary.	
___	___	___	10. Check the insertion-site dressing. Ensure that it is intact. Assess for leakage and dislodgement. Assess for redness, warmth, swelling, pain at site, and drainage.	
___	___	___	11. Review the device with the patient. Review the function of the device and reason for its use. Reinforce the purpose and action of the medication to the patient.	

Excellent	Satisfactory	Needs Practice	SKILL 10-6 **Caring for a Patient Receiving Continuous Wound Perfusion Pain Management** *(Continued)*	Comments
			To Remove the Catheter	
___	___	___	12. Check to ensure that infusion is complete. Infusion is complete when the delivery time has passed and the balloon is no longer inflated.	
___	___	___	13. Perform hand hygiene. Identify the patient. Put on gloves. Remove the catheter-site dressing. Loosen adhesive skin closure strips at the catheter site.	
___	___	___	14. Grasp the catheter close to the patient's skin at the insertion site. Gently pull catheter to remove. Catheter should be easy to remove and not painful. Do not tug or quickly pull on the catheter during removal. Check the distal end of the catheter for the black marking.	
___	___	___	15. Cover puncture site with a dry dressing, according to facility policy.	
___	___	___	16. Dispose of the balloon, tubing, and catheter, according to facility policy.	
___	___	___	17. Remove gloves and additional PPE, if used. Perform hand hygiene.	

Skill Checklists for Taylor's Clinical Nursing Skills. A Nursing Process Approach, 5th edition

Name ______________________ Date ______________

Unit ______________________ Position ______________

Instructor/Evaluator: ______________________ Position ______________

SKILL 11-1

Assisting a Patient With Eating

Excellent	Satisfactory	Needs Practice	**Goal:** The patient consumes a variety of food consistent with the prescribed diet and individual circumstances to attain and maintain ideal body weight.	Comments
___	___	___	1. Check the medical order for the type of diet prescribed for the patient.	
___	___	___	2. Perform hand hygiene and put on PPE, if indicated.	
___	___	___	3. Identify the patient.	
___	___	___	4. Explain the procedure to the patient.	
___	___	___	5. ***Assess level of consciousness, for any physical limitations, decreased hearing or visual acuity. If patient uses a hearing aid or wears glasses or dentures, provide, as needed. Ask if the patient has any cultural or religious preferences and food likes and dislikes, if possible.***	
___	___	___	6. Pull the patient's bedside curtain. Assess the abdomen. Ask the patient if he or she has any nausea. Ask the patient if he or she has any difficulty swallowing. Assess the patient for nausea or pain and administer an antiemetic or analgesic, as needed.	
___	___	___	7. Offer to assist the patient with any elimination needs.	
___	___	___	8. Provide hand hygiene and mouth care, as needed.	
___	___	___	9. Remove any bedpans or undesirable equipment and odors, if possible, from the vicinity where the meal will be eaten. Perform hand hygiene.	
___	___	___	10. Open the patient's bedside curtain. Assist to, or position the patient in, a high-Fowler's or sitting position in the bed or chair. Position the bed in the low position if the patient remains in bed.	
___	___	___	11. Place protective covering or towel over the patient if desired and as necessary.	
___	___	___	12. Check food tray to make sure that it is the correct tray before serving. Place tray on the overbed table so the patient can see the food, if able. Ensure that hot foods are hot and cold foods are cold. Use caution with hot beverages, allowing sufficient time for cooling, if needed. Ask the patient for his/her preference related to what foods are desired first. Cut food into small pieces, as needed. Observe swallowing ability throughout the meal.	

Excellent	Satisfactory	Needs Practice	SKILL 11-1 **Assisting a Patient With Eating** *(Continued)*	Comments
___	___	___	13. If possible, sit facing the patient at the patient's eye level while eating is taking place. If the patient is able, encourage him or her to hold finger foods and feed self as much as possible. Converse with patient during the meal and make eye contact, as appropriate. If, however, the patient has dysphagia, limit questioning or conversation that would require patient response during eating. Play relaxation music if patient desires.	
___	___	___	14. Allow enough time for the patient to chew and swallow the food adequately. The patient may need to rest for short periods during eating.	
___	___	___	15. When the meal is completed or the patient is unable to eat any more, remove the tray from the room. ***Note the amount and types of food consumed. Note the volume of liquid consumed.***	
___	___	___	16. Reposition the overbed table, remove the protective covering, offer hand hygiene, as needed, and offer the bedpan. Assist the patient to a position of comfort and relaxation.	
___	___	___	17. Remove PPE, if used. Perform hand hygiene.	

Skill Checklists for Taylor's Clinical Nursing Skills. A Nursing Process Approach, 5th edition

Name ______________________ Date ______________________

Unit ______________________ Position ______________________

Instructor/Evaluator: ______________________ Position ______________________

SKILL 11-2

Confirming Placement of a Nasogastric Tube

Goal: The tube is located in the patient's stomach without any complications and the patient does not exhibit signs and symptoms of aspiration.

Excellent	Satisfactory	Needs Practice		Comments
___	___	___	1. Gather equipment.	
___	___	___	2. Perform hand hygiene and put on PPE, if indicated.	
___	___	___	3. Identify the patient.	
___	___	___	4. Explain the procedure to the patient, including the rationale for confirming tube placement. Answer any questions as needed.	
___	___	___	5. Assemble equipment on overbed table or other surface within reach.	
___	___	___	6. Close the patient's bedside curtain or door. Raise the bed to a comfortable working position, usually elbow height of the caregiver (VHA Center for Engineering & Occupational Safety and Health [CEOSH], 2016). Perform abdominal assessments as described above. Drape chest with bath towel or disposable pad.	
___	___	___	7. Confirm placement of the nasogastric tube in the patient's stomach using at least two methods. The first method utilized should be measurement of the exposed length of tube.	
___	___	___	8. Put on gloves. Unsecure the tube from the patient's gown. Verify the position of the marking on the tube at the nostril. Measure length of exposed tube and compare with the documented length. Resecure the tube to the patient's gown.	
___	___	___	9. Check to ensure a 1-hour interval has elapsed since the patient has received medication or completed an intermittent feeding before testing pH of gastric fluid. Attach syringe to end of tube and aspirate a small amount of stomach contents. If unable to obtain a specimen, reposition the patient and flush the tube with 30 mL of air in a large syringe. Slowly apply negative pressure to withdraw fluid.	
___	___	___	10. Measure the pH of aspirated fluid using pH paper or a meter. Place a drop of gastric secretions onto pH paper or place small amount in a plastic cup and dip the pH paper into it. Within 30 seconds, compare the color on the paper with the chart supplied by the manufacturer.	

Excellent	Satisfactory	Needs Practice	SKILL 11-2 **Confirming Placement of a Nasogastric Tube** *(Continued)*	Comments
___	___	___	11. Examine aspirated contents, checking for color and consistency.	
___	___	___	12. If it is not possible to aspirate contents; assessments to check placement are inconclusive; the exposed tube length has changed; or there are any other indications that the tube is not in place, check placement by radiograph (x-ray) of placement of tube based on facility policy (and ordered by the primary health care provider).	
___	___	___	13. Flush tube with 30 to 50 mL of water for irrigation. Disconnect syringe from tubing and cap end of tubing.	
___	___	___	14. Clamp tube and remove the syringe. Cap the tube, reattach to the feeding delivery set, or attach tube to suction, based on the circumstances.	
___	___	___	15. Remove equipment and return patient to a position of comfort. Remove gloves. Raise side rail and lower bed.	
___	___	___	16. Remove additional PPE, if used. Perform hand hygiene.	

Skill Checklists for Taylor's Clinical Nursing Skills. A Nursing Process Approach, 5th edition

Name ______________________ Date ______________________

Unit ______________________ Position ______________________

Instructor/Evaluator: ______________________ Position ______________________

SKILL 11-3

Administering a Tube Feeding

Excellent	Satisfactory	Needs Practice	**Goal:** The patient receives the tube feeding without complaints of nausea, episodes of vomiting, gastric distention, or diarrhea.	Comments
___	___	___	1. Gather equipment. Check amount, concentration, type, and frequency of tube feeding in the patient's medical record. Check formula expiration date.	
___	___	___	2. Perform hand hygiene and put on PPE, if indicated.	
___	___	___	3. Identify the patient.	
___	___	___	4. Explain the procedure to the patient. Answer any questions, as needed.	
___	___	___	5. Assemble equipment on overbed table or other surface within reach.	
___	___	___	6. Close the patient's bedside curtain or door. Raise the bed to a comfortable working position, usually elbow height of the caregiver (VHACEOSH, 2016). Perform abdominal assessments as described above.	
___	___	___	7. ***Position the patient with HOB elevated at least 30 to 45 degrees or as near normal position for eating as possible.***	
___	___	___	8. Confirm placement of the nasogastric tube in the patient's stomach using at least two methods (refer to Skill 11-2). The first method utilized should be measurement of the exposed length of tube.	
___	___	___	9. Put on gloves. Unsecure the tube from the patient's gown. Verify the position of the marking on the tube at the nostril. Measure length of exposed tube and compare with the documented length.	
___	___	___	10. Check the pH of and visualize aspirated contents, checking for color and consistency as described in Skill 11-2, Steps 9–12.	
___	___	___	11. If it is not possible to aspirate contents; assessments to check placement are inconclusive; the exposed tube length has changed; or there are any other indications that the tube is not in place, check placement by radiograph (x-ray) of placement of tube, based on facility policy (and ordered by the primary health care provider).	

Excellent	Satisfactory	Needs Practice	SKILL 11-3 **Administering a Tube Feeding** *(Continued)*	Comments
___	___	___	12. After multiple steps have been taken to ensure that the feeding tube is located in the stomach or small intestine, ***aspirate all gastric contents with the syringe and measure to check for gastric residual—the amount of feeding remaining in the stomach.*** Return the residual based on facility policy. Proceed with feeding if amount of residual does not exceed facility policy or the limit indicated in the medical record.	
___	___	___	13. Flush tube with 30 to 50 mL of water for irrigation. Disconnect syringe from tubing and cap end of tubing while preparing the formula feeding equipment. Remove gloves.	
___	___	___	14. Put on gloves before preparing, assembling, and handling any part of the feeding system.	
___	___	___	15. Administer feeding.	
			When Using a Feeding Bag Administration System (Open System)	
___	___	___	a. Label bag and/or tubing with date and time. Hang bag on IV pole and adjust to about 12 in above the stomach. Clamp tubing.	
___	___	___	b. Check the expiration date of the formula. Cleanse top of feeding container with a disinfectant before opening it. Pour formula into feeding bag and allow solution to run through tubing. Close clamp.	
___	___	___	c. Attach feeding administration set to feeding tube, open clamp, and regulate drip according to the medical order, or allow feeding to run in over 30 minutes.	
___	___	___	d. ***Add 30 to 60 mL (1 to 2 oz) of water for irrigation to feeding bag when feeding is almost completed and allow it to run through the tube.***	
___	___	___	e. Clamp tubing immediately after water has been instilled. Disconnect feeding administration set from feeding tube. Clamp tube and cover end with cap.	
			When Using a Large Syringe (Open System)	
___	___	___	a. Remove plunger from 30- or 60-mL syringe.	
___	___	___	b. Attach syringe to feeding tube and pour premeasured amount of tube-feeding formula into syringe. Open the clamp on the feeding tube and allow formula to enter tube. Regulate rate, fast or slow, by height of the syringe. ***Do not push formula with syringe plunger.***	

SKILL 11-3

Administering a Tube Feeding *(Continued)*

Excellent	Satisfactory	Needs Practice		Comments
___	___	___	c. When feeding is almost completed, ***add 30 to 60 mL (1 to 2 oz) of water for irrigation to syringe*** and allow it to run through the tube.	
___	___	___	d. When syringe has emptied, hold syringe high, clamp the tube, and disconnect from tube. Cover end with cap.	
			When Using an Enteral Feeding Pump	
___	___	___	a. Close flow-regulator clamp on tubing and fill feeding bag with prescribed formula, as described in Steps 15a and 15b. Amount used depends on facility policy. Place label on container with patient's name, date, and time the feeding was hung.	
___	___	___	b. Hang feeding container on IV pole. Allow solution to flow through tubing.	
___	___	___	c. Connect to feeding pump, following manufacturer's directions. Set rate. Maintain the patient in the upright position throughout the feeding. If the patient needs to lie flat temporarily, pause the feeding. Resume the feeding after the patient's position has been changed back to at least 30 to 45 degrees (Bankhead et al., 2009).	
___	___	___	d. ***Check placement of tube and gastric residual every 4 to 6 hours (Bankhead et al., 2009). Flush tube with 30 to 50 mL of water at least every 4 hours during continuous feeding.***	
___	___	___	16. Observe the patient's response during and after tube feeding and assess the abdomen at least once a shift.	
___	___	___	17. ***Have patient remain in upright position for at least 1 hour after feeding.***	
___	___	___	18. Remove equipment and return patient to a position of comfort. Remove gloves. Raise side rail and lower bed.	
___	___	___	19. Put on gloves. Wash and clean equipment or replace according to facility policy. Remove gloves.	
___	___	___	20. Remove additional PPE, if used. Perform hand hygiene.	

Skill Checklists for Taylor's Clinical Nursing Skills. A Nursing Process Approach, 5th edition

Name ______________________ Date ______________________

Unit ______________________ Position ______________________

Instructor/Evaluator: ______________________ Position ______________________

SKILL 11-4

Caring for a Gastrostomy Tube

Goal: The patient does not exhibit signs and symptoms of irritation, excoriation, or infection at the tube insertion site.

Excellent	Satisfactory	Needs Practice		Comments
___	___	___	1. Gather equipment. Verify the medical order or facility policy and procedure regarding site care.	
___	___	___	2. Perform hand hygiene and put on PPE, if indicated.	
___	___	___	3. Identify the patient.	
___	___	___	4. Explain the procedure to the patient. Answer any questions, as needed.	
___	___	___	5. Assess for presence of pain at the tube-insertion site. If pain is present, offer the patient analgesic medication per the medical order and wait for medication absorption before beginning insertion site care.	
___	___	___	6. Pull the patient's bedside curtain. Assemble equipment on the bedside table, within reach. Raise bed to a comfortable working position, usually elbow height of the caregiver (VHACEOSH, 2016).	
___	___	___	7. Put on gloves. Assess the gastrostomy site, as described above.	
___	___	___	8. Measure the length of exposed tube, comparing it with the initial measurement after insertion. Alternately, examine the mark on the tube at the skin; mark should be at skin level at the insertion site.	
___	___	___	9. For the first 10 days when the gastrostomy tube is new and still has sutures holding it in place, dip a cotton-tipped applicator into sterile saline solution and gently clean around the insertion site, removing any crust or drainage. ***Avoid adjusting or lifting the external disk for the first few days after placement, except to clean the area.*** After the first 10 days, or when the gastric tube insertion site has healed and the sutures are removed, wet a washcloth and apply a small amount of skin cleanser onto washcloth. Gently cleanse around the insertion, removing any crust or drainage. Rinse site, removing all soap.	
___	___	___	10. Pat skin around insertion site dry.	

SKILL 11-4

Caring for a Gastrostomy Tube *(Continued)*

Excellent	Satisfactory	Needs Practice		Comments
____	____	____	11. If the sutures have been removed, ***gently push the tube forward toward the abdomen and rotate the tube. Gently rotate the guard or external bumper 90 degrees at least once a day. Assess that the guard or external bumper is not digging into the surrounding skin. Avoid placing any tension on the tube.***	
____	____	____	12. Leave the site open to air unless there is drainage. If drainage is present, place one thickness of a precut gauze pad or drain sponge under the external bumper and change, as needed, to keep the area dry. Use a skin protectant or barrier cream to prevent skin breakdown.	
____	____	____	13. If the tube is not in use, check that the cap is securely in place.	
____	____	____	14. Assess the integrity of the tape or device used to secure the tube to the stomach.	
____	____	____	15. Remove gloves. Lower the bed and assist the patient to a position of comfort, as needed.	
____	____	____	16. Remove additional PPE, if used. Perform hand hygiene.	

Skill Checklists for Taylor's Clinical Nursing Skills. A Nursing Process Approach, 5th edition

Name ______________________ Date ______________________

Unit ______________________ Position ______________________

Instructor/Evaluator: ______________________ Position ______________________

SKILL 12-1

Assisting With the Use of a Bedpan

Excellent	Satisfactory	Needs Practice	**Goal:** The patient is able to void with assistance.	Comments
___	___	___	1. Review the patient's medical record for any limitations in physical activity. Gather equipment.	
___	___	___	2. Perform hand hygiene and put on PPE, if indicated.	
___	___	___	3. Identify the patient.	
___	___	___	4. Assemble equipment on a chair next to the bed within reach.	
___	___	___	5. Close curtains around the bed and close the door to the room, if possible. Discuss the procedure with the patient and assess the patient's ability to assist with the procedure, as well as personal hygiene preferences.	
___	___	___	6. Unless contraindicated, apply powder to the rim of the bedpan. Place bedpan and cover on a chair next to the bed. Put on gloves.	
___	___	___	7. Adjust the bed to a comfortable working height, usually elbow height of the caregiver (VHACEOSH, 2016). Place the patient in a supine position, with the head of the bed elevated about 30 degrees, unless contraindicated.	
___	___	___	8. Fold top linen back just enough to allow placement of bedpan. If there is no waterproof pad on the bed and time allows, consider placing a waterproof pad under the patient's buttocks before placing the bedpan.	
___	___	___	9. Ask the patient to bend the knees. Have the patient lift his/her hips upward. Assist the patient, if necessary, by placing your hand that is closest to the patient palm up, under the lower back, and assist with lifting. Slip the bedpan into place with the other hand.	
___	___	___	10. ***Ensure that the bedpan is in proper position and the patient's buttocks are resting on the rounded shelf of the regular bedpan or the shallow rim of the fracture bedpan.***	
___	___	___	11. Raise the head of the bed as near to sitting position as tolerated, unless contraindicated. Cover the patient with bed linens.	

Excellent	Satisfactory	Needs Practice	SKILL 12-1 **Assisting With the Use of a Bedpan** *(Continued)*	Comments
___	___	___	12. ***Place the call bell and toilet tissue within easy reach. Place the bed in the lowest position.*** Leave the patient if it is safe to do so. Use side rails appropriately.	
___	___	___	13. Remove gloves and additional PPE, if used. Perform hand hygiene.	
			Removing the Bedpan	
___	___	___	14. Perform hand hygiene and put on gloves and additional PPE, as indicated. Adjust the bed to a comfortable working height, usually elbow height of the caregiver (VHACEOSH, 2016). Have a receptacle, such as plastic trash bag, handy for discarding tissue.	
___	___	___	15. Lower the head of the bed, if necessary, to about 30 degrees. Remove bedpan in the same manner in which it was offered, being careful to hold it steady. Ask the patient to bend the knees and lift the buttocks up from the bedpan. Assist the patient, if necessary, by placing your hand that is closest to the patient palm up, under the lower back, and assist with lifting. Place the bedpan on the bedside chair and cover it.	
___	___	___	16. If the patient needs assistance with hygiene, wrap tissue around the hand several times, and wipe the patient clean, using one stroke from the pubic area toward the anal area. Discard tissue. Use warm, moist disposable washcloth and skin cleanser to clean the perineal area. Place the patient on his or her side and spread buttocks to clean the anal area.	
___	___	___	17. Do not place toilet tissue in the bedpan if a specimen is required or if output is being recorded. Place toilet tissue in an appropriate receptacle.	
___	___	___	18. Return the patient to a comfortable position. Make sure the linens under the patient are dry. Replace or remove the pad under the patient, as necessary. Remove your gloves and ensure that the patient is covered.	
___	___	___	19. Raise side rail. Lower bed height and adjust the head of the bed to a comfortable position. Reattach call bell.	
___	___	___	20. Offer patient supplies to wash and dry his/her hands, assisting as necessary.	
___	___	___	21. Put on clean gloves. Empty and clean the bedpan, measuring urine in graduated container, as necessary. Discard the trash receptacle with used toilet paper per facility policy.	
___	___	___	22. Remove additional PPE, if used. Perform hand hygiene.	

Skill Checklists for Taylor's Clinical Nursing Skills. A Nursing Process Approach, 5th edition

Name ______________________________ Date ______________

Unit ______________________________ Position ______________

Instructor/Evaluator: ______________________________ Position ______________

SKILL 12-2

Assisting With the Use of a Urinal

Excellent	Satisfactory	Needs Practice	**Goal:** The patient is able to void with assistance.	Comments
___	___	___	1. Review the patient's medical record for any limitations in physical activity. Gather equipment.	
___	___	___	2. Perform hand hygiene and put on PPE, if indicated.	
___	___	___	3. Identify the patient.	
___	___	___	4. Assemble equipment on a chair next to the bed within reach.	
___	___	___	5. Close the curtains around the bed and close the door to the room, if possible. Discuss the procedure with the patient and assess the patient's ability to assist with the procedure, as well as personal hygiene preferences.	
___	___	___	6. Put on gloves.	
___	___	___	7. Assist the patient to an appropriate position, as necessary: standing at the bedside, lying on one side or back, sitting in bed with the head elevated, or sitting on the side of the bed.	
___	___	___	8. If the patient remains in the bed, fold the linens just enough to allow for proper placement of the urinal.	
___	___	___	9. If the patient is not standing, have him spread his legs slightly. ***Hold the urinal close to the penis and position the penis completely within the urinal. Keep the bottom of the urinal lower than the penis. If necessary, assist the patient to hold the urinal in place.***	
___	___	___	10. Cover the patient with the bed linens.	
___	___	___	11. Place the call bell and toilet tissue within easy reach. Have a receptacle, such as a plastic trash bag, handy for discarding tissue. Ensure the bed is in the lowest position. Leave patient if it is safe to do so. Use side rails appropriately.	
___	___	___	12. Remove gloves and additional PPE, if used. Perform hand hygiene.	
			Removing the Urinal	
___	___	___	13. Perform hand hygiene. Put on gloves and additional PPE, as indicated.	

Excellent	Satisfactory	Needs Practice	SKILL 12-2 **Assisting With the Use of a Urinal** *(Continued)*	Comments
____	____	____	14. Pull back the patient's bed linens just enough to remove the urinal. Remove the urinal. Cover the open end of the urinal. Place on the bedside chair. If the patient needs assistance with hygiene, wrap tissue around the hand several times, and wipe the patient dry. Place tissue in a receptacle. Use warm, moist disposable washcloth and skin cleanser to clean perineal area, as necessary, and as per patient request.	
____	____	____	15. Return the patient to a comfortable position. Make sure the linens under the patient are dry. Remove your gloves and ensure that the patient is covered.	
____	____	____	16. Ensure the patient call bell is in reach.	
____	____	____	17. Offer patient supplies to wash and dry his hands, assisting as necessary.	
____	____	____	18. Put on clean gloves. Empty and clean the urinal, measuring urine in a graduated container, as necessary. Discard the trash receptacle with used toilet paper per facility policy.	
____	____	____	19. Remove gloves and additional PPE, if used, and perform hand hygiene.	

Skill Checklists for Taylor's Clinical Nursing Skills. A Nursing Process Approach, 5th edition

Name ______________________ Date ______________________

Unit ______________________ Position ______________________

Instructor/Evaluator: ______________________ Position ______________________

SKILL 12-3

Assisting With the Use of a Bedside Commode

Goal: The patient is able to void with assistance.

Excellent	Satisfactory	Needs Practice		Comments
___	___	___	1. Review the patient's chart for any limitations in physical activity. Gather equipment.	
___	___	___	2. Obtain assistance for patient transfer from another staff member and/or appropriate transfer equipment, as indicated.	
___	___	___	3. Perform hand hygiene and put on PPE, if indicated.	
___	___	___	4. Identify the patient.	
___	___	___	5. Close the curtains around the bed and close the door to the room, if possible. Discuss the procedure with the patient and assess the patient's ability to assist with the procedure, as well as personal hygiene preferences.	
___	___	___	6. Place the commode close to, and parallel with, the bed. Raise or remove the seat cover.	
___	___	___	7. Assist the patient to a standing position and then help the patient pivot to the commode. ***While bracing one commode leg with your foot, ask the patient to place his/her hands one at a time on the armrests. Assist the patient to lower himself/herself slowly onto the commode seat.***	
___	___	___	8. Cover the patient with a blanket. Place call bell and toilet tissue within easy reach. Leave patient if it is safe to do so. Remove PPE, if used, and perform hand hygiene.	
			Assisting Patient Off Commode	
___	___	___	9. Perform hand hygiene. Put on gloves and additional PPE, as indicated.	
___	___	___	10. Assist the patient to a standing position. If the patient needs assistance with hygiene, wrap toilet tissue around your hand several times, and wipe the patient clean, using one stroke from the pubic area toward the anal area. Discard tissue in an appropriate receptacle, according to facility policy, and continue with additional tissue until patient is dry. Place tissue in receptacle. Use warm, moist disposable washcloth and skin cleanser to clean perineal area, as necessary, and as per patient request.	

Excellent	Satisfactory	Needs Practice	SKILL 12-3 **Assisting With the Use of a Bedside Commode** *(Continued)*	Comments
____	____	____	11. Do not place toilet tissue in the commode if a specimen is required or if output is being recorded. Replace or lower the seat cover.	
____	____	____	12. Remove your gloves. Return the patient to the bed or chair. If the patient returns to the bed, raise side rails, as appropriate. Ensure that the patient is covered and call bell is readily within reach.	
____	____	____	13. Offer patient supplies to wash and dry his or her hands, assisting as necessary.	
____	____	____	14. Put on clean gloves. Empty and clean the commode, measuring urine in graduated container, as necessary.	
____	____	____	15. Remove gloves and additional PPE, if used. Perform hand hygiene.	

Skill Checklists for Taylor's Clinical Nursing Skills. A Nursing Process Approach, 5th edition

Name ______________________ Date ______________________

Unit ______________________ Position ______________________

Instructor/Evaluator: ______________________ Position ______________________

SKILL 12-4

Assessing Bladder Volume Using an Ultrasound Bladder Scanner

Goal: The volume of urine in the bladder is accurately measured.

Excellent	Satisfactory	Needs Practice		Comments
___	___	___	1. Review the patient's medical record for any limitations in physical activity. Gather equipment.	
___	___	___	2. Perform hand hygiene and put on PPE, if indicated.	
___	___	___	3. Identify the patient.	
___	___	___	4. Close the curtains around the bed and close the door to the room, if possible. Discuss the procedure with the patient and assess the patient's ability to assist with the procedure, as well as personal hygiene preferences.	
___	___	___	5. Adjust the bed to a comfortable working height, usually elbow height of the caregiver (VHACEOSH, 2016). Place the patient in a supine position. Drape the patient. Stand on the patient's right side if you are right-handed, patient's left side if you are left-handed.	
___	___	___	6. Put on clean gloves.	
___	___	___	7. Press the ON button. Wait until the device warms up. Press the SCAN button to turn on the scanning screen.	
___	___	___	8. Press the appropriate biological sex button. The appropriate icon for male or female will appear on the screen.	
___	___	___	9. Clean the scanner head with the appropriate cleaner.	
___	___	___	10. Gently palpate the patient's symphysis pubis (anterior midline junction of pubic bones). Place a generous amount of ultrasound gel or gel pad midline on the patient's abdomen, about 1 to 1.5 in above the symphysis pubis.	
___	___	___	11. Place the scanner head on the gel or gel pad, ***with the directional icon on the scanner head toward the patient's head. Aim the scanner head toward the bladder (point the scanner head slightly downward toward the coccyx).*** Press and release the scan button.	
___	___	___	12. Observe the image on the scanner screen. ***Adjust the scanner head to center the bladder image on the crossbars.***	
___	___	___	13. Press and hold the DONE button until it beeps. Read the volume measurement on the screen. Print the results, if required, by pressing PRINT.	

Excellent	Satisfactory	Needs Practice	SKILL 12-4 **Assessing Bladder Volume Using an Ultrasound Bladder Scanner** *(Continued)*	Comments
___	___	___	14. Use a washcloth or paper towel to remove remaining gel from the patient's skin. Alternately, gently remove gel pad from patient's skin. Return the patient to a comfortable position. Remove your gloves and ensure that the patient is covered.	
___	___	___	15. Lower bed height and adjust the head of the bed to a comfortable position. Reattach call bell, if necessary.	
___	___	___	16. Put on gloves. Clean the scanner head according to the manufacturer's instructions and/or facility policy.	
___	___	___	17. Remove gloves and any additional PPE, if used. Perform hand hygiene.	

Skill Checklists for Taylor's Clinical Nursing Skills.
A Nursing Process Approach, 5th edition

Name ______________________ Date ______________________

Unit ______________________ Position ______________________

Instructor/Evaluator: ______________________ Position ______________________

SKILL 12-5

Applying an External Urinary Sheath (Condom Catheter)

Excellent	Satisfactory	Needs Practice	**Goal:** The patient's urinary elimination is maintained, with a urine output of at least 30 mL/hr, and the bladder is not distended.	**Comments**
____	____	____	1. Gather equipment.	
____	____	____	2. Perform hand hygiene and put on PPE, if indicated.	
____	____	____	3. Identify the patient.	
____	____	____	4. Close the curtains around the bed and close the door to the room, if possible. Discuss the procedure with the patient. Ask the patient if he has any allergies, especially to latex.	
____	____	____	5. Assemble equipment on overbed table or other surface within reach.	
____	____	____	6. Adjust the bed to a comfortable working height, usually elbow height of the caregiver (VHACEOSH, 2016). Stand on the patient's right side if you are right-handed, or on patient's left side if you are left-handed.	
____	____	____	7. Prepare urinary drainage setup or reusable leg bag for attachment to the external urinary sheath.	
____	____	____	8. Position the patient on his back with thighs slightly apart. Drape the patient so that only the area around the penis is exposed. Slide waterproof pad under the patient.	
____	____	____	9. Put on disposable gloves. Trim any long pubic hair that is in contact with the penis.	
____	____	____	10. Clean the genital area with washcloth, skin cleanser, and warm water. If patient is uncircumcised, retract foreskin and clean glans of penis. Replace foreskin. Clean the tip of the penis first, moving the washcloth in a circular motion from the meatus outward. Wash the shaft of the penis using downward strokes toward the pubic area. Rinse and dry. Remove gloves. Perform hand hygiene.	
____	____	____	11. Put on gloves. Apply skin protectant to the penis and allow to dry.	
____	____	____	12. Roll the external urinary sheath outward onto itself. Grasp the penis firmly with the nondominant hand. ***Apply the external urinary sheath by rolling it onto the penis with the dominant hand. Leave 1 to 2 in (2.5 to 5 cm) of space between the tip of the penis and the end of the external urinary sheath.***	

Excellent	Satisfactory	Needs Practice	SKILL 12-5 **Applying an External Urinary Sheath (Condom Catheter)** *(Continued)*	Comments
___	___	___	13. ***Apply pressure to the sheath at the base of the penis for 10 to 15 seconds.***	
___	___	___	14. Connect the external urinary sheath to drainage setup. Avoid kinking or twisting drainage tubing.	
___	___	___	15. Remove gloves. Secure drainage tubing to the patient's inner thigh with Velcro leg strap or tape. Leave some slack in tubing for leg movement.	
___	___	___	16. Assist the patient to a comfortable position. Cover the patient with bed linens. Place the bed in the lowest position.	
___	___	___	17. Secure the drainage bag below the level of the bladder. Check that drainage tubing is not kinked and that movement of side rails does not interfere with the drainage bag.	
___	___	___	18. Remove equipment. Remove gloves and additional PPE, if used. Perform hand hygiene.	

Skill Checklists for Taylor's Clinical Nursing Skills.
A Nursing Process Approach, 5th edition

Name ______________________ Date ______________________

Unit ______________________ Position ______________________

Instructor/Evaluator: ______________________ Position ______________________

SKILL 12-6

Catheterizing the Female Urinary Bladder

Goal: The catheter is successfully inserted without adverse effect; the patient's urinary elimination is maintained; and the patient's bladder is not distended.

Excellent	Satisfactory	Needs Practice		Comments
___	___	___	1. Review the patient's chart for any limitations in physical activity. Confirm the medical order for indwelling catheter insertion.	
___	___	___	2. Gather equipment. Obtain assistance from another staff member, if necessary.	
___	___	___	3. Perform hand hygiene and put on PPE, if indicated.	
___	___	___	4. Identify the patient.	
___	___	___	5. Close the curtains around the bed and close the door to the room, if possible. Discuss the procedure with the patient and assess the patient's ability to assist with the procedure. Ask the patient if she has any allergies, especially to latex or iodine.	
___	___	___	6. Provide good lighting. Artificial light is recommended (use of a flashlight requires an assistant to hold and position it). Place a trash receptacle within easy reach.	
___	___	___	7. Assemble equipment on overbed table or other surface within reach.	
___	___	___	8. Adjust the bed to a comfortable working height, usually elbow height of the caregiver (VHACEOSH, 2016). Stand on the patient's right side if you are right-handed, patient's left side if you are left-handed.	
___	___	___	9. Assist the patient to a dorsal recumbent position with knees flexed, feet about 2 ft apart, with her legs abducted. Drape the patient. Alternately, the Sims', or lateral, position can be used. Place the patient's buttocks near the edge of the bed with her shoulders at the opposite edge and her knees drawn toward her chest. Allow the patient to lie on either side, depending on which position is easiest for the nurse and best for the patient's comfort. Slide waterproof pad under the patient.	
___	___	___	10. Put on clean gloves. Clean the perineal area with washcloth, skin cleanser, and warm water, using a different corner of the washcloth with each stroke. Wipe from above orifice downward toward sacrum (front to back). Rinse and dry. Remove gloves. Perform hand hygiene again.	

Excellent	Satisfactory	Needs Practice	SKILL 12-6 **Catheterizing the Female Urinary Bladder** *(Continued)*	Comments
___	___	___	11. Prepare urine drainage setup if a separate urine collection system is to be used. Secure to bed frame, according to the manufacturer's directions.	
___	___	___	12. Open sterile catheterization tray on a clean overbed table using sterile technique.	
___	___	___	13. Put on sterile gloves. Grasp upper corners of drape and unfold drape without touching nonsterile areas. Fold back a corner on each side to make a cuff over gloved hands. Ask the patient to lift her buttocks and slide sterile drape under her with gloves protected by cuff.	
___	___	___	14. Based on facility policy, position the fenestrated sterile drape. Place a fenestrated sterile drape over the perineal area, exposing the labia.	
___	___	___	15. Place sterile tray on drape between the patient's thighs.	
___	___	___	16. Open all the supplies. Remove cap from the prefilled sterile saline syringe and attach to the balloon inflation port on the catheter. Open the package of antiseptic swabs. Alternately, fluff cotton balls in a tray before pouring antiseptic solution over them. Open specimen container if specimen is to be obtained.	
___	___	___	17. Lubricate 1 to 2 in of catheter tip.	
___	___	___	18. With thumb and one finger of nondominant hand, spread labia and identify meatus. ***Be prepared to maintain separation of labia with one hand until catheter is inserted and urine is flowing well and continuously.*** If the patient is in the side-lying position, lift the upper buttock and labia to expose the urinary meatus.	
___	___	___	19. Use the dominant hand to pick up an antiseptic swab or use forceps to pick up a cotton ball. ***Clean one labial fold, top to bottom (from above the meatus down toward the rectum), then discard the cotton ball. Using a new cotton ball/swab for each stroke, continue to clean the other labial fold, then directly over the meatus.***	
___	___	___	20. With your noncontaminated, dominant hand, place the drainage end of the catheter in a receptacle. If the catheter is preattached to sterile tubing and drainage container (closed drainage system), position the catheter and setup within easy reach on sterile field. Ensure that the clamp on the drainage bag is closed.	

Excellent	Satisfactory	Needs Practice	SKILL 12-6 **Catheterizing the Female Urinary Bladder** *(Continued)*	Comments
___	___	___	21. ***Using your dominant hand, hold the catheter 2 to 3 in from the tip and insert slowly into the urethra. Advance the catheter until there is a return of urine (approximately 2 to 3 in [4.8 to 7.2 cm]). Once urine drains, advance the catheter another 2 to 3 in (4.8 to 7.2 cm). Do not force the catheter through the urethra into the bladder.*** Ask the patient to breathe deeply, and rotate catheter gently if slight resistance is met as the catheter reaches the external sphincter.	
___	___	___	22. Hold the catheter securely at the meatus with your nondominant hand. Use your dominant hand to inflate the catheter balloon. Inject the entire volume of sterile water supplied in a prefilled syringe. Remove the syringe from the port.	
___	___	___	23. Pull gently on the catheter after the balloon is inflated to feel resistance.	
___	___	___	24. Attach the catheter to the drainage system if not already preattached.	
___	___	___	25. Remove equipment and dispose of it according to facility policy. Discard syringe in sharps container. Wash and dry the perineal area, as needed.	
___	___	___	26. Remove gloves. ***Secure catheter tubing to the patient's inner thigh with a catheter-securing device.*** Leave some slack in catheter for leg movement.	
___	___	___	27. Assist the patient to a comfortable position. Cover the patient with bed linens. Place the bed in the lowest position.	
___	___	___	28. Secure the drainage bag below the level of the bladder. Check that drainage tubing is not kinked and that movement of side rails does not interfere with the catheter or drainage bag.	
___	___	___	29. Put on clean gloves. Obtain urine specimen immediately, if needed, from the drainage bag. Label specimen. Send urine specimen to the laboratory promptly or refrigerate it.	
___	___	___	30. Remove gloves and additional PPE, if used. Perform hand hygiene.	

Skill Checklists for Taylor's Clinical Nursing Skills. A Nursing Process Approach, 5th edition

Name ______________________ Date ______________________

Unit ______________________ Position ______________________

Instructor/Evaluator: ______________________ Position ______________________

SKILL 12-7

Catheterizing the Male Urinary Bladder

Excellent	Satisfactory	Needs Practice	Goal: The catheter is successfully inserted without adverse effect; the patient's urinary elimination is maintained; and the patient's bladder is not distended.	Comments
___	___	___	1. Review chart for any limitations in physical activity. Confirm the medical order for indwelling catheter insertion.	
___	___	___	2. Gather equipment. Obtain assistance from another staff member, if necessary.	
___	___	___	3. Perform hand hygiene and put on PPE, if indicated.	
___	___	___	4. Identify the patient.	
___	___	___	5. Close the curtains around the bed and close the door to the room, if possible. Discuss the procedure with the patient and assess the patient's ability to assist with the procedure. Ask the patient if he has any allergies, especially to latex or iodine.	
___	___	___	6. Provide good lighting. Artificial light is recommended (use of a flashlight requires an assistant to hold and position it). Place a trash receptacle within easy reach.	
___	___	___	7. Assemble equipment on overbed table or other surface within reach.	
___	___	___	8. Adjust the bed to a comfortable working height, usually elbow height of the caregiver (VHACEOSH, 2016). Stand on the patient's right side if you are right-handed, patient's left side if you are left-handed.	
___	___	___	9. Position the patient on his back with thighs slightly apart. Drape the patient so that only the area around the penis is exposed. Slide waterproof pad under the patient.	
___	___	___	10. Put on clean gloves. Clean the genital area with washcloth, skin cleanser, and warm water. Clean the tip of the penis first, moving the washcloth in a circular motion from the meatus outward. Wash the shaft of the penis using downward strokes toward the pubic area. Rinse and dry. Remove gloves. Perform hand hygiene again.	
___	___	___	11. Prepare urine drainage setup if a separate urine collection system is to be used. Secure to bed frame according to the manufacturer's directions.	

Excellent	Satisfactory	Needs Practice	SKILL 12-7 **Catheterizing the Male Urinary Bladder** *(Continued)*	Comments
___	___	___	12. Open sterile catheterization tray on a clean overbed table or other flat surface, using sterile technique.	
___	___	___	13. Put on sterile gloves. Open sterile drape and place on patient's thighs. Place fenestrated drape with opening over the penis.	
___	___	___	14. Place the catheter setup on or next to the patient's legs on sterile drape.	
___	___	___	15. Open all the supplies. Remove cap from the prefilled sterile saline syringe and attach to the balloon inflation port on the catheter. Open package of antiseptic swabs. Alternately, fluff cotton balls in a tray before pouring antiseptic solution over them. Open specimen container if specimen is to be obtained. Remove cap from syringe prefilled with lubricant.	
___	___	___	16. Place the drainage end of the catheter in a receptacle. If the catheter is preattached to sterile tubing and drainage container (closed drainage system), position catheter and setup within easy reach on sterile field. Ensure that the clamp on drainage bag is closed. Lubricate 1 to 2 in of catheter tip.	
___	___	___	17. Lift the penis with the nondominant hand. Retract the foreskin in an uncircumcised patient. ***Be prepared to keep this hand in this position until the catheter is inserted and urine is flowing well and continuously. Use the dominant hand to pick up an antiseptic swab or use forceps to pick up a cotton ball. Using a circular motion, clean the penis, moving from the meatus down the glans of the penis. Repeat this cleansing motion two more times, using a new cotton ball/swab each time. Discard each cotton ball/swab after one use.***	
___	___	___	18. Hold the penis with slight upward tension and perpendicular to the patient's body. Use the dominant hand to pick up the lubricant syringe. ***Gently insert the tip of the syringe with a lubricant into the urethra and instill the 10 mL of lubricant.***	
___	___	___	19. Use the dominant hand to pick up the catheter and hold it an inch or two from the tip. Ask the patient to bear down as if voiding. ***Insert the catheter tip into the meatus. Ask the patient to take deep breaths. Advance the catheter to the bifurcation or "Y" level of the ports. Do not use force to introduce the catheter.*** If the catheter resists entry, ask the patient to breathe deeply and rotate the catheter slightly.	

SKILL 12-7

Catheterizing the Male Urinary Bladder *(Continued)*

Excellent	Satisfactory	Needs Practice		Comments
___	___	___	20. Hold the catheter securely at the meatus with your nondominant hand. Use your dominant hand to inflate the catheter balloon. ***Inject the entire volume of sterile water supplied in a prefilled syringe. Once the balloon is inflated, the catheter may be gently pulled back into place. Replace foreskin, if present, over the catheter.*** Lower the penis.	
___	___	___	21. Pull gently on the catheter after the balloon is inflated to feel resistance.	
___	___	___	22. Attach the catheter to drainage system, if necessary.	
___	___	___	23. Remove equipment and dispose of it according to facility policy. Discard syringe in sharps container. Wash and dry the perineal area, as needed.	
___	___	___	24. Remove gloves. Secure catheter tubing to the patient's inner thigh or lower abdomen (with the penis directed toward the patient's chest) with a catheter-securing device or tape. Leave some slack in the catheter for leg movement.	
___	___	___	25. Assist the patient to a comfortable position. Cover the patient with bed linens. Place the bed in the lowest position.	
___	___	___	26. Secure drainage bag below the level of the bladder. Check that drainage tubing is not kinked and that movement of side rails does not interfere with the catheter or drainage bag.	
___	___	___	27. Put on clean gloves. Obtain urine specimen immediately, if needed, from drainage bag. Label specimen. Send urine specimen to the laboratory promptly or refrigerate it.	
___	___	___	28. Remove gloves and additional PPE, if used. Perform hand hygiene.	

Skill Checklists for Taylor's Clinical Nursing Skills.
A Nursing Process Approach, 5th edition

Name ______________________ Date ______________

Unit ______________________ Position ______________

Instructor/Evaluator: ______________________ Position ______________

SKILL 12-8

Removing an Indwelling Urinary Catheter

Goal: The catheter is removed without difficulty and with minimal patient discomfort.

Excellent	Satisfactory	Needs Practice		Comments
___	___	___	1. Confirm the order for catheter removal in the medical record. Gather equipment.	
___	___	___	2. Perform hand hygiene and put on PPE, if indicated.	
___	___	___	3. Identify the patient.	
___	___	___	4. Close the curtains around the bed and close the door to the room, if possible. Discuss the procedure with the patient and assess the patient's ability to assist with the procedure.	
___	___	___	5. Adjust the bed to a comfortable working height, usually elbow height of the caregiver (VHACEOSH, 2016). Stand on the patient's right side if you are right-handed, patient's left side if you are left-handed.	
___	___	___	6. Position the patient as for catheter insertion. Drape the patient so that only the area around the catheter is exposed. Slide waterproof pad between the female patient's legs or over the male patient's thighs.	
___	___	___	7. Remove the device used to secure the catheter to the patient's thigh or abdomen.	
___	___	___	8. Insert the syringe into the balloon inflation port. Allow the pressure within the balloon to force the syringe plunger back and fill the syringe with water. Refer to manufacturer's instructions for deflation. ***Do not cut the inflation port.***	
___	___	___	9. Ask the patient to take several slow deep breaths. ***Slowly and gently remove the catheter.*** Place it on the waterproof pad and wrap it in the pad.	
___	___	___	10. Wash and dry the perineal area, as needed.	
___	___	___	11. Remove gloves. Assist the patient to a comfortable position. Cover the patient with bed linens. Place the bed in the lowest position.	
___	___	___	12. Put on clean gloves. Remove equipment and dispose of it according to facility policy. Note characteristics and amount of urine in drainage bag.	
___	___	___	13. Remove gloves and additional PPE, if used. Perform hand hygiene.	

Skill Checklists for Taylor's Clinical Nursing Skills. A Nursing Process Approach, 5th edition

Name ______________________ Date ______________________

Unit ______________________ Position ______________________

Instructor/Evaluator: ______________________ Position ______________________

SKILL 12-9

Performing Intermittent Closed Catheter Irrigation

Excellent	Satisfactory	Needs Practice	**Goal:** The catheter is irrigated without adverse effect and the patient exhibits the free flow of urine through the catheter.	**Comments**
____	____	____	1. Confirm the order for catheter irrigation and prescribed solution in the medical record.	
____	____	____	2. Gather equipment.	
____	____	____	3. Perform hand hygiene and put on PPE, if indicated.	
____	____	____	4. Identify the patient.	
____	____	____	5. Close the curtains around the bed and close the door to the room, if possible. Discuss the procedure with the patient.	
____	____	____	6. Assemble equipment on overbed table or other surface within reach.	
____	____	____	7. Adjust the bed to a comfortable working height, usually elbow height of the caregiver (VHACEOSH, 2016).	
____	____	____	8. Put on gloves. Empty the catheter drainage bag and measure the amount of urine, noting the amount and characteristics of the urine. Remove gloves. Perform hand hygiene.	
____	____	____	9. Assist the patient to a comfortable position and expose access port on catheter setup. Place waterproof pad under catheter and aspiration port. Remove catheter from device or tape anchoring catheter to the patient.	
____	____	____	10. Open supplies, using aseptic technique. Pour sterile solution into sterile basin. Aspirate the prescribed amount of irrigant (usually 30 to 60 mL) into sterile syringe. Put on gloves.	
____	____	____	11. ***Cleanse the access port on the catheter with antimicrobial swab.***	
____	____	____	12. Clamp or fold catheter tubing below the access port.	
____	____	____	13. Attach the syringe to the access port on the catheter using a twisting motion. ***Gently instill solution into catheter.***	
____	____	____	14. Remove syringe from access port. ***Unclamp or unfold tubing and allow irrigant and urine to flow into the drainage bag.*** Repeat procedure, as necessary.	
____	____	____	15. Remove gloves. Secure catheter tubing to the patient's inner thigh or lower abdomen (if a male patient) with anchoring device or tape. Leave some slack in the catheter for leg movement.	

Excellent	Satisfactory	Needs Practice	SKILL 12-9 **Performing Intermittent Closed Catheter Irrigation** *(Continued)*	**Comments**
___	___	___	16. Assist the patient to a comfortable position. Cover the patient with bed linens. Place the bed in the lowest position.	
___	___	___	17. Secure drainage bag below the level of the bladder. Check that drainage tubing is not kinked and that movement of side rails does not interfere with catheter or drainage bag.	
___	___	___	18. Remove equipment and discard syringe in appropriate receptacle. Remove gloves and additional PPE, if used. Perform hand hygiene.	
___	___	___	19. Assess the patient's response to the procedure and the quality and amount of drainage after the irrigation.	

Skill Checklists for Taylor's Clinical Nursing Skills. A Nursing Process Approach, 5th edition

Name ______________________ Date ______________________

Unit ______________________ Position ______________________

Instructor/Evaluator: ______________________ Position ______________________

SKILL 12-10

Administering a Continuous Closed Bladder or Catheter Irrigation

Goal: The irrigation is administered without adverse effect and the patient exhibits free-flowing urine through the catheter.

Excellent	Satisfactory	Needs Practice		Comments
___	___	___	1. Confirm the order for catheter irrigation in the medical record, including infusion parameters. If irrigation is to be implemented via gravity infusion, calculate the drip rate. Often, orders are to infuse to keep the urine clear of blood or clots.	
___	___	___	2. Gather equipment.	
___	___	___	3. Perform hand hygiene and put on PPE, if indicated.	
___	___	___	4. Identify the patient.	
___	___	___	5. Close the curtains around the bed and close the door to the room, if possible. Discuss the procedure with the patient.	
___	___	___	6. Assemble equipment on overbed table or other surface within reach.	
___	___	___	7. Adjust the bed to a comfortable working height, usually elbow height of the caregiver (VHACEOSH, 2016).	
___	___	___	8. Empty the catheter drainage bag and measure the amount of urine, noting the amount and characteristics of the urine.	
___	___	___	9. Assist the patient to a comfortable position and expose the irrigation port on the catheter setup. Place waterproof pad under the catheter and irrigation port.	
___	___	___	10. Prepare sterile irrigation bag for use as directed by manufacturer. Clearly label the solution as "Bladder Irrigant." Include the date and time on the label. Hang bag on IV pole 2.5 to 3 ft above the level of the patient's bladder. Close tubing clamp and insert sterile tubing with drip chamber to container using aseptic technique. Release clamp and remove protective cover on end of tubing without contaminating it. Allow solution to flush tubing and remove air. Clamp tubing and replace end cover.	

Excellent	Satisfactory	Needs Practice	SKILL 12-10 **Administering a Continuous Closed Bladder or Catheter Irrigation** *(Continued)*	Comments
___	___	___	11. Put on gloves. ***Cleanse the irrigation port on the catheter with an alcohol swab. Using aseptic technique, attach irrigation tubing to irrigation port of three-way indwelling catheter.***	
___	___	___	12. Check the drainage tubing to make sure clamp, if present, is open.	
___	___	___	13. ***Release clamp on irrigation tubing and regulate flow at determined drip rate, according to the ordered rate.*** If the bladder irrigation is to be done with a medicated solution, use an electronic infusion device to regulate the flow.	
___	___	___	14. Remove gloves. Assist the patient to a comfortable position. Cover the patient with bed linens. Place the bed in the lowest position.	
___	___	___	15. Assess the patient's response to the procedure, and the quality and amount of drainage.	
___	___	___	16. Remove equipment. Remove additional PPE, if used. Perform hand hygiene.	
___	___	___	17. As irrigation fluid container nears empty, clamp the administration tubing. Do not allow drip chamber to empty. Disconnect empty bag and attach a new full irrigation solution bag.	
___	___	___	18. Put on gloves and empty drainage collection bag as each new container is hung. Record initiation of new container and volume of drainage.	

Skill Checklists for Taylor's Clinical Nursing Skills.
A Nursing Process Approach, 5th edition

Name ______________________ Date ______________________

Unit ______________________ Position ______________________

Instructor/Evaluator: ______________________ Position ______________________

SKILL 12-11

Emptying and Changing a Stoma Appliance on a Urinary Diversion

Excellent	Satisfactory	Needs Practice	**Goal:** The stoma appliance is applied correctly to the skin to allow urine to drain freely.	**Comments**
___	___	___	1. Gather equipment.	
___	___	___	2. Perform hand hygiene and put on PPE, if indicated.	
___	___	___	3. Identify the patient.	
___	___	___	4. Close the curtains around the bed and close the door to the room, if possible. Explain what you are going to do and why you are going to do it to the patient. Encourage the patient to observe or participate, if possible.	
___	___	___	5. Assemble equipment on overbed table or other surface within reach.	
___	___	___	6. Assist the patient to a comfortable sitting or lying position in bed or a standing or sitting position in the bathroom. If the patient is in bed, adjust the bed to a comfortable working height, usually elbow height of the caregiver (VHACEOSH, 2016). Place waterproof pad under the patient at the stoma site.	
			Emptying the Appliance	
___	___	___	7. Put on gloves. Hold end of appliance over a bedpan, toilet, or measuring device. Remove the end cap from the spout. Open the spout and empty the contents into the bedpan, toilet, or measuring device.	
___	___	___	8. Close the spout. Wipe the spout with toilet tissue. Replace the cap.	
___	___	___	9. Remove equipment. Remove gloves. Assist the patient to a comfortable position.	
___	___	___	10. If appliance is not to be changed, place bed in lowest position. Remove additional PPE, if used. Perform hand hygiene.	
			Changing the Appliance	
___	___	___	11. Place a disposable waterproof pad on the overbed table or other work area. Open the premoistened disposable washcloths or set up the washbasin with warm water and the rest of the supplies. Place a trash bag within reach.	

Excellent	Satisfactory	Needs Practice	SKILL 12-11 **Emptying and Changing a Stoma Appliance on a Urinary Diversion** *(Continued)*	Comments
___	___	___	12. Put on clean gloves. Place waterproof pad under the patient at the stoma site. Empty the appliance, if necessary, as described in Steps 6 to 8.	
___	___	___	13. Put on gloves. Gently remove the appliance faceplate, starting at the top and keeping the abdominal skin taut. Remove appliance faceplate from skin by pushing skin from appliance rather than pulling appliance from skin. Apply a silicone-based adhesive remover by spraying or wiping with the remover wipe, as needed.	
___	___	___	14. Place the appliance in the trash bag, if disposable. If reusable, set aside to wash in lukewarm soap and water and allow to air dry after the new appliance is in place.	
___	___	___	15. Clean skin around stoma with mild skin cleanser and water or a cleansing agent and a washcloth. Remove all old adhesive from the skin; additional adhesive remover may be used. Do not apply lotion to the peristomal area.	
___	___	___	16. Gently pat area dry. ***Make sure skin around stoma is thoroughly dry.*** Assess stoma and condition of surrounding skin.	
___	___	___	17. Place one or two gauze squares over the stoma opening.	
___	___	___	18. Apply skin protectant to a 2-in (5-cm) radius around the stoma, and allow it to dry completely, which takes about 30 seconds.	
___	___	___	19. Lift the gauze squares for a moment and measure the stoma opening, using the measurement guide. Replace the gauze. Trace the same-size opening on the back center of the appliance. Cut the opening 1/8 in larger than the stoma size. Use a finger to gently smooth the wafer edges after cutting. Check that the spout is closed and the end cap is in place.	
___	___	___	20. Remove the paper backing from the appliance faceplate. Quickly remove the gauze squares and discard appropriately; ease the appliance over the stoma. Gently press onto the skin while smoothing over the surface. Apply gentle, even pressure to the appliance for approximately 30 seconds.	
___	___	___	21. Secure optional belt to appliance and around the patient.	
___	___	___	22. Remove gloves. Assist the patient to a comfortable position. Cover the patient with bed linens. Place the bed in the lowest position.	
___	___	___	23. Put on clean gloves. Remove or discard any remaining equipment and assess the patient's response to the procedure.	
___	___	___	24. Remove gloves and additional PPE, if used. Perform hand hygiene.	

Skill Checklists for Taylor's Clinical Nursing Skills. A Nursing Process Approach, 5th edition

Name ______________________ Date ______________________

Unit ______________________ Position ______________________

Instructor/Evaluator: ______________________ Position ______________________

SKILL 12-12

Caring for a Suprapubic Urinary Catheter

Goal: The patient's skin remains clean, dry, intact, and without evidence of irritation or breakdown; and the patient verbalizes an understanding of the purpose for, and care of the catheter, as appropriate.

Excellent	Satisfactory	Needs Practice		Comments
___	___	___	1. Gather equipment.	
___	___	___	2. Perform hand hygiene and put on PPE, if indicated.	
___	___	___	3. Identify the patient.	
___	___	___	4. Close the curtains around the bed and close the door to the room, if possible. Explain what you are going to do, and why you are going to do it, to the patient. Encourage the patient to observe or participate, if possible.	
___	___	___	5. Assemble equipment on overbed table or other surface within reach.	
___	___	___	6. Adjust the bed to a comfortable working height, usually elbow height of the caregiver (VHACEOSH, 2016). Assist the patient to a supine position. Place waterproof pad under the patient at the stoma site.	
___	___	___	7. Put on clean gloves. Gently remove old dressing, if one is in place. Place dressing in trash bag. Remove gloves. Perform hand hygiene.	
___	___	___	8. Assess the insertion site and surrounding skin.	
___	___	___	9. Remove one disposable washcloth from package or wet washcloth with warm water and apply skin cleanser. ***Gently cleanse around suprapubic exit site.*** Remove any encrustations. Alternately, if this is a new suprapubic catheter, use sterile cotton-tipped applicators and sterile saline to clean the site until the incision has healed. Moisten the applicators with the saline. ***Clean in circular motion from the insertion site outward.***	
___	___	___	10. Rinse area of all cleanser. Pat dry.	
___	___	___	11. If the exit site has been draining, place a small drain sponge around the catheter to absorb any drainage. Be prepared to change this sponge throughout the day, depending on the amount of drainage. Do not cut a 4×4 gauze to make a drain sponge.	
___	___	___	12. Remove gloves. Form a loop in the tubing and anchor it on the patient's abdomen.	

Excellent	Satisfactory	Needs Practice	SKILL 12-12 **Caring for a Suprapubic Urinary Catheter** *(Continued)*	**Comments**
___	___	___	13. Assist the patient to a comfortable position. Cover the patient with bed linens. Place the bed in the lowest position.	
___	___	___	14. Put on clean gloves. Remove or discard equipment and assess the patient's response to the procedure.	
___	___	___	15. Remove gloves and additional PPE, if used. Perform hand hygiene.	

Skill Checklists for Taylor's Clinical Nursing Skills. A Nursing Process Approach, 5th edition

Name ____________________ Date ____________________

Unit ____________________ Position ____________________

Instructor/Evaluator: ____________________ Position ____________________

SKILL 12-13

Caring for a Peritoneal Dialysis Catheter

Goal: The peritoneal dialysis catheter dressing change is completed using aseptic technique without trauma to the site or patient; the site is clean, dry, and intact, without evidence of inflammation or infection; and the patient participates in self-care, as appropriate.

Excellent	Satisfactory	Needs Practice		Comments
___	___	___	1. Review the patient's medical record for orders related to catheter site care. Gather equipment.	
___	___	___	2. Perform hand hygiene and put on PPE, if indicated.	
___	___	___	3. Identify the patient.	
___	___	___	4. Close the curtains around the bed and close the door to the room, if possible. Explain what you are going to do and why you are going to do it to the patient. Encourage the patient to observe or participate, if possible.	
___	___	___	5. Assemble equipment on overbed table or other surface within reach.	
___	___	___	6. Adjust the bed to a comfortable working height, usually elbow height of the caregiver (VHACEOSH, 2016). Assist the patient to a supine position. Expose the abdomen, draping the patient's chest with the bath blanket, exposing only the catheter site.	
___	___	___	7. Put on nonsterile gloves. Put on one of the facemasks; have patient put on the other mask.	
___	___	___	8. Gently remove old dressing, noting odor, amount, and color of drainage; leakage and condition of skin around the catheter. Discard dressing in appropriate container.	
___	___	___	9. Remove gloves and discard. Set up sterile field. Open packages. Using aseptic technique, place two sterile gauze squares in basin with antimicrobial agent. Leave two sterile gauze squares opened on sterile field. Alternately (based on facility's policy), place sterile antimicrobial swabs on the sterile field. Place sterile applicator on field. Squeeze a small amount of the topical antibiotic on one of the gauze squares on the sterile field.	
___	___	___	10. Put on sterile gloves. Pick up dialysis catheter with the nondominant hand. ***With the antimicrobial-soaked gauze/swab, cleanse the skin around the exit site using a circular motion, starting at the exit site and then slowly going outward 3 to 4 in. Gently remove crusted scabs, if necessary.***	

SKILL 12-13

Caring for a Peritoneal Dialysis Catheter *(Continued)*

Excellent	Satisfactory	Needs Practice		Comments
___	___	___	11. ***Continue to hold the catheter with your nondominant hand. After skin has dried, clean the catheter with an antimicrobial-soaked gauze, beginning at the exit site, going around catheter, and then moving up to end of the catheter. Gently remove crusted secretions on the tube, if necessary.***	
___	___	___	12. Using the sterile applicator, apply the topical antibiotic to the catheter exit site, if prescribed.	
___	___	___	13. Place sterile drain sponge around the exit site. Then place a 4 × 4 gauze over the exit site. Cover with transparent, occlusive dressing. Remove gloves and then masks.	
___	___	___	14. Label dressing with date, time of change, and initials.	
___	___	___	15. Coil the exposed length of tubing and secure to the dressing or the patient's abdomen with tape.	
___	___	___	16. Assist the patient to a comfortable position. Cover the patient with bed linens. Place the bed in the lowest position.	
___	___	___	17. Put on clean gloves. Remove or discard equipment and assess the patient's response to the procedure.	
___	___	___	18. Remove gloves and additional PPE, if used. Perform hand hygiene.	

Skill Checklists for Taylor's Clinical Nursing Skills.
A Nursing Process Approach, 5th edition

Name ______________________________ Date ______________

Unit ______________________________ Position ______________

Instructor/Evaluator: ______________________________ Position ______________

SKILL 12-14

Caring for a Hemodialysis Access (Arteriovenous Fistula or Graft)

Goal: The graft or fistula remains patent; the patient verbalizes appropriate care measures and observations to be made, and demonstrates appropriate care measures.

Excellent	Satisfactory	Needs Practice		Comments
___	___	___	1. Perform hand hygiene and put on PPE, if indicated.	
___	___	___	2. Identify the patient.	
___	___	___	3. Close the curtains around the bed and close the door to the room, if possible. Explain what you are going to do, and why you are going to do it, to the patient.	
___	___	___	4. Question the patient about the presence of muscle weakness and cramping; changes in temperature; sensations, such as numbness, tingling, pain, burning, itchiness; and pain.	
___	___	___	5. Inspect the area over the access site for continuity of skin color. Inspect for any redness, warmth, tenderness, edema, rash, blemishes, bleeding, tremors, and twitches. Inspect the muscle strength, and the patient's ability to perform range of motion in the extremity/body part with the hemodialysis access.	
___	___	___	6. Palpate over the access site, feeling for a thrill or vibration. Palpate pulses above and below the site. Palpate the continuity of the skin temperature along and around the extremity. Check capillary refill in fingers or toes of extremity with the fistula or graft.	
___	___	___	7. Auscultate over the access site with bell of stethoscope, listening for a bruit or vibration.	
___	___	___	8. Ensure that a sign is placed over the head of the bed informing the health care team which arm is affected. ***Do not measure blood pressure, perform a venipuncture, or start an IV on the access arm.***	
___	___	___	9. Instruct the patient not to sleep with the arm with the access site under the head or body.	
___	___	___	10. Instruct the patient not to lift heavy objects with, or put pressure on, the arm with the access site. Advise the patient not to carry heavy bags (including purses) on the shoulder of that arm.	
___	___	___	11. Remove PPE, if used. Perform hand hygiene.	

Skill Checklists for Taylor's Clinical Nursing Skills. A Nursing Process Approach, 5th edition

Name ______________________ Date ______________

Unit ______________________ Position ______________

Instructor/Evaluator: ______________________ Position ______________

SKILL 13-1
Administering a Large-Volume Cleansing Enema

Excellent	Satisfactory	Needs Practice	**Goal:** The patient expels feces.	Comments
___	___	___	1. Verify the order for the enema. Gather equipment.	
___	___	___	2. Perform hand hygiene and put on PPE, if indicated.	
___	___	___	3. Identify the patient.	
___	___	___	4. Explain the procedure to the patient and provide the rationale as to why the enema is needed. Discuss the associated discomforts that may be experienced and possible interventions that may allay this discomfort. Answer any questions, as needed.	
___	___	___	5. Assemble equipment on overbed table or other surface within reach.	
___	___	___	6. Close the curtains around the bed and close the door to the room, if possible. Discuss where the patient will defecate. Have a bedpan, commode, or nearby bathroom ready for use.	
___	___	___	7. Warm the enema solution in the amount ordered, and check the temperature with a thermometer, if available. If a thermometer is not available, warm to room temperature or slightly higher, and test on inner wrist. If tap water is used, adjust the temperature as it flows from the faucet.	
___	___	___	8. Add enema solution to a container. Release clamp and allow fluid to progress through the tube before reclamping.	
___	___	___	9. Adjust the bed to a comfortable working height, usually elbow height of the caregiver (VHACEOSH, 2016). Position the patient on the left side (Sims position), with the upper thigh pulled toward the abdomen, if possible, or the knee–chest position, as dictated by patient comfort and condition. Fold top linen back just enough to allow access to the patient's rectal area. Drape the patient with the bath blanket, as necessary, to maintain privacy and warmth. Place a waterproof pad under the patient's hip.	
___	___	___	10. Put on gloves.	
___	___	___	11. Elevate solution so that it is no higher than 18 in (45 cm) above level of anus. Plan to give the solution slowly over a period of 5 to 10 minutes. Hang the container on an IV pole or hold it at the proper height.	

Excellent	Satisfactory	Needs Practice	SKILL 13-1 **Administering a Large-Volume Cleansing Enema** *(Continued)*	Comments
___	___	___	12. Generously lubricate end of the rectal tube 2 to 3 in (5 to 7 cm). A disposable enema set may have a prelubricated rectal tube.	
___	___	___	13. Lift buttock to expose anus. Ask patient to take several deep breaths. Slowly and gently insert the enema tube 3 to 4 in (7 to 10 cm) for an adult. Direct it at an angle pointing toward the umbilicus, not the bladder.	
___	___	___	14. If resistance is met while inserting the tube, permit a small amount of solution to enter, withdraw the tube slightly, and then continue to insert it. ***Do not force entry of the tube.*** Ask the patient to take several deep breaths.	
___	___	___	15. Introduce solution slowly over a period of 5 to 10 minutes. Hold tubing all the time that solution is being instilled. Assess for dizziness, lightheadedness, nausea, diaphoresis, and clammy skin during administration. ***If the patient experiences any of these symptoms, stop the procedure immediately, monitor the patient's heart rate and blood pressure, and notify the primary care provider.***	
___	___	___	16. Clamp tubing or lower container if the patient has the urge to defecate or cramping occurs. Instruct the patient to take small, fast breaths or to pant.	
___	___	___	17. After the solution has been given, clamp tubing and remove the tube. Have paper towel ready to receive the tube as it is withdrawn.	
___	___	___	18. Return the patient to a comfortable position. Encourage the patient to hold the solution until the urge to defecate is strong, usually in about 5 to 15 minutes. Make sure the linens under the patient are dry. Remove your gloves and ensure that the patient is covered.	
___	___	___	19. Raise side rail. Lower bed height and adjust head of bed to a comfortable position.	
___	___	___	20. Remove additional PPE, if used. Perform hand hygiene.	
___	___	___	21. When patient has a strong urge to defecate, place him or her in a sitting position on a bedpan or assist to a commode or bathroom. Offer toilet tissues, if not in the patient's reach. Stay with the patient or have call bell readily accessible.	
___	___	___	22. Remind the patient not to flush the commode before you inspect results of enema.	

Excellent	Satisfactory	Needs Practice	SKILL 13-1 **Administering a Large-Volume Cleansing Enema** *(Continued)*	Comments
___	___	___	23. Put on gloves and assist patient, if necessary, with cleaning anal area. Offer washcloths, skin cleanser, and water for handwashing. Remove gloves.	
___	___	___	24. Leave the patient clean and comfortable. Care for equipment properly.	
___	___	___	25. Perform hand hygiene.	

Skill Checklists for Taylor's Clinical Nursing Skills.
A Nursing Process Approach, 5th edition

Name ______________________ Date ______________________

Unit ______________________ Position ______________________

Instructor/Evaluator: ______________________ Position ______________________

SKILL 13-2

Administering a Small-Volume Cleansing Enema

Goal: The patient expels feces and reports a decrease in pain and discomfort.

Excellent	Satisfactory	Needs Practice		Comments
___	___	___	1. Verify the order for the enema. Gather equipment.	
___	___	___	2. Perform hand hygiene and put on PPE, if indicated.	
___	___	___	3. Identify the patient.	
___	___	___	4. Explain the procedure to the patient and provide the rationale why the tube is needed. Discuss the associated discomforts that may be experienced and possible interventions that may allay this discomfort. Answer any questions, as needed.	
___	___	___	5. Assemble equipment on overbed table or other surface within reach.	
___	___	___	6. Close the curtains around the bed and close the door to the room, if possible. Discuss where the patient will defecate. Have a bedpan, commode, or nearby bathroom ready for use.	
___	___	___	7. Adjust the bed to a comfortable working height, usually elbow height of the caregiver (VHACEOSH, 2016). Position the patient on the left side (Sims position), with the upper thigh pulled toward the abdomen, if possible, or the knee–chest position, as dictated by patient comfort and condition. Fold top linen back just enough to allow access to the patient's rectal area. Drape the patient with the bath blanket, as necessary, to maintain privacy and provide warmth. Place a waterproof pad under the patient's hip.	
___	___	___	8. Put on gloves.	
___	___	___	9. Remove the cap and generously lubricate end of rectal tube 2 to 3 in (5 to 7 cm).	
___	___	___	10. Lift buttock to expose anus. Ask the patient to take several deep breaths. Slowly and gently insert the rectal tube 3 to 4 in (7 to 10 cm) for an adult. Direct it at an angle pointing toward the umbilicus, not bladder. ***Do not force entry of the tube.***	

Excellent	Satisfactory	Needs Practice	SKILL 13-2 **Administering a Small-Volume Cleansing Enema** *(Continued)*	Comments
___	___	___	11. Compress the container with your hands. Roll the end up on itself, toward the rectal tip. Administer all the solution in the container. Assess for dizziness, lightheadedness, nausea, diaphoresis, and clammy skin during administration. ***If the patient experiences any of these symptoms, stop the procedure immediately, monitor the patient's heart rate and blood pressure, and notify the primary care provider.***	
___	___	___	12. After the solution has been given, remove the tube, ***keeping the container compressed.*** Have paper towel ready to receive tube as it is withdrawn. Encourage the patient to hold the solution until the urge to defecate is strong, usually in about 5 to 15 minutes.	
___	___	___	13. Remove gloves. Return the patient to a comfortable position. Make sure the linens under the patient are dry. Ensure that the patient is covered.	
___	___	___	14. Raise side rail. Lower bed height and adjust head of bed to a comfortable position.	
___	___	___	15. Remove additional PPE, if used. Perform hand hygiene.	
___	___	___	16. When the patient has a strong urge to defecate, place him or her in a sitting position on a bedpan or assist to commode or bathroom. Stay with patient or have call bell readily accessible.	
___	___	___	17. Remind the patient not to flush the toilet or empty the commode before you inspect the results of the enema.	
___	___	___	18. Put on gloves and assist patient, if necessary, with cleaning of anal area. Offer washcloths, skin cleanser, and water for handwashing. Remove gloves.	
___	___	___	19. Leave the patient clean and comfortable. Care for equipment properly.	
___	___	___	20. Perform hand hygiene.	

Skill Checklists for Taylor's Clinical Nursing Skills. A Nursing Process Approach, 5th edition

Name ______________________ Date ______________________

Unit ______________________ Position ______________________

Instructor/Evaluator: ______________________ Position ______________________

SKILL 13-3

Administering a Retention Enema

Goal: The patient retains the solution for the prescribed, appropriate length of time and experiences the expected therapeutic effect of the solution.

Excellent	Satisfactory	Needs Practice		Comments
___	___	___	1. Verify the order for the enema. Gather equipment.	
___	___	___	2. Perform hand hygiene and put on PPE, if indicated.	
___	___	___	3. Identify the patient.	
___	___	___	4. Explain the procedure to the patient and provide the rationale as to why the tube is needed. Discuss the associated discomforts that may be experienced and possible interventions that may allay this discomfort. Answer any questions, as needed.	
___	___	___	5. Assemble equipment on overbed table or other surface within reach.	
___	___	___	6. Close the curtains around the bed and close the door to the room, if possible. Discuss where the patient will defecate. Have a bedpan, commode, or nearby bathroom ready for use.	
___	___	___	7. Adjust the bed to a comfortable working height, usually elbow height of the caregiver (VHACEOSH, 2016). Position the patient on the left side (Sims position), with the upper thigh pulled toward the abdomen, if possible, or the knee–chest position, as dictated by patient comfort and condition. Fold top linen back just enough to allow access to the patient's rectal area. Drape the patient with the bath blanket, as necessary, to maintain privacy and provide warmth. Place a waterproof pad under the patient's hip.	
___	___	___	8. Put on gloves.	
___	___	___	9. Remove cap of prepackaged enema solution. Apply a generous amount of lubricant to the tube.	
___	___	___	10. Lift buttock to expose anus. Ask the patient to take several deep breaths. Slowly and gently insert the rectal tube 3 to 4 in (7 to 10 cm) for an adult. Direct it at an angle pointing toward the umbilicus.	

SKILL 13-3

Administering a Retention Enema *(Continued)*

Excellent	Satisfactory	Needs Practice		Comments
___	___	___	11. Compress the container with your hands. Roll the end up on itself, toward the rectal tip. Administer all the solution in the container. Assess for dizziness, lightheadedness, nausea, diaphoresis, and clammy skin during administration. ***If the patient experiences any of these symptoms, stop the procedure immediately, monitor the patient's heart rate and blood pressure, and notify the primary care provider.***	
___	___	___	12. ***Remove the container while keeping it compressed.*** Have paper towel ready to receive tube as it is withdrawn.	
___	___	___	13. ***Instruct the patient to retain the enema solution for at least 30 minutes or as indicated, per manufacturer's direction.***	
___	___	___	14. Remove gloves. Return the patient to a comfortable position. Make sure the linens under the patient are dry and ensure that the patient is covered.	
___	___	___	15. Raise side rail. Lower bed height and adjust head of bed to a comfortable position.	
___	___	___	16. Remove additional PPE, if used. Perform hand hygiene.	
___	___	___	17. When the patient has a strong urge to dispel the solution, place him or her in a sitting position on bedpan or assist to commode or bathroom. Stay with the patient or have call bell readily accessible.	
___	___	___	18. Remind the patient not to flush the commode before you inspect the results of the enema, if used for bowel evacuation. Record character of stool, as appropriate, and patient's reaction to the enema.	
___	___	___	19. Put on gloves and assist patient, if necessary, with cleaning of anal area. Offer washcloths, skin cleanser, and water for handwashing. Remove gloves.	
___	___	___	20. Leave patient clean and comfortable. Care for equipment properly.	
___	___	___	21. Perform hand hygiene.	

Skill Checklists for Taylor's Clinical Nursing Skills. A Nursing Process Approach, 5th edition

Name ______________________ Date ______________________

Unit ______________________ Position ______________________

Instructor/Evaluator: ______________________ Position ______________________

SKILL 13-4

Digital Removal of Stool

Goal: The patient expels feces with assistance.

Excellent	Satisfactory	Needs Practice		Comments
___	___	___	1. Verify the order for digital removal of stool. Gather equipment.	
___	___	___	2. Perform hand hygiene and put on PPE, if indicated.	
___	___	___	3. Identify the patient.	
___	___	___	4. Explain the procedure to the patient and provide the rationale why the procedure is needed. Discuss the associated discomforts that may be experienced. Discuss signs and symptoms of a slow heart rate. Instruct the patient to alert you if any of these symptoms are felt during the procedure. Have a bedpan ready for use.	
___	___	___	5. Assemble equipment on overbed table or other surface within reach.	
___	___	___	6. Close the curtains around the bed and close the door to the room, if possible. Discuss where the patient will defecate, if necessary. Have a bedpan, commode, or nearby bathroom ready for use.	
___	___	___	7. Adjust the bed to a comfortable working height, usually elbow height of the caregiver (VHACEOSH, 2016). Position the patient on the left side (Sims position), with the upper thigh pulled toward the abdomen, if possible, or the knee–chest position, as dictated by patient comfort and condition. Fold top linen back just enough to allow access to the patient's rectal area. Drape the patient with the bath blanket, as necessary, to maintain privacy and provide warmth. Place a waterproof pad under the patient's hip.	
___	___	___	8. Put on nonsterile gloves.	
___	___	___	9. Generously lubricate index finger of dominant hand with water-soluble lubricant and insert finger gently into anal canal, pointing toward the umbilicus.	
___	___	___	10. Gently work the finger around and into the hardened mass to break it up and then remove pieces of it. Instruct patient to bear down, if possible, while extracting feces to ease in removal. Place extracted stool in bedpan.	

Excellent	Satisfactory	Needs Practice	SKILL 13-4 **Digital Removal of Stool** *(Continued)*	Comments
___	___	___	11. Remove impaction at intervals if it is severe. ***Instruct the patient to alert you if he or she begins to feel lightheaded or nauseated. If patient reports either symptom, stop removal and assess the patient.***	
___	___	___	12. When the procedure is completed, put on clean gloves. Assist the patient, if necessary, with cleaning of anal area. Offer washcloth, skin cleanser, and water for handwashing. If the patient is able, offer sitz bath.	
___	___	___	13. Remove gloves. Return the patient to a comfortable position. Make sure the linens under the patient are dry. Ensure that the patient is covered.	
___	___	___	14. Raise side rail. Lower bed height and adjust head of bed to a comfortable position.	
___	___	___	15. Remove additional PPE, if used. Perform hand hygiene.	

Skill Checklists for Taylor's Clinical Nursing Skills. A Nursing Process Approach, 5th edition

Name ______________________ Date ______________

Unit ______________________ Position ______________

Instructor/Evaluator: ______________________ Position ______________

SKILL 13-5
Applying a Fecal Incontinence Collection Device

Excellent	Satisfactory	Needs Practice	**Goal:** The patient expels feces into the device and maintains intact perianal skin.	Comments
___	___	___	1. Gather equipment.	
___	___	___	2. Perform hand hygiene and put on PPE, if indicated.	
___	___	___	3. Identify the patient.	
___	___	___	4. Close the curtains around the bed and close the door to the room, if possible. Explain what you are going to do and why you are going to do it to the patient.	
___	___	___	5. Assemble equipment on overbed table or other surface within reach.	
___	___	___	6. Adjust the bed to a comfortable working height, usually elbow height of the caregiver (VHACEOSH, 2016). Position the patient on the left side (Sims position), as dictated by patient comfort and condition. Fold top linen back just enough to allow access to the patient's rectal area. Drape the patient with the bath blanket, as necessary, to maintain privacy and provide warmth. Place a waterproof pad under the patient's hip.	
___	___	___	7. Put on gloves. Cleanse perianal area. Pat dry thoroughly.	
___	___	___	8. Trim perianal hair with scissors, if needed.	
___	___	___	9. Apply the skin protectant or barrier and allow it to dry. Skin protectant may be contraindicated for use with some devices. Check manufacturer's recommendations before use.	
___	___	___	10. If necessary, enlarge the opening in the adhesive skin barrier to fit the patient's anatomy. Do not cut beyond the printed line on the barrier. Remove paper backing from adhesive of device.	
___	___	___	11. With nondominant hand, separate buttocks. Apply fecal device to anal area with dominant hand, ensuring that the bag opening is over anus. Hold the device in place for 30 seconds to achieve good adhesion.	
___	___	___	12. Release buttocks. Attach connector of fecal incontinence device to drainage bag. Hang drainage bag below level of the patient.	

Excellent	Satisfactory	Needs Practice	SKILL 13-5 **Applying a Fecal Incontinence Collection Device** *(Continued)*	Comments
____	____	____	13. Remove gloves. Return the patient to a comfortable position. Make sure the linens under the patient are dry. Ensure that the patient is covered.	
____	____	____	14. Raise side rail. Lower bed height and adjust head of bed to a comfortable position.	
____	____	____	15. Remove additional PPE, if used. Perform hand hygiene.	

Skill Checklists for Taylor's Clinical Nursing Skills. A Nursing Process Approach, 5th edition

Name ____________________ Date ____________________

Unit ____________________ Position ____________________

Instructor/Evaluator: ____________________ Position ____________________

SKILL 13-6

Emptying and Changing an Ostomy Appliance

Goal: The stoma appliance is applied correctly to the skin to allow stool to drain freely.

Excellent	Satisfactory	Needs Practice		Comments
___	___	___	1. Gather equipment.	
___	___	___	2. Perform hand hygiene and put on PPE, if indicated.	
___	___	___	3. Identify the patient.	
___	___	___	4. Close the curtains around the bed and close the door to the room, if possible. Explain what you are going to do and why you are going to do it to the patient. Encourage the patient to observe or participate, if possible.	
___	___	___	5. Assemble equipment on overbed table or other surface within reach.	
___	___	___	6. Assist the patient to a comfortable sitting or lying position in bed or a standing or sitting position in the bathroom. If the patient is in bed, adjust the bed to a comfortable working height, usually elbow height of the caregiver (VHACEOSH, 2016). Place waterproof pad under the patient at the stoma site.	
			Emptying an Appliance	
___	___	___	7. Put on gloves. Remove clamp and fold end of appliance or pouch upward like a cuff.	
___	___	___	8. Empty contents into bedpan, toilet, or measuring device.	
___	___	___	9. Wipe the lower 2 in of the appliance or pouch with toilet tissue or paper towel.	
___	___	___	10. Uncuff edge of appliance or pouch and apply clip or clamp, or secure Velcro closure. Ensure the curve of the clamp follows the curve of the patient's body. Remove gloves. Assist the patient to a comfortable position.	
___	___	___	11. If appliance is not to be changed, place bed in lowest position. Remove additional PPE, if used. Perform hand hygiene.	
			Changing an Appliance	
___	___	___	12. Place a disposable pad on the work surface. Open the premoistened disposable washcloths or set up the washbasin with warm water and the rest of the supplies. Place a trash bag within reach.	
___	___	___	13. Put on clean gloves. Place waterproof pad under the patient at the stoma site. Empty the appliance as described in Steps 7–10.	

Excellent	Satisfactory	Needs Practice	SKILL 13-6 **Emptying and Changing an Ostomy Appliance** *(Continued)*	Comments
___	___	___	14. Put on gloves. Start at the top of the appliance and keep the abdominal skin taut. Gently remove pouch faceplate from skin by pushing skin from the appliance rather than pulling the appliance from skin. Apply a silicone-based adhesive remover by spraying or wiping with the remover wipe.	
___	___	___	15. Place the appliance in the trash bag, if disposable. If reusable, set aside to wash in lukewarm soap and water and allow to air dry after the new appliance is in place.	
___	___	___	16. Use toilet tissue to remove any excess stool from the stoma. Cover the stoma with gauze pad. Clean the skin around the stoma with skin cleanser and water or a cleansing agent and a washcloth. Remove all old adhesive from the skin; use an adhesive remover, as necessary. Do not apply lotion to the peristomal area.	
___	___	___	17. Gently pat area dry. ***Make sure the skin around the stoma is thoroughly dry.*** Assess the stoma and the condition of the surrounding skin.	
___	___	___	18. Apply skin protectant to a 2-in (5 cm) radius around the stoma, and allow it to dry completely, which takes about 30 seconds.	
___	___	___	19. Lift the gauze squares for a moment and measure the stoma opening, using the measurement guide. Replace the gauze. Trace the same-size opening on the back center of the appliance. Cut the opening 1/8 in larger than the stoma size. Using a finger, gently smooth the wafer edges after cutting.	
___	___	___	20. Remove the paper backing from the appliance faceplate. Quickly remove the gauze squares and ease the appliance over the stoma. Gently press onto the skin while smoothing over the surface. Apply gentle, even pressure to the appliance for approximately 30 seconds.	
___	___	___	21. Close the bottom of the appliance or pouch by folding the end upward and using the clamp or clip that comes with the product, or secure the Velcro closure. Ensure the curve of the clamp follows the curve of the patient's body.	
___	___	___	22. Remove gloves. Assist the patient to a comfortable position. Cover the patient with bed linens. Place the bed in the lowest position.	
___	___	___	23. Put on clean gloves. Remove or discard equipment and assess the patient's response to the procedure.	
___	___	___	24. Remove gloves and additional PPE, if used. Perform hand hygiene.	

Skill Checklists for Taylor's Clinical Nursing Skills.
A Nursing Process Approach, 5th edition

Name ____________________ Date ____________________

Unit ____________________ Position ____________________

Instructor/Evaluator: ____________________ Position ____________________

SKILL 13-7

Irrigating a Colostomy

Excellent	Satisfactory	Needs Practice	**Goal:** The patient expels soft, formed stool.	**Comments**
____	____	____	1. Verify the order for the irrigation. Gather equipment.	
____	____	____	2. Perform hand hygiene and put on PPE, if indicated.	
____	____	____	3. Identify the patient.	
____	____	____	4. Close the curtains around the bed and close the door to the room, if possible. Explain what you are going to do and why you are going to do it to the patient. Plan where the patient will receive irrigation. Assist the patient onto bedside commode or into nearby bathroom.	
____	____	____	5. Assemble equipment on overbed table or other surface within reach.	
____	____	____	6. Warm solution in amount ordered and check temperature with a bath thermometer, if available. If bath thermometer is not available, warm to room temperature or slightly higher, and test on inner wrist. Water should feel lukewarm (Clow, Disley, Greening, & Harker, 2015). If tap water is used, adjust temperature as it flows from faucet.	
____	____	____	7. Add irrigation solution to container. Release clamp and allow fluid to progress through tube before reclamping.	
____	____	____	8. Hang container on IV pole so that bottom of bag will be at the patient's shoulder level when seated.	
____	____	____	9. Put on gloves.	
____	____	____	10. Remove ostomy appliance and attach irrigation sleeve. Place drainage end into toilet bowl or commode.	
____	____	____	11. Lubricate end of cone with water-soluble lubricant.	
____	____	____	12. Insert the cone through the top of the irrigation sleeve and into the stoma. Introduce solution slowly over a period of 5 to 10 minutes. Hold cone and tubing (or if patient is able, allow patient to hold) all the time that solution is being instilled. Control rate of flow by closing or opening the clamp.	
____	____	____	13. Hold cone in place for an additional 10 seconds after the fluid is infused.	
____	____	____	14. Remove cone. Patient should remain seated on toilet or bedside commode.	

SKILL 13-7

Irrigating a Colostomy *(Continued)*

Excellent	Satisfactory	Needs Practice		Comments
___	___	___	15. After majority of solution has returned, allow the patient to clip (close) the bottom of irrigating sleeve and continue with daily activities.	
___	___	___	16. After solution has stopped flowing from stoma, put on clean gloves. Remove irrigating sleeve and cleanse skin around stoma opening with skin cleanser and water. Gently pat peristomal skin dry.	
___	___	___	17. Attach new appliance to stoma or stoma cover, as needed.	
___	___	___	18. Remove gloves. Return the patient to a comfortable position. Make sure the linens under the patient are dry, if appropriate. Ensure that the patient is covered.	
___	___	___	19. Raise side rail. Lower bed height and adjust head of bed to a comfortable position, as necessary.	
___	___	___	20. Remove additional PPE, if used. Perform hand hygiene.	

Skill Checklists for Taylor's Clinical Nursing Skills. A Nursing Process Approach, 5th edition

Name ______________________ Date ______________________

Unit ______________________ Position ______________________

Instructor/Evaluator: ______________________ Position ______________________

SKILL 13-8

Inserting a Nasogastric Tube

Goal: The tube is passed into the patient's stomach without any complications.

Excellent	Satisfactory	Needs Practice		Comments
___	___	___	1. Verify the medical order for insertion of an NG tube. Gather equipment, including selection of the appropriate NG tube.	
___	___	___	2. Perform hand hygiene and put on PPE, if indicated.	
___	___	___	3. Identify the patient.	
___	___	___	4. Explain the procedure to the patient, including the rationale for why the tube is needed. Discuss the associated discomforts that may be experienced and possible interventions that may allay this discomfort. Answer any questions, as needed.	
___	___	___	5. Assemble equipment on overbed table or other surface within reach.	
___	___	___	6. Close the patient's bedside curtain or door. Raise the bed to a comfortable working position, usually elbow height of the caregiver (VHACEOSH, 2016). Assist the patient to high-Fowler's position or elevate the head of the bed 45 degrees if the patient is unable to maintain an upright position. Drape chest with a bath towel or disposable pad. Have emesis basin and tissues within reach.	
___	___	___	7. ***Measure the distance to insert the tube by placing the tube tip at the patient's nostril and extending it to the tip of the earlobe and then to tip of the xiphoid process.*** Add any extra length based on facility policy. Mark the tube with an indelible marker.	
___	___	___	8. Put on gloves. Lubricate the tip of the tube (at least 2 to 4 in) with water-soluble lubricant. Apply topical anesthetic to the nostril and oropharynx, as appropriate.	
___	___	___	9. After selecting the appropriate nostril, ask the patient to flex the head slightly back against the pillow. Gently insert the tube into the nostril while directing the tube upward and backward along the floor of the nose. The patient may gag when the tube reaches the pharynx. Provide tissues for tearing or watering of eyes. Offer comfort and reassurance to the patient.	

SKILL 13-8

Inserting a Nasogastric Tube *(Continued)*

Excellent	Satisfactory	Needs Practice		Comments
___	___	___	10. When pharynx is reached, instruct the patient to touch chin to chest. Encourage the patient to sip water through a straw or swallow. Advance the tube in downward and backward direction when patient swallows. Stop when the patient breathes. ***If gagging and coughing persist, stop advancing the tube and check placement of the tube with a tongue blade and flashlight.*** If the tube is curled, straighten the tube and attempt to advance again. Keep advancing the tube until pen marking is reached. ***Do not use force.*** Rotate the tube if it meets resistance.	
___	___	___	11. ***Discontinue the procedure and remove the tube if there are signs of distress, such as gasping, coughing, cyanosis, and inability to speak or hum.***	
___	___	___	12. Secure the tube loosely to the nose or cheek until it is determined that the tube is in the patient's stomach. Confirm placement of the NG tube in the patient's stomach using at least two methods, based on the type of tube in place.	
___	___	___	a. Obtain radiograph (x-ray) of placement of the tube, based on facility policy and as ordered by the primary care provider.	
___	___	___	b. Put on gloves. Attach the syringe to end of the tube and aspirate a small amount of stomach contents. If unable to obtain a specimen, reposition the patient and flush the tube with 30 mL of air in a large syringe. Slowly apply negative pressure to withdraw fluid.	
___	___	___	c. Measure the pH of aspirated fluid using pH paper or a meter. Place a drop of gastric secretions onto pH paper or place small amount in a plastic cup and dip the pH paper into it. Within 30 seconds, compare the color on the paper with the chart supplied by the manufacturer.	
___	___	___	d. Visualize aspirated contents, checking for color and consistency.	
___	___	___	e. Measure the length of the exposed tube at the nostril. Mark the tube with an indelible marker.	

SKILL 13-8

Inserting a Nasogastric Tube *(Continued)*

Excellent	Satisfactory	Needs Practice		Comments
___	___	___	13. After confirmation of the tube placement, secure the tube. Apply skin barrier to the tip and end of the nose and allow to dry. Remove gloves and secure the tube with a commercially prepared device (follow manufacturer's directions) or tape to the patient's nose. To secure with tape:	
___	___	___	a. Cut a 4-in piece of tape and split bottom 2 in or use packaged nose tape for NG tubes.	
___	___	___	b. Place unsplit end over the bridge of the patient's nose.	
___	___	___	c. Wrap split ends under and around the NG tube. ***Be careful not to pull the tube too tightly against the nose.***	
___	___	___	14. Put on gloves. Clamp the tube and remove the syringe. Cap or attach the tube to suction according to the medical orders. Remove gloves.	
___	___	___	15. Measure the length of the exposed tube. Reinforce marking on the tube at the nostril with indelible ink. Ask the patient to turn his/her head to the side opposite the nostril in which the tube is inserted. Secure the tube to the patient's gown by using rubber band or tape and safety pin. For additional support, tape the tube onto the patient's cheek using a piece of tape. ***If a double-lumen tube (e.g., Salem sump) is used, secure the vent above stomach level.*** Attach the vent at shoulder level.	
___	___	___	16. Put on gloves. Assist with or provide oral hygiene at 2- to 4-hour intervals. Lubricate the lips generously and clean nares and lubricate, as needed. Offer analgesic throat lozenges or anesthetic spray for throat irritation, if needed.	
___	___	___	17. Remove equipment and return patient to a position of comfort. Remove gloves. Raise side rail and lower bed.	
___	___	___	18. Remove additional PPE, if used. Perform hand hygiene.	

Skill Checklists for Taylor's Clinical Nursing Skills. A Nursing Process Approach, 5th edition

Name ______________________ Date ______________________

Unit ______________________ Position ______________________

Instructor/Evaluator: ______________________ Position ______________________

SKILL 13-9

Irrigating a Nasogastric Tube Connected to Suction

Goal: The tube maintains patency with irrigation.

Excellent	Satisfactory	Needs Practice		Comments
___	___	___	1. Gather equipment. Verify the medical order or facility policy and procedure regarding frequency of irrigation, solution type, and amount of irrigant. Check expiration dates on irrigating solution and irrigation set.	
___	___	___	2. Perform hand hygiene and put on PPE, if indicated.	
___	___	___	3. Identify the patient.	
___	___	___	4. Explain the procedure to the patient and why this intervention is needed. Answer any questions, as needed. Perform key abdominal assessments as described above.	
___	___	___	5. Assemble equipment on overbed table or other surface within reach.	
___	___	___	6. Pull the patient's bedside curtain. Raise bed to a comfortable working position, usually elbow height of the caregiver (VHACEOSH, 2016). Assist the patient to 30- to 45-degree position, unless this is contraindicated. Pour the irrigating solution into container.	
___	___	___	7. Put on gloves. Place waterproof pad on the patient's chest, under connection of the NG tube and suction tubing. ***Check placement of the NG tube.*** (Refer to Skill 13-8.)	
___	___	___	8. Draw up 30 mL of irrigation solution (or amount indicated in the order or policy) into the syringe.	
___	___	___	9. Clamp the NG tube near connection site. Disconnect the tube from the suction apparatus and lay on a disposable pad or towel, or hold both tubes upright in nondominant hand.	
___	___	___	10. Place tip of the syringe in the tube. ***If Salem sump or double-lumen tube is used, make sure that the syringe tip is placed in the drainage port and not in blue air vent.*** Hold the syringe upright and gently insert the irrigant (or allow solution to flow in by gravity if facility policy or medical order indicates). ***Do not force solution into the tube.***	
___	___	___	11. ***If unable to irrigate the tube, reposition patient and attempt irrigation again. Inject 10 to 20 mL of air and aspirate again. If repeated attempts to irrigate the tube fail, consult with primary care provider or follow facility policy.***	

Excellent	Satisfactory	Needs Practice	SKILL 13-9 **Irrigating a Nasogastric Tube Connected to Suction** *(Continued)*	Comments
___	___	___	12. After irrigant has been instilled, hold the end of the NG tube over irrigation tray or emesis basin. Observe for return flow of NG drainage into an available container. Alternately, you may reconnect the NG tube to suction and observe the return drainage as it drains into the suction container.	
___	___	___	13. If not already done, reconnect drainage port to suction, if ordered.	
___	___	___	14. Inject air into blue air vent after irrigation is complete. Position the blue air vent above the patient's stomach.	
___	___	___	15. Remove gloves. Lower the bed and raise side rails, as necessary. Assist the patient to a position of comfort. Perform hand hygiene.	
___	___	___	16. Put on gloves. Measure returned solution, if collected outside of suction apparatus. Rinse equipment if it will be reused. Label with the date, patient's name, room number, and purpose (for NG tube/irrigation).	
___	___	___	17. Remove gloves and additional PPE, if used. Perform hand hygiene.	

Skill Checklists for Taylor's Clinical Nursing Skills.
A Nursing Process Approach, 5th edition

Name ______________________ Date ______________________

Unit ______________________ Position ______________________

Instructor/Evaluator: ______________________ Position ______________________

SKILL 13-10
Removing a Nasogastric Tube

Goal: The tube is removed with minimal discomfort to the patient; the patient does not aspirate; and the patient maintains an adequate nutritional intake.

Excellent	Satisfactory	Needs Practice		Comments
___	___	___	1. Check medical record for the order for removal of the NG tube.	
___	___	___	2. Perform hand hygiene and put on PPE, if indicated.	
___	___	___	3. Identify the patient.	
___	___	___	4. Explain the procedure to the patient and why this intervention is warranted. Describe that it will entail a quick few moments of discomfort. Perform key abdominal assessments as described above.	
___	___	___	5. Pull the patient's bedside curtain. Raise the bed to a comfortable working position; usually elbow height of the caregiver (VHACEOSH, 2016). Assist the patient to a 30- to 45-degree position. Place a towel or disposable pad across the patient's chest. Give tissues and emesis basin to the patient.	
___	___	___	6. Put on gloves. Discontinue suction and separate the tube from suction. Detach the tube from the patient's gown and carefully remove adhesive tape from the patient's nose.	
___	___	___	7. Check placement (as outlined in Skill 13-8) and ***flush with 10 mL of water or normal saline solution (optional) or clear with 30 to 50 mL of air.***	
___	___	___	8. Clamp the tube with fingers by doubling the tube on itself. ***Instruct the patient to take a deep breath and hold it. Quickly and carefully remove the tube while the patient holds breath.*** Coil the tube in the disposable pad as you remove it from the patient.	
___	___	___	9. Dispose of the tube per facility policy. Remove gloves. Perform hand hygiene.	
___	___	___	10. Offer mouth care to the patient and facial tissue to blow nose. Lower the bed and assist the patient to a position of comfort, as needed.	
___	___	___	11. Remove equipment and raise side rail and lower bed.	

SKILL 13-10

Removing a Nasogastric Tube *(Continued)*

Excellent	Satisfactory	Needs Practice		Comments
____	____	____	12. Put on gloves and measure the amount of NG drainage in the collection device. Record the measurement on the output flow record, subtracting irrigant fluids if necessary. Add solidifying agent to NG drainage and dispose of drainage according to facility policy.	
____	____	____	13. Remove additional PPE, if used. Perform hand hygiene.	

Skill Checklists for Taylor's Clinical Nursing Skills.
A Nursing Process Approach, 5th edition

Name ____________________ Date ____________________

Unit ____________________ Position ____________________

Instructor/Evaluator: ____________________ Position ____________________

SKILL 14-1
Using a Pulse Oximeter

Goal: The patient exhibits oxygen saturation within a range of 95% to 100%, or within acceptable parameters for the person, and the heart rate displayed on the oximeter correlates with the pulse measurement.

Excellent	Satisfactory	Needs Practice	Step	Comments
___	___	___	1. Review health record for any health problems that would affect the patient's oxygenation status. Gather equipment.	
___	___	___	2. Perform hand hygiene and put on PPE, if indicated.	
___	___	___	3. Identify the patient.	
___	___	___	4. Assemble equipment to the bedside stand or overbed table or other surface within reach.	
___	___	___	5. Close the curtains around the bed and close the door to the room, if possible. Explain what you are going to do and why you are going to do it to the patient.	
___	___	___	6. Select an appropriate site for application of the sensor.	
___	___	___	a. Use the patient's index, middle, or ring finger.	
___	___	___	b. Check the proximal pulse and capillary refill closest to the site.	
___	___	___	c. If circulation to the site is inadequate, consider using the earlobe, forehead, or bridge of the nose. Use the appropriate oximetry sensor for the chosen site.	
___	___	___	d. Use a toe only if lower extremity circulation is not compromised.	
___	___	___	7. Select proper equipment:	
___	___	___	a. If one finger is too large for the probe, use a smaller finger.	
___	___	___	b. Use probes appropriate for the patient's age and size. Use a pediatric probe for a small adult, if necessary.	
___	___	___	c. Check if the patient is allergic to adhesive. A nonadhesive finger clip or reflectance sensor is available.	
___	___	___	8. Prepare the monitoring site. Cleanse the selected area with the alcohol wipe or disposable cleansing cloth, as necessary. Allow the area to dry. If necessary, remove the nail polish and artificial nails after checking pulse oximeter's manufacturer's instructions.	
___	___	___	9. Attach the probe securely to the skin. *Make sure that the light-emitting sensor and the light-receiving sensor are aligned opposite each other (not necessary to check if placed on the forehead or bridge of the nose).*	

SKILL 14-1

Using a Pulse Oximeter *(Continued)*

Excellent	Satisfactory	Needs Practice		Comments
___	___	___	10. Connect the sensor probe to the pulse oximeter, turn the oximeter on, and check operation of the equipment (audible beep, fluctuation of the bar of light or waveform on the face of the oximeter).	
___	___	___	11. Set alarms on the pulse oximeter. Check the manufacturer's alarm limits for high and low pulse rate settings.	
___	___	___	12. Check oxygen saturation at regular intervals, as ordered by the primary care provider, nursing assessment, and signaled by alarms. Monitor the hemoglobin level.	
___	___	___	13. Remove the sensor on a regular basis and check for skin irritation or signs of pressure (every 2 hours for spring-tension sensor or every 4 hours for adhesive finger or toe sensor).	
___	___	___	14. Clean nondisposable sensors according to the manufacturer's directions. Remove PPE, if used. Perform hand hygiene.	

Skill Checklists for Taylor's Clinical Nursing Skills. A Nursing Process Approach, 5th edition

Name ______________________ Date ______________

Unit ______________________ Position ______________

Instructor/Evaluator: ______________________ Position ______________

SKILL 14-2

Teaching a Patient to Use an Incentive Spirometer

Excellent	Satisfactory	Needs Practice	**Goal:** The patient accurately demonstrates the procedure for using the spirometer.	Comments
___	___	___	1. Review the patient's health record for any health problems that would affect the patient's oxygenation status. Gather equipment.	
___	___	___	2. Perform hand hygiene and put on PPE, if indicated.	
___	___	___	3. Identify the patient.	
___	___	___	4. Assemble equipment on the overbed table or other surface within reach.	
___	___	___	5. Close the curtains around the bed and close the door to the room, if possible. Explain what you are going to do and why you are going to do it to the patient. Using the chart provided with the device by the manufacturer, note the patient's inspiration target, based on the patient's height and age.	
___	___	___	6. Assist the patient to an upright or semi-Fowler's position, if possible. Remove dentures if they fit poorly. Assess the patient's level of pain. Administer pain medication, as prescribed, if needed. Wait the appropriate amount of time for the medication to take effect. ***If the patient has recently undergone abdominal or chest surgery, place a pillow or folded blanket over a chest or abdominal incision for splinting.***	
___	___	___	7. Demonstrate how to steady the device with one hand and hold the mouthpiece with the other hand. If the patient cannot use hands, assist the patient with the incentive spirometer.	
___	___	___	8. Instruct the patient to exhale normally and then place lips securely around the mouthpiece.	
___	___	___	9. ***Instruct the patient to inhale slowly and as deeply as possible through the mouthpiece without using nose (if desired, a nose clip may be used).*** Note the movement of the inhalation indicator on the spirometer.	
___	___	___	10. When the patient cannot inhale anymore, ***the patient should hold his or her breath and count to three.*** Check position of gauge to determine progress and level attained. If patient begins to cough, splint an abdominal or chest incision.	

Excellent	Satisfactory	Needs Practice	SKILL 14-2 **Teaching a Patient to Use an Incentive Spirometer** *(Continued)*	Comments
____	____	____	11. Instruct the patient to remove lips from mouthpiece and exhale normally. ***If patient becomes lightheaded during the process, tell him or her to stop and take a few normal breaths before resuming incentive spirometry.***	
____	____	____	12. Encourage the patient to perform incentive spirometry 5 to 10 times every 1 to 2 hours, if possible.	
____	____	____	13. Clean the mouthpiece with water and shake to dry. Remove PPE, if used. Perform hand hygiene.	

Skill Checklists for Taylor's Clinical Nursing Skills.
A Nursing Process Approach, 5th edition

Name ______________________ Date ______________________

Unit ______________________ Position ______________________

Instructor/Evaluator: ______________________ Position ______________________

SKILL 14-3

Administering Oxygen by Nasal Cannula

Goal: The patient exhibits an oxygen saturation level within acceptable parameters.

Excellent	Satisfactory	Needs Practice		Comments
___	___	___	1. Review the medical order to verify the use of the nasal cannula, flow rate, and administration parameters. Gather equipment.	
___	___	___	2. Perform hand hygiene and put on PPE, if indicated.	
___	___	___	3. Identify the patient.	
___	___	___	4. Assemble equipment on the overbed table or other surface within reach.	
___	___	___	5. Close the curtains around the bed and close the door to the room, if possible.	
___	___	___	6. Explain what you are going to do and the reason for doing it to the patient. Review safety precautions necessary when oxygen is in use.	
___	___	___	7. Connect the nasal cannula to the oxygen source, with humidification, if appropriate. Adjust the flow rate as ordered. Check that oxygen is flowing out of prongs.	
___	___	___	8. Place prongs in the patient's nostrils. Place tubing over and behind each ear with adjuster comfortably under chin. Alternatively, the tubing may be placed around the patient's head, with the adjuster at the back or base of the head. Place gauze pads at ear beneath the tubing or commercially available ear pads, as necessary.	
___	___	___	9. Adjust the fit of the cannula, as necessary. Tubing should be snug but not tight against the skin.	
___	___	___	10. ***Encourage patients to breathe through the nose, with the mouth closed.***	
___	___	___	11. Reassess the patient's respiratory status, including the respiratory rate, effort, and lung sounds. Note any signs of respiratory distress, such as tachypnea, nasal flaring, use of accessory muscles, or dyspnea.	
___	___	___	12. Remove PPE, if used. Perform hand hygiene.	
___	___	___	13. Put on clean gloves. Remove and clean the cannula and assess nares at least every 8 hours, or according to facility recommendations. Check nares for evidence of irritation or bleeding.	

Skill Checklists for Taylor's Clinical Nursing Skills. A Nursing Process Approach, 5th edition

Name ______________________ Date ______________________

Unit ______________________ Position ______________________

Instructor/Evaluator: ______________________ Position ______________________

SKILL 14-4

Administering Oxygen by Mask

Goal: The patient exhibits an oxygen saturation level within acceptable parameters.

Excellent	Satisfactory	Needs Practice		Comments
___	___	___	1. Review the medical order to verify the use of the particular mask, flow rate/concentration, and administration parameters. Gather equipment.	
___	___	___	2. Perform hand hygiene and put on PPE, if indicated.	
___	___	___	3. Identify the patient.	
___	___	___	4. Assemble equipment on the overbed table or other surface within reach.	
___	___	___	5. Close the curtains around the bed and close the door to the room, if possible.	
___	___	___	6. Explain what you are going to do and the reason for doing it to the patient. Review safety precautions necessary when oxygen is in use.	
___	___	___	7. Attach the face mask to the oxygen source (with humidification, if appropriate, for the specific mask). Start the flow of oxygen at the specified rate. For a mask with a reservoir, be sure to allow oxygen to fill the bag before proceeding to the next step.	
___	___	___	8. Position face mask over the patient's nose and mouth. ***Adjust the elastic strap so that the mask fits snugly but comfortably on the face.*** Adjust to the prescribed flow rate.	
___	___	___	9. If the patient reports irritation or you note redness, use gauze pads under the elastic strap at pressure points to reduce irritation to ears and scalp.	
___	___	___	10. Reassess the patient's respiratory status, including respiratory rate, effort, and lung sounds. Note any signs of respiratory distress, such as tachypnea, nasal flaring, use of accessory muscles, or dyspnea.	
___	___	___	11. Remove PPE, if used. Perform hand hygiene.	
___	___	___	12. ***Remove the mask and dry the skin every 2 to 3 hours if the oxygen is running continuously. Do not use powder around the mask.***	

Skill Checklists for Taylor's Clinical Nursing Skills. A Nursing Process Approach, 5th edition

Name ________________ Date ________________

Unit ________________ Position ________________

Instructor/Evaluator: ________________ Position ________________

SKILL 14-5

Suctioning the Oropharyngeal and Nasopharyngeal Airways

Goal: The patient exhibits improved breath sounds and a clear, patent airway.

Excellent	Satisfactory	Needs Practice		Comments
___	___	___	1. Gather equipment.	
___	___	___	2. Perform hand hygiene and put on PPE, if indicated.	
___	___	___	3. Identify the patient.	
___	___	___	4. Assemble equipment on the overbed table or other surface within reach.	
___	___	___	5. Close the curtains around the bed and close the door to the room, if possible.	
___	___	___	6. Determine the need for suctioning. Verify the suction order in the patient's medical record, if necessary. ***Assess for pain or the potential to cause pain. Administer pain medication, as prescribed, before suctioning.***	
___	___	___	7. Explain what you are going to do and the reason for suctioning to the patient, even if the patient does not appear to be alert. Reassure the patient you will interrupt the procedure if he or she indicates respiratory difficulty.	
___	___	___	8. Adjust the bed to a comfortable working height, usually elbow height of the caregiver (VHACEOSH, 2016). Lower the side rail closest to you. ***If conscious, place the patient in a semi-Fowler's position. If unconscious, place the patient in the lateral position, facing you.*** Move the bedside table close to your work area and raise it to waist height.	
___	___	___	9. Place towel or waterproof pad across the patient's chest.	
___	___	___	10. ***Adjust suction to appropriate pressure.***	
___	___	___	• Using a wall unit for adults and adolescents: no more than 150 mm Hg; neonates: no more than 80 mm Hg; infants: no more than 100 mm Hg; children: no more than 125 mm Hg (Hess et al., 2016).	
___	___	___	• For a portable unit for an adult: 10 to 15 cm Hg; neonates: 6 to 8 cm Hg; infants: 8 to 10 cm Hg; children: 8 to 10 cm Hg; adolescents: 8 to 15 cm Hg. ***Put on a disposable, clean glove and occlude the end of the connecting tubing to check suction pressure.*** Place the connecting tubing in a convenient location.	

Excellent	Satisfactory	Needs Practice	SKILL 14-5 **Suctioning the Oropharyngeal and Nasopharyngeal Airways** *(Continued)*	Comments
___	___	___	11. Open sterile suction package using aseptic technique. The open wrapper or container becomes a sterile field to hold other supplies. Carefully remove the sterile container, touching only the outside surface. Set it up on the work surface and pour sterile saline into it.	
___	___	___	12. Place a small amount of water-soluble lubricant on the sterile field, taking care to avoid touching the sterile field with the lubricant package.	
___	___	___	13. Increase the patient's supplemental oxygen level or apply supplemental oxygen per facility policy or primary care provider order.	
___	___	___	14. Put on face shield or goggles and mask. Put on sterile gloves. ***The dominant hand will manipulate the catheter and must remain sterile. The nondominant hand is considered clean rather than sterile and will control the suction valve (Y-port) on the catheter.*** In the home setting and other community-based settings, maintenance of sterility is not necessary.	
___	___	___	15. With the dominant gloved hand, pick up the sterile catheter. Pick up the connecting tubing with the nondominant hand and connect the tubing and suction catheter.	
___	___	___	16. Moisten the catheter by dipping it into the container of sterile saline. Occlude Y-tube to check suction.	
___	___	___	17. Encourage the patient to take several deep breaths.	
___	___	___	18. Apply lubricant to the first 2 to 3 in of the catheter, using the lubricant that was placed on the sterile field.	
___	___	___	19. Remove the oxygen delivery device, if appropriate. Do not apply suction as the catheter is inserted. Hold the catheter between your thumb and forefinger.	
___	___	___	20. Insert the catheter:	
___	___	___	a. **For nasopharyngeal suctioning,** gently insert the catheter through the naris and along the floor of the nostril toward the trachea. Roll the catheter between your fingers to help advance it. Advance the catheter approximately 5 to 6 in to reach the pharynx.	
___	___	___	b. **For oropharyngeal suctioning,** insert catheter through the mouth, along the side of the mouth toward the trachea. Advance the catheter 3 to 4 in to reach the pharynx.	

SKILL 14-5

Suctioning the Oropharyngeal and Nasopharyngeal Airways *(Continued)*

Excellent	Satisfactory	Needs Practice		Comments
___	___	___	21. ***Apply suction by intermittently occluding the Y-port on the catheter with the thumb of your nondominant hand and gently rotating the catheter as it is being withdrawn. Do not suction for more than 10 to 15 seconds at a time.***	
___	___	___	22. Replace the oxygen delivery device using your nondominant hand, if appropriate, and have the patient take several deep breaths.	
___	___	___	23. Flush the catheter with saline. Assess the effectiveness of suctioning and repeat, as needed, and according to the patient's tolerance. Wrap the suction catheter around your dominant hand between attempts.	
___	___	___	24. ***Allow at least a 30-second to 1-minute interval if additional suctioning is needed. No more than three suction passes should be made per suctioning episode. Alternate the naris, unless contraindicated, if repeated suctioning is required.*** Do not force the catheter through the naris. Encourage the patient to cough and deep breathe between suctioning. ***Suction the oropharynx after suctioning the nasopharynx.***	
___	___	___	25. When suctioning is completed, remove gloves from the dominant hand over the coiled catheter, pulling them off inside out. Remove the glove from the nondominant hand and dispose of gloves, catheter, and container with solution in the appropriate receptacle. Assist the patient to a comfortable position. Raise bed rail and place bed in the lowest position.	
___	___	___	26. Turn off suction. Remove supplemental oxygen placed for suctioning, if appropriate. Remove face shield or goggles and mask. Perform hand hygiene.	
___	___	___	27. Perform oral hygiene after suctioning.	
___	___	___	28. Reassess the patient's respiratory status, including respiratory rate, effort, oxygen saturation, and lung sounds.	
___	___	___	29. Remove additional PPE, if used. Perform hand hygiene.	

Skill Checklists for Taylor's Clinical Nursing Skills.
A Nursing Process Approach, 5th edition

Name ______________________ Date ______________

Unit ______________________ Position ______________

Instructor/Evaluator: ______________________ Position ______________

SKILL 14-6
Inserting an Oropharyngeal Airway

Goal: The patient maintains a patent airway and exhibits oxygen saturation within acceptable parameters.

Excellent	Satisfactory	Needs Practice		Comments
___	___	___	1. Gather equipment.	
___	___	___	2. Perform hand hygiene and put on PPE, if indicated.	
___	___	___	3. Identify the patient.	
___	___	___	4. Assemble equipment on the overbed table or other surface within reach.	
___	___	___	5. Close the curtains around the bed and close the door to the room, if possible.	
___	___	___	6. Explain to the patient what you are going to do and the reason for doing it, even if the patient does not appear to be alert.	
___	___	___	7. Put on disposable gloves; put on goggles and mask or face shield, as indicated.	
___	___	___	8. Measure the oropharyngeal airway for correct size. Measure the oropharyngeal airway by holding the airway on the side of the patient's face. The airway should reach from the opening of the mouth to the back angle of the jaw.	
___	___	___	9. ***Check mouth for any loose teeth, dentures, or other foreign material. Remove dentures or material, if present.***	
___	___	___	10. Position patient in semi-Fowler's position.	
___	___	___	11. Suction the patient, if necessary.	
___	___	___	12. Open the patient's mouth by using your thumb and index finger to gently pry teeth apart. ***Insert the airway with the curved tip pointing up toward the roof of the mouth.***	
___	___	___	13. Slide the airway across the tongue to the back of the mouth. Rotate the airway 180 degrees as it passes the uvula. The tip should point down and the curvature should follow the contour of the roof of the mouth. Use a flashlight to confirm the position of the airway with the curve fitting over the tongue.	
___	___	___	14. Ensure accurate placement and adequate ventilation by auscultating breath sounds.	
___	___	___	15. Position the patient on his or her side when the airway is in place.	

Excellent	Satisfactory	Needs Practice	SKILL 14-6 **Inserting an Oropharyngeal Airway** *(Continued)*	**Comments**
____	____	____	16. Remove gloves and additional PPE, if used. Perform hand hygiene.	
____	____	____	17. Remove the airway for a brief period every 4 hours, or according to facility policy. Assess mouth; provide mouth care and clean the airway according to facility policy before reinserting it.	

Skill Checklists for Taylor's Clinical Nursing Skills. A Nursing Process Approach, 5th edition

Name ______________________ Date ______________________

Unit ______________________ Position ______________________

Instructor/Evaluator: ______________________ Position ______________________

SKILL 14-7

Suctioning an Endotracheal Tube: Open System

Excellent	Satisfactory	Needs Practice	**Goal:** The patient exhibits a clear, patent airway.	Comments
___	___	___	1. Gather equipment.	
___	___	___	2. Perform hand hygiene and put on PPE, if indicated.	
___	___	___	3. Identify the patient.	
___	___	___	4. Assemble equipment on the overbed table or other surface within reach.	
___	___	___	5. Close the curtains around the bed and close the door to the room, if possible.	
___	___	___	6. Determine the need for suctioning. Verify the suction order in the patient's medical record. ***Assess for pain or the potential to cause pain. Administer pain medication, as prescribed, before suctioning.***	
___	___	___	7. Explain what you are going to do and the reason for doing it to the patient, even if the patient does not appear to be alert. Reassure the patient you will interrupt the procedure if he or she indicates respiratory difficulty.	
___	___	___	8. Adjust the bed to a comfortable working position, usually elbow height of the caregiver (VHACEOSH, 2016). Lower the side rail closest to you. ***If conscious, place in a semi-Fowler's position. If unconscious, place the patient in the lateral position, facing you.*** Move the overbed table close to your work area and raise it to waist height.	
___	___	___	9. Place towel or waterproof pad across the patient's chest.	
___	___	___	10. ***Adjust suction to appropriate pressure.***	
___	___	___	• Using a wall unit for adults and adolescents: no more than 150 mm Hg; neonates: no more than 80 mm Hg; infants: no more than 100 mm Hg; children: no more than 125 mm Hg (Hess et al., 2016).	
___	___	___	• For a portable unit for an adult: 10 to 15 cm Hg; neonates: 6 to 8 cm Hg; infants: 8 to 10 cm Hg; children: 8 to 10 cm Hg; adolescents: 8 to 15 cm Hg.	
___	___	___	11. Put on a disposable, clean glove and occlude the end of the connecting tubing to check suction pressure. Place the connecting tubing in a convenient location. Place the resuscitation bag connected to oxygen within convenient reach, if using.	

SKILL 14-7

Suctioning an Endotracheal Tube: Open System *(Continued)*

Excellent	Satisfactory	Needs Practice		Comments
___	___	___	12. Open sterile suction package using aseptic technique. The open wrapper becomes a sterile field to hold other supplies. Carefully remove the sterile container, touching only the outside surface. Set it up on the work surface and pour sterile saline into it.	
___	___	___	13. Put on face shield or goggles and mask. Put on sterile gloves. ***The dominant hand will manipulate the catheter and must remain sterile. The nondominant hand is considered clean rather than sterile and will control the suction valve (Y-port) on the catheter.***	
___	___	___	14. With dominant gloved hand, pick up sterile catheter. Pick up the connecting tubing with the nondominant hand and connect the tubing and suction catheter.	
___	___	___	15. Moisten the catheter by dipping it into the container of sterile saline, unless it is a silicone catheter. Occlude Y-tube to check suction.	
___	___	___	16. Using your nondominant hand, remove the ventilator tubing from the endotracheal tube and attach the manual resuscitation bag. Hyperventilate the patient using your nondominant hand and the manual resuscitation bag, delivering three to six breaths. Alternatively, use the sigh mechanism on a mechanical ventilator.	
___	___	___	17. Open the adapter on the mechanical ventilator tubing or remove the manual resuscitation bag with your nondominant hand.	
___	___	___	18. Using your dominant hand, gently and quickly insert the catheter into the endotracheal tube. ***Advance the catheter to the predetermined length. Do not occlude Y-port when inserting the catheter.***	
___	___	___	19. Apply suction by intermittently occluding the Y-port on the catheter with the thumb of your nondominant hand, and gently rotate the catheter as it is being withdrawn. ***Do not suction for more than 10 to 15 seconds at a time.***	
___	___	___	20. Hyperventilate the patient using your nondominant hand and a manual resuscitation bag and deliver three to six breaths. Replace the oxygen delivery device, if applicable, using your nondominant hand and have the patient take several deep breaths. If the patient is mechanically ventilated, close the adapter on the mechanical ventilator tubing or replace the ventilator tubing and use the sigh mechanism on a mechanical ventilator.	

SKILL 14-7

Suctioning an Endotracheal Tube: Open System *(Continued)*

Excellent	Satisfactory	Needs Practice		Comments
___	___	___	21. Flush catheter with saline. Assess the effectiveness of suctioning and repeat, as needed, and according to patient's tolerance. Wrap the suction catheter around your dominant hand between attempts.	
___	___	___	22. ***Allow at least a 30-second to 1-minute interval if additional suctioning is needed. Do not make more than three suction passes per suctioning episode.*** Suction the oropharynx after suctioning the trachea. Do not reinsert in the endotracheal tube after suctioning the mouth.	
___	___	___	23. Perform oral hygiene after tracheal suctioning.	
___	___	___	24. When suctioning is completed, remove gloves from dominant hand over the coiled catheter, pulling off inside out. Remove glove from nondominant hand and dispose of gloves, catheter, and container with solution in the appropriate receptacle. Assist patient to a comfortable position. Raise bed rail and place bed in the lowest position.	
___	___	___	25. Turn off suction. Remove face shield or goggles and mask. Perform hand hygiene.	
___	___	___	26. Reassess the patient's respiratory status, including respiratory rate, effort, oxygen saturation, lung sounds, tracheal sounds, and presence/absence of secretions in artificial airway.	
___	___	___	27. Remove additional PPE, if used. Perform hand hygiene.	

Skill Checklists for Taylor's Clinical Nursing Skills. A Nursing Process Approach, 5th edition

Name ______________________ Date ______________________

Unit ______________________ Position ______________________

Instructor/Evaluator: ______________________ Position ______________________

SKILL 14-8

Suctioning an Endotracheal Tube: Closed System

Excellent	Satisfactory	Needs Practice	**Goal:** The patient exhibits a clear, patent airway.	**Comments**
___	___	___	1. Gather equipment.	
___	___	___	2. Perform hand hygiene and put on PPE, if indicated.	
___	___	___	3. Identify the patient.	
___	___	___	4. Assemble equipment on the overbed table or other surface within reach.	
___	___	___	5. Close the curtains around the bed and close the door to the room, if possible.	
___	___	___	6. Determine the need for suctioning. Verify the suction order in the patient's medical record. ***Assess for pain or the potential to cause pain. Administer pain medication, as prescribed, before suctioning.***	
___	___	___	7. Explain what you are going to do and the reason for doing it to the patient, even if the patient does not appear to be alert. Reassure the patient you will interrupt the procedure if he or she indicates respiratory difficulty.	
___	___	___	8. Adjust the bed to a comfortable working position, usually elbow height of the caregiver (VHACEOSH, 2016). Lower the side rail closest to you. ***If conscious, place the patient in a semi-Fowler's position. If unconscious, place the patient in the lateral position, facing you.*** Move the overbed table close to your work area and raise to waist height.	
___	___	___	9. ***Adjust suction to appropriate pressure.***	
___	___	___	• Using a wall unit for adults and adolescents: no more than 150 mm Hg; neonates: no more than 80 mm Hg; infants: no more than 100 mm Hg; children: no more than 125 mm Hg (Hess et al., 2016).	
___	___	___	• For a portable unit for an adult: 10 to 15 cm Hg; neonates: 6 to 8 cm Hg; infants: 8 to 10 cm Hg; children: 8 to 10 cm Hg; adolescents: 8 to 15 cm Hg.	
___	___	___	10. Open the package of the closed suction device using aseptic technique. Make sure that the device remains sterile.	
___	___	___	11. Put on sterile gloves.	
___	___	___	12. If a closed suctioning device is not in place, continue with Step 13. If this device is already in place, continue with Step 16.	

Excellent	Satisfactory	Needs Practice	SKILL 14-8 **Suctioning an Endotracheal Tube: Closed System** *(Continued)*	Comments
___	___	___	13. Using nondominant hand, disconnect ventilator from endotracheal tube. Place ventilator tubing in a convenient location so that the inside of the tubing remains sterile, or continue to hold the tubing in your nondominant hand.	
___	___	___	14. ***Using dominant hand and keeping device sterile, connect the closed suctioning device so that the suctioning catheter is in line with the endotracheal tube.***	
___	___	___	15. ***Keeping the inside of the ventilator tubing sterile, attach ventilator tubing to port perpendicular to the endotracheal tube.*** Attach suction tubing to suction catheter.	
___	___	___	16. Pop top off sterile normal saline dosette. Open plug to port by suction catheter and insert saline dosette or syringe.	
___	___	___	17. Hyperventilate the patient by using the sigh button on the ventilator before suctioning. Turn safety cap on suction button of catheter so that button is depressed easily.	
___	___	___	18. Grasp suction catheter through protective sheath, about 6 in (15 cm) from the endotracheal tube. Gently insert the catheter into the endotracheal tube. Release the catheter while holding on to the protective sheath. Move hand farther back on catheter. ***Grasp catheter through sheath and repeat movement, advancing the catheter to the predetermined length. Do not occlude Y-port when inserting the catheter.***	
___	___	___	19. Apply intermittent suction by depressing the suction button with thumb of nondominant hand. Gently rotate the catheter with thumb and index finger of dominant hand as catheter is being withdrawn. ***Do not suction for more than 10 to 15 seconds at a time.*** Hyperoxygenate or hyperventilate with sigh button on ventilator, as ordered.	
___	___	___	20. Once the catheter is withdrawn back into the sheath, depress the suction button while gently squeezing the normal saline dosette until the catheter is clean. ***Allow at least a 30-second to 1-minute interval if additional suctioning is needed. No more than three suction passes should be made per suctioning episode.***	
___	___	___	21. When the procedure is completed, ***ensure that the catheter is withdrawn into the sheath***, and turn the safety button. Remove normal saline dosette and apply cap to port.	
___	___	___	22. Suction the oral cavity with a separate single-use, disposable catheter and perform oral hygiene. Remove gloves. Turn off suction.	

Excellent	Satisfactory	Needs Practice	SKILL 14-8 **Suctioning an Endotracheal Tube: Closed System** *(Continued)*	Comments
___	___	___	23. Assist the patient to a comfortable position. Raise the bed rail and place the bed in the lowest position.	
___	___	___	24. Reassess the patient's respiratory status, including respiratory rate, effort, oxygen saturation, lung sounds, tracheal sounds, and presence/absence of secretions in artificial airway.	
___	___	___	25. Remove additional PPE, if used. Perform hand hygiene.	

Skill Checklists for Taylor's Clinical Nursing Skills. A Nursing Process Approach, 5th edition

Name ______________________ Date ______________________

Unit ______________________ Position ______________________

Instructor/Evaluator: ______________________ Position ______________________

SKILL 14-9

Securing an Endotracheal Tube

Excellent	Satisfactory	Needs Practice	**Goal:** The tube remains in place, and the patient maintains bilaterally equal and clear lung sounds.	Comments
___	___	___	1. Gather equipment.	
___	___	___	2. Perform hand hygiene and put on PPE, if indicated.	
___	___	___	3. Identify the patient.	
___	___	___	4. Assemble equipment on the overbed table or other surface within reach.	
___	___	___	5. Close the curtains around the bed and close the door to the room, if possible.	
___	___	___	6. Assess the need for endotracheal tube retaping. ***Administer pain medication or sedation, as prescribed, before attempting to retape endotracheal tube.*** Explain what you are going to do and the reason for doing it to the patient, even if the patient does not appear to be alert.	
___	___	___	7. Obtain the assistance of a second person to hold the endotracheal tube in place while the old tape is removed and the new tape is placed.	
___	___	___	8. Adjust the bed to a comfortable working position, usually elbow height of the caregiver (VHACEOSH, 2016). Lower the side rail closest to you. ***If conscious, place the patient in a semi-Fowler's position. If unconscious, place the patient in the lateral position, facing you.*** Move the overbed table close to your work area and raise to waist height. Place a trash receptacle within easy reach of the work area.	
___	___	___	9. Put on face shield or goggles and mask. Suction patient as described in Skill 14-7 or 14-8.	
___	___	___	10. Measure a piece of tape for the length needed to reach around the patient's neck to the mouth plus 8 in. Cut tape. Lay it adhesive side up on the table.	
___	___	___	11. Cut another piece of tape long enough to reach from one jaw around the back of the neck to the other jaw. Lay this piece on the center of the longer piece on the table, matching the tapes' adhesive sides together.	
___	___	___	12. Take one 3-mL syringe or tongue blade and wrap the sticky tape around the syringe until the nonsticky area is reached. Do this for the other side as well.	

Excellent	Satisfactory	Needs Practice	SKILL 14-9 **Securing an Endotracheal Tube** *(Continued)*	Comments
___	___	___	13. Take one of the 3-mL syringes or tongue blades and pass it under the patient's neck so that there is a 3-mL syringe on either side of the patient's head.	
___	___	___	14. Put on disposable gloves. Have the assistant put on gloves as well.	
___	___	___	15. Provide oral care, including suctioning the oral cavity.	
___	___	___	16. Take note of the "cm" position markings on the tube. Begin to unwrap old tape from around the endotracheal tube. After one side is unwrapped, have assistant hold the endotracheal tube as close to the lips or naris as possible to offer stabilization.	
___	___	___	17. Carefully remove the remaining tape from the endotracheal tube. ***After tape is removed, have assistant gently and slowly move endotracheal tube (if orally intubated) to the other side of the mouth. Assess mouth for any skin breakdown. Before applying new tape, make sure that markings on endotracheal tube are at same spot as when retaping began.***	
___	___	___	18. Remove old tape from cheeks and side of face. Use adhesive remover to remove excess adhesive from tape. Clean the face and neck with washcloth and cleanser. If patient has facial hair, consider shaving cheeks. Pat cheeks dry with the towel.	
___	___	___	19. Apply the skin barrier to the patient's face (under nose, on cheeks, and lower lip) where the tape will sit. Unroll one side of the tape. Ensure that nonstick part of tape remains behind the patient's neck while pulling firmly on the tape. Place adhesive portion of tape snugly against the patient's cheek. Keep track of the pilot balloon from the endotracheal tube, to avoid taping it to the patient's face. Split the tape in half from the end to the corner of the mouth.	
___	___	___	20. Place the top-half piece of tape under the patient's nose. Wrap the lower half around the tube in one direction, such as over and around the tube. Fold over tab on end of tape.	
___	___	___	21. Unwrap second side of tape. Split to corner of the mouth. Place the bottom-half piece of tape along the patient's lower lip. Wrap the top half around the tube in the opposite direction, such as below and around the tube. Fold over tab on end of tape. Apply pressure to the tape on the endotracheal tube to ensure the tape is secure. Remove gloves.	

Excellent	Satisfactory	Needs Practice	SKILL 14-9 **Securing an Endotracheal Tube** *(Continued)*	Comments
___	___	___	22. ***Auscultate lung sounds. Assess for cyanosis, oxygen saturation, chest symmetry, and endotracheal tube stability. Again check to ensure that the tube is at the correct depth.***	
___	___	___	23. ***If the endotracheal tube is cuffed, check pressure of the balloon by attaching a handheld pressure gauge to the pilot balloon of the endotracheal tube.***	
___	___	___	24. Assist the patient to a comfortable position. Raise the bed rail and place the bed in the lowest position.	
___	___	___	25. Remove face shield or goggles and mask. Remove additional PPE, if used. Perform hand hygiene.	

Skill Checklists for Taylor's Clinical Nursing Skills. A Nursing Process Approach, 5th edition

Name ______________________ Date ______________________

Unit ______________________ Position ______________________

Instructor/Evaluator: ______________________ Position ______________________

SKILL 14-10

Suctioning a Tracheostomy: Open System

Excellent	Satisfactory	Needs Practice	**Goal:** The patient exhibits a clear, patent airway.	**Comments**
____	____	____	1. Gather equipment.	
____	____	____	2. Perform hand hygiene and put on PPE, if indicated.	
____	____	____	3. Identify the patient.	
____	____	____	4. Assemble equipment on the overbed table or other surface within reach.	
____	____	____	5. Close the curtains around the bed and close the door to the room, if possible.	
____	____	____	6. Determine the need for suctioning. Verify the suction order in the patient's medical record. ***Assess for pain or the potential to cause pain. Administer pain medication, as prescribed, before suctioning.***	
____	____	____	7. Explain to the patient what you are going to do and the reason for doing it, even if the patient does not appear to be alert. Reassure the patient you will interrupt the procedure if he or she indicates respiratory difficulty.	
____	____	____	8. Adjust the bed to a comfortable working position, usually elbow height of the caregiver (VHACEOSH, 2016). Lower the side rail closest to you. ***If conscious, place the patient in a semi-Fowler's position. If unconscious, place the patient in the lateral position, facing you.***	
____	____	____	9. Place a towel or waterproof pad across the patient's chest.	
____	____	____	10. ***Adjust suction to appropriate pressure.***	
____	____	____	• Using a wall unit for adults and adolescents: no more than 150 mm Hg; neonates: no more than 80 mm Hg; infants: no more than 100 mm Hg; children: no more than 125 mm Hg (Hess et al., 2016).	
____	____	____	• For a portable unit for an adult: 10 to 15 cm Hg; neonates: 6 to 8 cm Hg; infants: 8 to 10 cm Hg; children: 8 to 10 cm Hg; adolescents: 8 to 15 cm Hg. Put on a disposable, clean glove and occlude the end of the connecting tubing to check suction pressure. Place the connecting tubing in a convenient location. If using, place the resuscitation bag connected to oxygen within convenient reach.	

Excellent	Satisfactory	Needs Practice	SKILL 14-10 **Suctioning a Tracheostomy: Open System** *(Continued)*	Comments
___	___	___	11. Open the sterile suction package using aseptic technique. The open wrapper or container becomes a sterile field to hold other supplies. Carefully remove the sterile container, touching only the outside surface. Set it up on the work surface and pour sterile saline into it.	
___	___	___	12. Put on face shield or goggles and mask. Put on sterile gloves. ***The dominant hand will manipulate the catheter and must remain sterile. The nondominant hand is considered clean rather than sterile and will control the suction valve (Y-port) on the catheter.***	
___	___	___	13. With the dominant gloved hand, pick up the sterile catheter. Pick up the connecting tubing with the nondominant hand and connect the tubing and suction catheter.	
___	___	___	14. Moisten the catheter by dipping it into the container of sterile saline, unless it is a silicone catheter. Occlude Y-tube to check suction.	
___	___	___	15. Using your nondominant hand and a manual resuscitation bag, hyperventilate the patient, delivering three to six breaths or use the sigh mechanism on a mechanical ventilator.	
___	___	___	16. Remove the manual resuscitation bag or open the adapter on the mechanical ventilator tubing with your nondominant hand.	
___	___	___	17. Using your dominant hand, gently and quickly insert the catheter into the trachea. ***Advance the catheter to the predetermined length. Do not occlude the Y-port when inserting the catheter.***	
___	___	___	18. Apply suction by intermittently occluding the Y-port on the catheter with the thumb of your nondominant hand, and gently rotate the catheter as it is being withdrawn. ***Do not suction for more than 10 to 15 seconds at a time.***	
___	___	___	19. Hyperventilate the patient using your nondominant hand and a manual resuscitation bag, delivering three to six breaths. Replace the oxygen delivery device, if applicable, using your nondominant hand and have the patient take several deep breaths. If the patient is mechanically ventilated, close the adapter on the mechanical ventilator tubing and use the sigh mechanism on a mechanical ventilator.	
___	___	___	20. Flush the catheter with saline. Assess the effectiveness of suctioning and repeat, as needed, according to the patient's tolerance. Wrap the suction catheter around your dominant hand between attempts.	

Excellent	Satisfactory	Needs Practice	SKILL 14-10 **Suctioning a Tracheostomy: Open System** *(Continued)*	Comments
___	___	___	21. ***Allow at least a 30-second to 1-minute interval if additional suctioning is needed. Do not make more than three suction passes per suctioning episode. Encourage the patient to cough and deep breathe between suctioning attempts.*** Suction the oropharynx after suctioning the trachea. Do not reinsert in the tracheostomy after suctioning the mouth.	
___	___	___	22. Perform oral hygiene after tracheal suctioning.	
___	___	___	23. When suctioning is completed, coil the catheter in one hand. Remove the glove from the hand over the coiled catheter (catheter remains inside glove), pulling the glove off inside out. Remove the glove from the other hand, pulling inside out, and dispose of gloves, catheter, and container with solution in the appropriate receptacle. Assist the patient to a comfortable position. Raise the bed rail and place the bed in the lowest position.	
___	___	___	24. Turn off suction. Remove supplemental oxygen placed for suctioning, if appropriate. Remove face shield or goggles and mask. Perform hand hygiene.	
___	___	___	25. Reassess the patient's respiratory status, including respiratory rate, effort, oxygen saturation, and lung sounds.	
___	___	___	26. Remove additional PPE, if used. Perform hand hygiene.	

Skill Checklists for Taylor's Clinical Nursing Skills. A Nursing Process Approach, 5th edition

Name ______________________ Date ______________________

Unit ______________________ Position ______________________

Instructor/Evaluator: ______________________ Position ______________________

SKILL 14-11

Providing Care of a Tracheostomy Tube

Excellent	Satisfactory	Needs Practice	**Goal:** The patient exhibits a tracheostomy tube and site free from drainage, secretions, and skin irritation or breakdown and a patent airway.	Comments
___	___	___	1. Gather equipment.	
___	___	___	2. Perform hand hygiene and put on PPE, if indicated.	
___	___	___	3. Identify the patient.	
___	___	___	4. Assemble equipment on the overbed table or other surface within reach.	
___	___	___	5. Close the curtains around the bed and close the door to the room, if possible.	
___	___	___	6. Determine the need for tracheostomy care. ***Assess the patient's pain and administer pain medication, if indicated.***	
___	___	___	7. Explain what you are going to do and the reason for doing it to the patient, even if the patient does not appear to be alert. Reassure the patient you will interrupt the procedure if he or she indicates respiratory difficulty.	
___	___	___	8. Adjust the bed to a comfortable working position, usually elbow height of the caregiver (VHACEOSH, 2016). Lower the side rail closest to you. ***If conscious, place the patient in a semi-Fowler's position. If unconscious, place the patient in the lateral position, facing you.*** Move the overbed table close to your work area and raise it to waist height. Place a trash receptacle within easy reach of the work area.	
___	___	___	9. Put on face shield or goggles and mask. Suction tracheostomy, if necessary. If tracheostomy has just been suctioned, remove soiled site dressing and discard before removal of gloves used to perform suctioning.	
			Cleaning the Tracheostomy: Disposable Inner Cannula	
___	___	___	10. Carefully open the package with the new disposable inner cannula, taking care not to contaminate the cannula or the inside of the package. Carefully open the package with the sterile cotton-tipped applicators, taking care not to contaminate them. Open the sterile cup or basin and fill 0.5 in deep with saline. Open the plastic disposable bag and place within reach on work surface.	

SKILL 14-11

Providing Care of a Tracheostomy Tube *(Continued)*

Excellent	Satisfactory	Needs Practice		Comments
___	___	___	11. Put on disposable gloves.	
___	___	___	12. Remove the oxygen source if one is present. Stabilize the outer cannula and faceplate of the tracheostomy with your nondominant hand. Grasp the locking mechanism of the inner cannula with your dominant hand. Press the tabs and release the lock. Gently remove the inner cannula and place in disposal bag. If not already removed, remove site dressing and dispose of it in the trash.	
___	___	___	13. Working quickly, discard gloves and put on sterile gloves. Pick up the new inner cannula with your dominant hand; stabilize the faceplate with your nondominant hand and gently insert the new inner cannula into the outer cannula. Press the tabs to allow the lock to grab the outer cannula. Reapply oxygen source, if needed.	
			Applying Clean Dressing and Holder	
___	___	___	14. Remove oxygen source, if necessary. Dip cotton-tipped applicator or gauze sponge in cup or basin with sterile saline and clean stoma under faceplate. Use each applicator or sponge only once, moving from stoma site outward.	
___	___	___	15. Pat skin gently with dry 4 × 4 gauze sponge.	
___	___	___	16. Slide commercially prepared tracheostomy dressing or prefolded non–cotton-filled 4 × 4-in dressing under the faceplate.	

Excellent	Satisfactory	Needs Practice	SKILL 14-11 **Providing Care of a Tracheostomy Tube** *(Continued)*	Comments
___	___	___	17. Change the tracheostomy holder:	
___	___	___	a. ***Obtain the assistance of a second person to hold the tracheostomy tube in place while the old collar is removed and the new collar is placed.***	
___	___	___	b. Open the package for the new tracheostomy collar.	
___	___	___	c. Both nurses should put on clean gloves.	
___	___	___	d. One nurse holds the faceplate while the other pulls up the Velcro tabs. Gently remove the collar.	
___	___	___	e. The first nurse continues to hold the tracheostomy faceplate.	
___	___	___	f. The other nurse places the collar around the patient's neck and inserts first one tab, then the other, into the openings on the faceplate and secures the Velcro tabs on the tracheostomy holder.	
___	___	___	g. Check the fit of the tracheostomy collar. You should be able to fit one finger between the neck and the collar. Check to make sure that the patient can flex the neck comfortably. Reapply the oxygen source, if necessary.	
___	___	___	18. Remove gloves. Remove face shield or goggles and mask. Assist the patient to a comfortable position. Raise the bed rail and place the bed in the lowest position.	
___	___	___	19. Reassess the patient's respiratory status, including respiratory rate, effort, oxygen saturation, and lung sounds.	
___	___	___	20. Remove additional PPE, if used. Perform hand hygiene.	

Skill Checklists for Taylor's Clinical Nursing Skills.
A Nursing Process Approach, 5th edition

Name ______________________ Date ______________

Unit ______________________ Position ______________

Instructor/Evaluator: ______________________ Position ______________

SKILL 14-12

Providing Care of a Chest Drainage System

Goal: The patient does not experience any complications related to the chest drainage system or respiratory distress.

Excellent	Satisfactory	Needs Practice		Comments
___	___	___	1. Gather equipment.	
___	___	___	2. Perform hand hygiene and put on PPE, if indicated.	
___	___	___	3. Identify the patient.	
___	___	___	4. Assemble equipment on the overbed table or other surface within reach.	
___	___	___	5. Close the curtains around the bed and close the door to the room, if possible.	
___	___	___	6. Explain what you are going to do, and the reason for doing it, to the patient.	
___	___	___	7. ***Assess the patient's level of pain. Administer prescribed medication, as needed.***	
___	___	___	8. Put on clean gloves.	
			Assessing the Drainage System	
___	___	___	9. Move the patient's gown to expose the chest tube insertion site. Keep the patient covered as much as possible, using a bath blanket to drape the patient, if necessary. Observe the dressing at the chest tube insertion site and confirm that it is dry, intact, and occlusive.	
___	___	___	10. Check that all connections are securely taped. Gently palpate around the insertion site, feeling for crepitus, a result of air or gas collecting under the skin (subcutaneous emphysema). This may feel crunchy or spongy, or like "popping" under your fingers.	
___	___	___	11. Check drainage tubing to ensure that there are no dependent loops or kinks. Position the drainage collection device below the tube insertion site.	
___	___	___	12. If the chest tube is ordered to be connected to suction, note the fluid level in the suction chamber and check it with the amount of ordered suction. Look for bubbling in the suction chamber. Temporarily disconnect the suction to check the level of water in the chamber. Add sterile water or saline, if necessary, to maintain correct amount of suction.	

Excellent	Satisfactory	Needs Practice	SKILL 14-12 **Providing Care of a Chest Drainage System** *(Continued)*	Comments
___	___	___	13. Observe the water seal chamber for fluctuations of the water level with the patient's inspiration and expiration (tidaling). If suction is used, temporarily disconnect the suction to observe for fluctuation. Assess for the presence of bubbling in the water seal chamber. Add water, if necessary, to maintain the level at the 2-cm mark, or the mark recommended by the manufacturer.	
___	___	___	14. Assess the amount and type of fluid drainage. Measure drainage output at the end of each shift by marking the level on the container or placing a small piece of tape at the drainage level to indicate date and time. The amount should be a running total, because the drainage system is never emptied. If the drainage system fills, remove and replace it.	
___	___	___	15. Remove gloves. Assist the patient to a comfortable position. Raise the bed rail and place the bed in the lowest position, as necessary.	
___	___	___	16. Remove additional PPE, if used. Perform hand hygiene.	
			Changing the Drainage System	
___	___	___	17. Some drainage systems have a clamp on the drainage tubing. If present, there is no need to use other clamps. Otherwise, obtain two-padded Kelly clamps, a new drainage system, and a bottle of sterile water. Add water to the water seal chamber in the new system until it reaches the 2-cm mark or the mark recommended by the manufacturer. Follow manufacturer's directions to add water to the suction system, if suction is ordered.	
___	___	___	18. Put on clean gloves and additional PPE, as indicated.	
___	___	___	19. ***Engage the clamp on the drainage tubing.*** Alternatively, ***apply Kelly clamps 1.5 to 2.5 in from insertion site and 1 in apart, going in opposite directions.***	
___	___	___	20. Remove the suction from the current drainage system by unrolling or use scissors to carefully cut away any foam tape on the connection of the chest tube and drainage system. Using a slight twisting motion, remove the drainage system. ***Do not pull on the chest tube.***	

Excellent	Satisfactory	Needs Practice	SKILL 14-12 **Providing Care of a Chest Drainage System** *(Continued)*	Comments
___	___	___	21. Keeping the end of the chest tube sterile, insert the end of the new drainage system into the chest tube. ***Unclamp the tubing clamp or remove Kelly clamps.*** Reconnect suction, if ordered. Apply foam tape to chest tube/drainage system connection site.	
___	___	___	22. Assess the patient and the drainage system as outlined (Steps 5 to 15).	
___	___	___	23. Remove additional PPE, if used. Perform hand hygiene.	

Skill Checklists for Taylor's Clinical Nursing Skills. A Nursing Process Approach, 5th edition

Name ______________________ Date ______________________

Unit ______________________ Position ______________________

Instructor/Evaluator: ______________________ Position ______________________

SKILL 14-13

Assisting With Removal of a Chest Tube

Goal: The chest tube is removed without patient injury and the patient remains free from respiratory distress.

Excellent	Satisfactory	Needs Practice		Comments
____	____	____	1. Gather equipment.	
____	____	____	2. Perform hand hygiene and put on PPE, if indicated.	
____	____	____	3. Identify the patient.	
____	____	____	4. Assemble equipment on the overbed table or other surface within reach.	
____	____	____	5. Administer pain medication, as prescribed. ***Premedicate patient before the chest tube removal, at a sufficient interval to allow for the medication to take effect, based on the medication prescribed.***	
____	____	____	6. Close the curtains around the bed and close the door to the room, if possible.	
____	____	____	7. Explain what you are going to do and the reason for doing it to the patient. Explain any nonpharmacologic pain interventions the patient may use to decrease discomfort during tube removal.	
____	____	____	8. Explain that the patient will be required to take and hold a deep breath or exhale during chest tube removal. Instruct the patient to practice taking deep breaths and holding them. Alternately, the patient may be asked to take a deep breath and hum during removal of the tube (Muzzy & Butler, 2015).	
____	____	____	9. Put on clean gloves.	
____	____	____	10. Provide reassurance to the patient while the practitioner removes the dressing and then the tube.	
____	____	____	11. ***After the practitioner has removed the chest tube and secured the occlusive dressing, assess patient's lung sounds, vital signs, oxygen saturation, and pain level.***	
____	____	____	12. Anticipate an order for a chest x-ray.	
____	____	____	13. Dispose of equipment appropriately.	
____	____	____	14. Remove gloves and additional PPE, if used. Perform hand hygiene.	
____	____	____	15. Continue to monitor the patient's cardiopulmonary status and comfort level. Monitor the site and dressing.	

Skill Checklists for Taylor's Clinical Nursing Skills. A Nursing Process Approach, 5th edition

Name ______________________ Date ______________________

Unit ______________________ Position ______________________

Instructor/Evaluator: ______________________ Position ______________________

SKILL 14-14

Using a Manual Resuscitation Bag and Mask

Excellent	Satisfactory	Needs Practice	**Goal:** The patient exhibits signs and symptoms of adequate oxygen saturation.	Comments
___	___	___	1. If not a crisis situation, perform hand hygiene.	
___	___	___	2. Put on PPE, as indicated.	
___	___	___	3. If not a crisis situation, identify the patient.	
___	___	___	4. Explain what you are going to do and the reason for doing it to the patient, even if the patient does not appear to be alert.	
___	___	___	5. Put on disposable gloves. Put on face shield or goggles and mask.	
___	___	___	6. ***Ensure that the mask is connected to the bag device, the oxygen tubing is connected to the oxygen source, and the oxygen is turned on, at a flow rate of 10 to 15 L/min.*** This may be done by visualizing or by listening to the open end of the reservoir or tail: if air is heard flowing, the oxygen tubing is attached and on.	
___	___	___	7. Initiate CPR, if indicated. Refer to Skill 16-1.	
___	___	___	8. If possible, get behind head of bed and remove headboard. ***Slightly hyperextend the patient's neck (unless contraindicated). If unable to hyperextend, use jaw-thrust maneuver to open airway.***	
___	___	___	9. Place mask over the patient's face with opening over oral cavity. If mask is teardrop-shaped, the narrow portion should be placed over the bridge of the nose.	
___	___	___	10. ***Use the thumb and index finger of one hand to make a "C" on the side of the mask, pressing the edges of the mask to the face to form a seal around the patient's face. Use the remaining three fingers on the same hand to lift the angles of the jaw to open the airway and press the mask to the face.***	
___	___	___	11. Using the remaining hand, squeeze the bag to give a breath over 1 second, watching the chest for symmetric rise.	

SKILL 14-14

Using a Manual Resuscitation Bag and Mask *(Continued)*

Excellent	Satisfactory	Needs Practice		Comments
____	____	____	12. Deliver the breaths with the patient's own inspiratory effort, if present. Avoid delivering breaths when the patient exhales. Deliver one breath every 5 to 6 seconds (about 10 to 12 breaths/min, adults) (American Heart Association [AHA], 2015a), if the patient's own respiratory drive is absent. Continue delivering breaths until the patient's drive returns or until the patient is intubated and attached to mechanical ventilation.	
____	____	____	13. When use of the manual resuscitation bag and mask is no longer required, dispose of equipment appropriately.	
____	____	____	14. Remove face shield or goggles and mask. Remove gloves and additional PPE, if used. Perform hand hygiene.	

Skill Checklists for Taylor's Clinical Nursing Skills.
A Nursing Process Approach, 5th edition

Name ______________________ Date ______________________

Unit ______________________ Position ______________________

Instructor/Evaluator: ______________________ Position ______________________

SKILL 15-1

Initiating a Peripheral Venous Access IV Infusion

Excellent	Satisfactory	Needs Practice	**Goal:** The access device is inserted using sterile technique on the first attempt.	**Comments**
___	___	___	1. Verify the IV solution order on the eMAR/MAR with the medical order. Consider the appropriateness of the prescribed therapy in relation to the patient. Clarify any inconsistencies. Check the patient's chart for allergies. Check solution for color, leaking, and expiration date. Know techniques for IV insertion, precautions, and purpose of the IV solution administration, if ordered. Gather necessary supplies.	
___	___	___	2. Perform hand hygiene and put on PPE, if indicated.	
___	___	___	3. Identify the patient.	
___	___	___	4. Assemble equipment to the bedside stand or overbed table or other surface within reach.	
___	___	___	5. Close the curtains around the bed and close the door to the room, if possible. Explain what you are going to do and why you are going to do it to the patient. Ask the patient about allergies to medications, tape, or skin antiseptics, as appropriate. If considering using a local anesthetic, inquire about allergies for these substances as well.	
___	___	___	6. If using a local anesthetic, explain the rationale and procedure to the patient. Apply the anesthetic to a few potential insertion sites. Allow sufficient time for the anesthetic to take effect.	
			Prepare the IV Solution and Administration Set	
___	___	___	7. Compare the IV container label with the eMAR/MAR. Remove IV bag from outer wrapper, if indicated. Check expiration dates. Scan bar code on container, if necessary. Compare patient identification band with the eMAR/MAR. Alternately, label the solution container with the patient's name, solution type, additives, date, and time. Complete a time strip for the infusion and apply to IV container.	
___	___	___	8. Maintain aseptic technique when opening sterile packages and IV solution. Remove administration set from the package. Apply label to the tubing reflecting the day/date for next set change, per facility guidelines.	

Excellent	Satisfactory	Needs Practice	SKILL 15-1 **Initiating a Peripheral Venous Access IV Infusion** *(Continued)*	Comments
___	___	___	9. Close the roller clamp or slide the clamp on the IV administration set. Invert the IV solution container and remove the cap on the entry site, taking care not to touch the exposed entry site. Remove the cap from the spike on the administration set. Using a twisting and pushing motion, insert the administration set spike into the entry site of the IV container. Alternately, follow the manufacturer's directions for insertion.	
___	___	___	10. Hang the IV container on the IV pole. Squeeze the drip chamber and fill at least halfway.	
___	___	___	11. Open the IV tubing clamp, and allow fluid to move through the tubing. Follow the additional manufacturer's instructions for specific electronic infusion pump, as indicated. ***Allow fluid to flow until all air bubbles have disappeared and the entire length of the tubing is primed (filled) with IV solution.*** Close the clamp. Alternately, some brands of tubing may require removal of the cap at the end of the IV tubing to allow fluid to flow. Maintain its sterility. After fluid has filled the tubing, recap the end of the tubing.	
___	___	___	12. If an electronic device is to be used, follow the manufacturer's instructions for inserting the tubing into the device.	
			Initiate Peripheral Venous Access	
___	___	___	13. Place the patient in low-Fowler's position in bed. Place a protective towel or pad under the patient's arm.	
___	___	___	14. Provide emotional support, as needed.	
___	___	___	15. Open the short extension tubing package. Attach the needleless connector or end cap, if not in place. Clean the needleless connector or end cap with alcohol wipe. Insert a syringe with normal saline into the extension tubing. Fill the extension tubing with normal saline and place the extension tubing and syringe back on the package, within easy reach.	
___	___	___	16. Select and palpate for an appropriate vein. Refer to the guidelines in the previous Assessment section. If the intended insertion site is visibly soiled, clean the area with soap and water.	
___	___	___	17. If the site is hairy and facility policy permits, clip a 2-in area around the intended entry site.	
___	___	___	18. Put on gloves.	

Excellent	Satisfactory	Needs Practice	SKILL 15-1 **Initiating a Peripheral Venous Access IV Infusion** *(Continued)*	Comments
___	___	___	19. Apply a tourniquet 3 to 4 in above the venipuncture site to obstruct venous blood flow and distend the vein. Direct the ends of the tourniquet away from the entry site. Make sure the radial pulse is still present.	
___	___	___	20. Instruct the patient to hold the arm lower than the heart.	
___	___	___	21. Ask the patient to open and close the fist. Observe and palpate for a suitable vein. Try the following techniques if a vein cannot be felt:	
___	___	___	a. Lightly stroke the vein downward.	
___	___	___	b. Remove tourniquet and place warm, dry compresses over intended vein for 10 to 15 minutes.	
___	___	___	22. ***Cleanse the site with >5% chlorhexidine, or according to facility policy. Press the applicator against the skin and apply chlorhexidine using a gentle back and forth motion. Do not wipe or blot. Allow to dry completely for at least 30 seconds*** (INS, 2016a).	
___	___	___	23. Using the nondominant hand placed about 1 or 2 in below the entry site, hold the skin taut against the vein. ***Avoid touching the prepared site.*** Ask the patient to remain still while performing the venipuncture.	
___	___	___	24. Align the IV catheter on top of the vein; enter the skin gently, holding the catheter by the hub in your dominant hand, bevel side up, at a 10- to 15-degree angle. Insert the catheter from directly over the vein or from the side of the vein. While following the course of the vein, advance the needle or catheter into the vein. A sensation of "give" can be felt when the needle enters the vein.	
___	___	___	25. Continue to hold the skin taut. When blood returns through the catheter and/or the flashback chamber of the catheter, use the push-off tab to separate the catheter from the needle stylet and advance the catheter into the vein until the hub is at the venipuncture site. The exact technique depends on the type of device used.	
___	___	___	26. Release the tourniquet. Activate the safety mechanism on the needle stylet. Compress the skin well above the catheter tip to stop the flow of blood. Quickly remove the protective cap from the extension tubing and attach it to the catheter hub and tighten the Luer lock. Stabilize the catheter or needle with your nondominant hand.	
___	___	___	27. Continue to stabilize the catheter or needle and pull back on the syringe to assess for blood return, then, flush gently with the saline, observing the site for infiltration and leaking. Remove the syringe from the end cap.	

Excellent	Satisfactory	Needs Practice	SKILL 15-1 **Initiating a Peripheral Venous Access IV Infusion** *(Continued)*	Comments
___	___	___	28. Open the skin protectant wipe. Apply the skin protectant to the site, making sure to apply—at minimum—the area to be covered with the dressing. Place a sterile transparent dressing and/or catheter securing/stabilization device over the venipuncture site. Loop the tubing near the entry site, and anchor with tape (nonallergenic) close to the site.	
___	___	___	29. Label the IV dressing with the date, time, site, and type and size of the catheter placed.	
___	___	___	30. Using an antimicrobial swab, vigorously scrub the needleless connector or end cap on the extension tubing and allow to dry. Remove the end cap from the administration set. Insert the end of the administration set into the needleless connector or end cap. Loop the administration set tubing near the entry site, and anchor with tape (nonallergenic) close to the site. Remove gloves.	
___	___	___	31. Open the clamp on the administration set. Set the flow rate and begin the fluid infusion. Alternately, start the flow of solution by releasing the clamp on the tubing and counting the drops. Adjust until the correct drop rate is achieved. Assess the flow of the solution and function of the infusion device. Inspect the insertion site for signs of infiltration.	
___	___	___	32. Apply an IV securement/stabilization device if not already in place as part of the dressing, as indicated, based on facility policy. Explain to the patient the purpose of the device and the importance of safeguarding the site when using the extremity.	
___	___	___	33. Apply a passive disinfection cap to each access site on the administration set. Using an antimicrobial swab, vigorously scrub each access site cap on the administration set tubing and allow to dry. Attach a passive disinfection cap to each site.	
___	___	___	34. Remove equipment and return the patient to a position of comfort. Lower the bed, if not in the lowest position.	
___	___	___	35. Remove additional PPE, if used. Perform hand hygiene.	
___	___	___	36. Return to check the flow rate and observe the IV site for infiltration and/or other complications 30 minutes after starting infusion, and at least hourly thereafter. Ask the patient if he/she is experiencing any pain or discomfort related to the IV infusion.	

Skill Checklists for Taylor's Clinical Nursing Skills. A Nursing Process Approach, 5th edition

Name ______________________ Date ______________________

Unit ______________________ Position ______________________

Instructor/Evaluator: ______________________ Position ______________________

SKILL 15-2

Changing an IV Solution Container and Administration Set

Excellent	Satisfactory	Needs Practice	**Goal:** The prescribed IV infusion continues without interruption and with infusion complications identified.	**Comments**
___	___	___	1. Verify the IV solution order on the eMAR/MAR with the medical order. Consider the appropriateness of the prescribed therapy in relation to the patient. Clarify any inconsistencies. Check the patient's chart for allergies. Check solution for color, leaking, and expiration date. Know the purpose of the IV solution administration. Gather necessary supplies.	
___	___	___	2. Perform hand hygiene and put on PPE, if indicated.	
___	___	___	3. Identify the patient.	
___	___	___	4. Assemble equipment to the bedside stand or overbed table or other surface within reach.	
___	___	___	5. Close the curtains around the bed and close the door to the room, if possible. Explain what you are going to do and why you are going to do it to the patient. Ask the patient about allergies to medications or tape, as appropriate.	
___	___	___	6. Compare IV container label with the eMAR/MAR. Remove IV bag from the outer wrapper, if indicated. Check expiration dates. Scan bar code on container, if necessary. Compare patient identification band with the eMAR/MAR. Alternately, label the solution container with the patient's name, solution type, additives, date, and time. Complete a time strip for the infusion and apply to IV container.	
___	___	___	7. Maintain aseptic technique when opening sterile packages and IV solution. Remove administration set from the package. Apply label to the tubing reflecting the day/date for next set change, per facility guidelines.	
			To Change IV Solution Container	
___	___	___	8. If using an electronic infusion device, pause the device or put on "hold." Close the slide clamp on the administration set closest to the drip chamber. If using gravity infusion, close the roller clamp on the administration set.	
___	___	___	9. Carefully remove the cap on the entry site of the new IV solution container and expose the entry site, ***taking care not to touch the exposed entry site.***	

Excellent	Satisfactory	Needs Practice	SKILL 15-2 **Changing an IV Solution Container and Administration Set** *(Continued)*	Comments
___	___	___	10. Lift completed container off IV pole and invert it. Quickly remove the spike from the old IV container, ***being careful not to contaminate it.*** Discard old IV container.	
___	___	___	11. Using a twisting and pushing motion, insert the administration set spike into the entry site of the IV container. Alternately, follow the manufacturer's directions for insertion. Hang the container on the IV pole.	
___	___	___	12. Alternately, hang the new IV fluid container on an open hook on the IV pole. Carefully remove the cap on the entry site of the new IV solution container and expose the entry site, ***taking care not to touch the exposed entry site.*** Lift completed container off the IV pole and invert it. Quickly remove the spike from the old IV container, **being careful not to contaminate it**. Discard old IV container. Using a twisting and pushing motion, insert the administration set spike into the entry port of the new IV container as it hangs on the IV pole.	
___	___	___	13. If using an electronic infusion device, open the slide clamp, check the drip chamber of the administration set, verify the flow rate programmed in the infusion device, and turn the device to "run" or "infuse."	
___	___	___	14. If using gravity infusion, slowly open the roller clamp on the administration set and count the drops. Adjust until the correct drop rate is achieved.	
			To Change IV Solution Container and Administration Set	
___	___	___	15. Prepare the IV solution and administration set. Refer to Skill 15-1, Steps 7–11.	
___	___	___	16. Hang the new IV container on an open hook on the IV pole. Close the clamp on the existing IV administration set. Also, close the clamp on the short extension tubing connected to the IV catheter in the patient's arm.	
___	___	___	17. If using an electronic infusion device, remove the current administration set from the device. Following the manufacturer's directions, insert a new administration set into the infusion device.	

SKILL 15-2

Changing an IV Solution Container and Administration Set *(Continued)*

Excellent	Satisfactory	Needs Practice		Comments
___	___	___	18. Put on gloves. Remove the current infusion tubing from the needleless connector or end cap on the short extension IV tubing. Using an antimicrobial swab, vigorously scrub the needleless connector or end cap on the extension tubing and allow to dry. Remove the cap from the new administration set. Insert the end of the administration set into the needleless connector or end cap. Loop the administration set tubing near the entry site, and anchor with tape (nonallergenic) close to the site.	
___	___	___	19. Open the clamp on the extension tubing. Open the clamp on the administration set.	
___	___	___	20. If using an electronic infusion device, open the slide clamp, check the drip chamber of the administration set, verify the flow rate programmed in the infusion device, and turn the device to "run" or "infuse."	
___	___	___	21. If using gravity infusion, slowly open the roller clamp on the administration set and count the drops. Adjust until the correct drop rate is achieved.	
___	___	___	22. Apply a passive disinfection cap to each access site on the administration set. Using an antimicrobial swab, vigorously scrub each access site cap on the administration set tubing and allow to dry. Attach a passive disinfection cap to each site.	
___	___	___	23. Remove equipment. Ensure the patient's comfort. Remove gloves. Lower the bed, if not in the lowest position.	
___	___	___	24. Remove additional PPE, if used. Perform hand hygiene.	
___	___	___	25. Return to check the flow rate and observe the IV site for infiltration and/or other complications 30 minutes after starting infusion, and at least hourly thereafter. Ask the patient if he/she is experiencing any pain or discomfort related to the IV infusion.	

Skill Checklists for Taylor's Clinical Nursing Skills. A Nursing Process Approach, 5th edition

Name ______________________ Date ______________________

Unit ______________________ Position ______________________

Instructor/Evaluator: ______________________ Position ______________________

SKILL 15-3

Monitoring an IV Site and Infusion

Excellent	Satisfactory	Needs Practice	**Goal:** The patient remains free of complications related to IV therapy, exhibits a patent IV site, and the IV solution infuses at the prescribed flow rate.	Comments
___	___	___	1. Verify IV solution order on the eMAR/MAR with the medical order. Consider the appropriateness of the prescribed therapy in relation to the patient. Clarify any inconsistencies. Check the patient's medical record for allergies. Check for color, leaking, and expiration date. Know the purpose of the IV administration.	
___	___	___	2. ***Monitor IV infusion every hour or per facility policy. More frequent checks may be necessary if medication is being infused.***	
___	___	___	3. Perform hand hygiene and put on PPE, if indicated.	
___	___	___	4. Identify the patient.	
___	___	___	5. Close the curtains around the bed and close the door to the room, if possible. Explain what you are going to do and why you are doing it to the patient.	
___	___	___	6. If an electronic infusion device is being used, check settings, alarm, and indicator lights. Check set infusion rate. Note position of fluid in IV container in relation to time tape. Teach the patient about the alarm features on the electronic infusion device.	
___	___	___	7. If IV is infusing via gravity, check the drip chamber and time the drops.	
___	___	___	8. Check the tubing for anything that might interfere with the flow. Be sure clamps are in the open position.	
___	___	___	9. Observe the dressing for leakage of IV solution.	
___	___	___	10. Inspect the site for swelling, leakage at the site, coolness, or pallor, which may indicate infiltration. Ask if the patient is experiencing any pain or discomfort. If any of these symptoms are present, the IV will need to be removed and restarted at another site. Check facility policy for treating infiltration.	

Excellent	Satisfactory	Needs Practice	SKILL 15-3 **Monitoring an IV Site and Infusion** *(Continued)*	Comments
___	___	___	11. Inspect the site for redness, swelling, and heat. Palpate for induration. Ask if the patient is experiencing pain. These findings may indicate phlebitis, making it necessary to discontinue and restart the IV at another site. Grade phlebitis. Check facility policy for treatment of phlebitis. Notify the primary health care provider for severe (Grade 3 or 4) phlebitis (INS, 2016a).	
___	___	___	12. Check for local manifestations (redness, pus, warmth, induration, and pain) that may indicate an infection is present at the site. Also check for systemic manifestations (chills, fever, tachycardia, hypotension) that may accompany local infection at the site. If signs of infection are present, discontinue the IV and notify the primary care provider. Be careful not to disconnect the IV tubing when putting on the patient's hospital gown or assisting the patient with movement.	
___	___	___	13. Be alert for additional complications of IV therapy, such as fluid overload or bleeding.	
___	___	___	a. Fluid overload can result in signs of cardiac and/or respiratory failure. Monitor intake and output and vital signs. Assess for edema and auscultate lung sounds. Ask if the patient is experiencing any shortness of breath.	
___	___	___	b. Check for bleeding at the site.	
___	___	___	14. If appropriate, instruct the patient to call for assistance if any discomfort is noted at the site, solution container is nearly empty, flow has changed in any way, or if the electronic pump alarm sounds.	
___	___	___	15. Remove PPE, if used. Perform hand hygiene.	

Skill Checklists for Taylor's Clinical Nursing Skills. A Nursing Process Approach, 5th edition

Name ______________________ Date ______________________

Unit ______________________ Position ______________________

Instructor/Evaluator: ______________________ Position ______________________

SKILL 15-4

Changing a Peripheral Venous Access Site Dressing

Goal: The patient exhibits an access site that is clean, dry, and without evidence of any signs and symptoms of infection, infiltration, or phlebitis.

Excellent	Satisfactory	Needs Practice		Comments
___	___	___	1. Determine the need for a dressing change. Check facility policy. Gather equipment.	
___	___	___	2. Perform hand hygiene and put on PPE, if indicated.	
___	___	___	3. Identify the patient.	
___	___	___	4. Assemble equipment to the bedside stand or overbed table or other surface within reach.	
___	___	___	5. Close the curtains around the bed and close the door to the room, if possible. Explain what you are going to do and why you are going to do it to the patient. Ask the patient about allergies to tape and skin antiseptics.	
___	___	___	6. Put on gloves. Place a towel or disposable pad under the arm with the venous access. If the solution is currently infusing, temporarily stop the infusion. Hold the catheter in place with your nondominant hand. Beginning at the device hub, ***gently pull the dressing perpendicular to the skin toward the insertion site, carefully removing the old dressing and/or stabilization/securing device.*** Avoid inadvertently dislodging the catheter, as it may be adhered to the dressing (INS, 2016a). Use adhesive remover as necessary. Discard the dressing.	
___	___	___	7. ***Inspect the IV site for the presence of phlebitis (inflammation), infection, or infiltration.*** If noted, discontinue and relocate IV.	
___	___	___	8. ***Cleanse the site with an antiseptic solution, such as chlorhexidine, or according to facility policy. Press the applicator against the skin and apply chlorhexidine using a gentle back and forth motion. Do not wipe or blot. Allow to dry completely for at least 30 seconds (INS, 2016a).***	
___	___	___	9. Open the skin protectant wipe. Apply it to the site, making sure to cover at minimum the area to be covered with the dressing. Allow to dry. Place the sterile transparent dressing and/or catheter securing/stabilization device over the venipuncture site.	

Excellent	Satisfactory	Needs Practice	SKILL 15-4 **Changing a Peripheral Venous Access Site Dressing** *(Continued)*	Comments
____	____	____	10. Label the dressing with date, time of change, and initials. Loop the tubing near the entry site, and anchor with tape (nonallergenic) close to the site. Resume fluid infusion, if indicated. Check that IV flow is accurate and system is patent. Refer to Skill 15-3.	
____	____	____	11. Apply an IV securement/stabilization device if not already in place as part of the dressing, as indicated, based on facility policy. Explain to the patient the purpose of the device and the importance of safeguarding the site when using the extremity.	
____	____	____	12. Remove equipment. Ensure the patient's comfort. Remove gloves. Lower the bed, if not in the lowest position.	
____	____	____	13. Remove additional PPE, if used. Perform hand hygiene.	

Skill Checklists for Taylor's Clinical Nursing Skills. A Nursing Process Approach, 5th edition

Name ______________________ Date ______________________

Unit ______________________ Position ______________________

Instructor/Evaluator: ______________________ Position ______________________

SKILL 15-5

Capping for Intermittent Use and Flushing a Peripheral Venous Access Device

Goal: The IV is converted for intermittent use; the patient remains free of injury and any signs and symptoms of IV complications.

Excellent	Satisfactory	Needs Practice		Comments
___	___	___	1. Determine the need for conversion to an intermittent access. Verify medical order. Check facility policy. Gather equipment.	
___	___	___	2. Perform hand hygiene and put on PPE, if indicated.	
___	___	___	3. Identify the patient.	
___	___	___	4. Assemble equipment to the bedside stand or overbed table or other surface within reach.	
___	___	___	5. Close the curtains around the bed and close the door to the room, if possible. Explain what you are going to do and why you are going to do it to the patient. Ask the patient about allergies to tape and skin antiseptics.	
___	___	___	6. Assess the IV site. Refer to Skill 15-3.	
___	___	___	7. If using an electronic infusion device, stop the device. Close the roller clamp on the administration set. If using gravity infusion, close the roller clamp on the administration set.	
___	___	___	8. Put on gloves. Close the clamp on the short extension tubing connected to the IV catheter in the patient's arm.	
___	___	___	9. Remove the administration set tubing from the needleless connector or end cap on the extension set. Using an antimicrobial swab, vigorously scrub the needleless connector or end cap on the extension tubing and allow to dry.	
___	___	___	10. Insert the saline flush syringe into the needleless connector or end cap on the extension tubing. Pull back on the syringe to aspirate the catheter for positive blood return. If positive, instill the solution over 1 minute or flush the line according to facility policy. Remove the syringe and reclamp the extension tubing.	
___	___	___	11. If necessary, loop the extension tubing near the entry site and anchor it with tape (nonallergenic) close to the site.	
___	___	___	12. Using an antimicrobial swab, vigorously scrub the needleless connector or end cap on the extension tubing and allow to dry. Attach a passive disinfection cap.	
___	___	___	13. Remove equipment. Ensure the patient's comfort. Remove gloves. Lower the bed, if not in the lowest position.	
___	___	___	14. Remove additional PPE, if used. Perform hand hygiene.	

Skill Checklists for Taylor's Clinical Nursing Skills. A Nursing Process Approach, 5th edition

Name ______________________ Date ______________________

Unit ______________________ Position ______________________

Instructor/Evaluator: ______________________ Position ______________________

SKILL 15-6

Administering a Blood Transfusion

Goal: The patient receives the blood transfusion without any evidence of a transfusion reaction or complications.

Excellent	Satisfactory	Needs Practice		Comments
___	___	___	1. Verify the medical order for transfusion of a blood product. Verify the completion of informed consent documentation in the medical record. Verify any medical order for pretransfusion medication. If ordered, administer medication at least 30 minutes before initiating transfusion.	
___	___	___	2. Gather all equipment.	
___	___	___	3. Perform hand hygiene and put on PPE, if indicated.	
___	___	___	4. Identify the patient.	
___	___	___	5. Assemble equipment to the bedside stand or overbed table or other surface within reach.	
___	___	___	6. Close the curtains around the bed and close the door to the room, if possible. Explain what you are going to do and why you are going to do it to the patient. Ask the patient about previous experience with a transfusion and any reactions. Advise the patient to report any chills, itching, rash, or unusual symptoms.	
___	___	___	7. Prime blood administration set with the normal saline IV fluid. Refer to Skill 15-2.	
___	___	___	8. Put on gloves. If the patient does not have a venous access device in place, initiate peripheral venous access. (Refer to Skill 15-1.) Connect the administration set to the venous access device via the extension tubing. (Refer to Skill 15-1.) Infuse the normal saline per facility policy.	
___	___	___	9. Obtain blood product from blood bank according to facility policy. Scan the bar codes on blood products if required.	

SKILL 15-6

Administering a Blood Transfusion *(Continued)*

Excellent	Satisfactory	Needs Practice		Comments
___	___	___	10. Two registered nurses (or other licensed practitioner [hospital/outpatient setting], or responsible adult [home setting]) compare and validate the following information in the presence of the patient with the medical record, patient identification band (hospital/outpatient setting), and the label of the blood product:	
___	___	___	• Medical order for transfusion of blood product	
___	___	___	• Informed consent	
___	___	___	• Patient identification number	
___	___	___	• Patient name	
___	___	___	• Blood group and type	
___	___	___	• Expiration date	
___	___	___	• Inspection of blood product for clots, clumping, gas bubbles	
___	___	___	11. ***Obtain baseline set of vital signs before beginning the transfusion.***	
___	___	___	12. Put on gloves. If using an electronic infusion device, put the device on "hold." Close the roller clamp closest to the drip chamber on the saline side of the administration set. Close the roller clamp on the administration set below the infusion device. Alternately, if infusing via gravity, close the roller clamp on the administration set.	
___	___	___	13. Close the roller clamp closest to the drip chamber on the blood product side of the administration set. Remove the protective cap from the access port on the blood container. Remove the cap from the access spike on the administration set. Using a pushing and twisting motion, insert the spike into the access port on the blood container, taking care not to contaminate the spike. Hang the blood container on the IV pole. Open the roller clamp on the blood side of the administration set. Squeeze drip chamber until the in-line filter is saturated. Remove gloves.	
___	___	___	14. ***Start administration slowly (approximately 2 mL per minute for the first 15 minutes) (INS, 2016b). Stay with the patient for the first 5 to 15 minutes of transfusion.*** Open the roller clamp on the administration set below the infusion device. Set the flow rate and begin the transfusion. Alternately, start the flow of solution by releasing the clamp on the tubing and counting the drops. Adjust until the correct drop rate is achieved. Assess the flow of the blood and function of the infusion device. Inspect the insertion site for signs of infiltration.	

Excellent	Satisfactory	Needs Practice	SKILL 15-6 **Administering a Blood Transfusion** *(Continued)*	Comments
___	___	___	15. Observe the patient for flushing, dyspnea, itching, hives or rash, or any unusual comments.	
___	___	___	16. Reassess vital signs after 15 minutes. Obtain vital signs thereafter according to facility policy and nursing assessment.	
___	___	___	17. After the observation period (5 to 15 minutes) increase the infusion rate to the calculated rate to complete the infusion within the prescribed time frame, no more than 4 hours.	
___	___	___	18. Maintain the prescribed flow rate as ordered or as deemed appropriate based on the patient's overall condition, keeping in mind the outer limits for safe administration. Ongoing monitoring is crucial throughout the entire duration of the blood transfusion for early identification of any adverse reactions.	
___	___	___	19. ***During transfusion, assess frequently for transfusion reaction. Stop blood transfusion if you suspect a reaction. Quickly replace the blood tubing with a new administration set primed with normal saline for IV infusion. Initiate an infusion of normal saline for IV at an open rate, usually 40 mL/hr. Obtain vital signs. Notify primary care provider and blood bank.***	
___	___	___	20. When transfusion is complete, close the roller clamp on blood side of the administration set and open the roller clamp on the normal saline side of the administration set. Initiate infusion of normal saline. When all of blood has infused into the patient, clamp the administration set. Obtain vital signs. Put on gloves. Cap the access site or resume previous IV infusion. (Refer to Skills 15-1 and 15-5.) Dispose of blood-transfusion equipment or return to blood bank, according to facility policy.	
___	___	___	21. Remove equipment. Ensure the patient's comfort. Remove gloves. Lower the bed, if not in the lowest position.	
___	___	___	22. Remove additional PPE, if used. Perform hand hygiene.	
___	___	___	23. Monitor and assess the patient after the transfusion for signs and symptoms of delayed transfusion reaction. Provide patient education about signs and symptoms of delayed transfusion reactions.	

Skill Checklists for Taylor's Clinical Nursing Skills.
A Nursing Process Approach, 5th edition

Name ______________________ Date ______________

Unit ______________________ Position ______________

Instructor/Evaluator: ______________________ Position ______________

SKILL 15-7

Changing the Dressing and Flushing Central Venous Access Devices

Excellent	Satisfactory	Needs Practice	**Goal:** Site care is provided and the dressing is replaced.	Comments
___	___	___	1. Verify the medical order and/or facility policy and procedure. Determine the need for a dressing change. Often, the procedure for CVAD flushing and dressing changes will be a standing protocol. Gather equipment.	
___	___	___	2. Perform hand hygiene and put on PPE, if indicated.	
___	___	___	3. Identify the patient.	
___	___	___	4. Assemble equipment to the bedside stand or overbed table or other surface within reach.	
___	___	___	5. Close the curtains around the bed and close the door to the room, if possible. Explain what you are going to do and why you are going to do it to the patient. Ask the patient about allergies to tape and skin antiseptics.	
___	___	___	6. Place a waste receptacle or bag at a convenient location for use during the procedure.	
___	___	___	7. Adjust the bed to a comfortable working height, usually elbow height of the caregiver (VHACEOSH, 2016).	
___	___	___	8. Assist the patient to a comfortable position that provides easy access to the CVAD insertion site and dressing. If the patient has a PICC, position the patient with the arm extended from the body below heart level. Use the bath blanket to cover any exposed area other than the site.	
___	___	___	9. Apply a mask. Ask the patient to turn his/her head away from the access site. Alternately, have the patient put on a mask, depending on facility policy. Move the overbed table to a convenient location within easy reach. Set up a sterile field on the table. Open dressing supplies and add to sterile field. If IV solution is infusing via CVAD, interrupt and place on hold during dressing change. Apply slide clamp on each lumen of the CVAD.	

Excellent	Satisfactory	Needs Practice	SKILL 15-7 **Changing the Dressing and Flushing Central Venous Access Devices** *(Continued)*	Comments
___	___	___	10. Put on clean gloves. Assess the CVAD insertion site through the old dressing. Palpate the site, noting pain, tenderness, or discomfort. Remove the old dressing, beginning at the device hub. Stabilize the catheter. Gently pull the dressing perpendicular to the skin toward the insertion site (INS, 2016b). Take care to avoid inadvertently dislodging the catheter/needle. Discard the dressing in a trash receptacle.	
___	___	___	11. Based on the device in use, remove the stabilization device according to the manufacturer's directions. A subcutaneous external stabilization device is not removed with each dressing change (INS, 2016b). Note the status of any sutures or staples that may be present. Remove gloves and discard.	
___	___	___	12. Perform hand hygiene. Put on sterile gloves. Starting at the insertion site and continuing in a circle, wipe off any old blood or drainage with a sterile antimicrobial wipe. Using the chlorhexidine swab, cleanse the site, covering at least a 2- to 3-in area. ***Apply chlorhexidine using a gentle back and forth motion for at least 30 seconds (INS, 2016b). Do not wipe or blot. Allow to dry completely.***	
___	___	___	13. Apply antimicrobial dressing, based on facility policy. Apply the skin protectant to the same 2- to 3-in area, avoiding direct application to the antimicrobial pad or gel component of the dressing or the insertion site, and allow to dry. Apply the securement/stabilization device, if used, and/or the TSM dressing, centering over the insertion site. Measure the length of the catheter that extends out from the insertion site.	
___	___	___	14. Based on facility policy, replace end caps, as indicated. Working with one lumen at a time, remove the needleless connector or end cap. Using an antimicrobial swab, vigorously scrub the end of the lumen and apply a new needleless connector or end cap. Repeat for each lumen.	
___	___	___	15. If required, flush each lumen of the CVAD. Amount of saline and heparin flushes varies depending on specific CVAD and facility policy.	

Excellent	Satisfactory	Needs Practice	SKILL 15-7 **Changing the Dressing and Flushing Central Venous Access Devices** *(Continued)*	Comments
___	___	___	16. Using an antimicrobial swab, vigorously scrub the needleless connector or end cap on one of the lumens and allow to dry. Insert the saline flush syringe into the needleless connector. Open the clamp on the lumen. Slowly inject the saline flush, noting any resistance or sluggishness, and slowly pull back on the syringe to aspirate for positive blood return. If positive, instill the solution over 1 minute or by using a pulsatile flushing technique of 10 short boluses of 1 mL interrupted by brief pauses; flush the line according to facility policy. Remove the syringe. Insert the locking solution syringe and instill the volume of solution designated by facility policy over 1 minute or according to facility policy. Remove the syringe and reclamp the lumen. Remove gloves.	
___	___	___	17. Apply a passive disinfection cap to each needleless connector or end cap. Using an antimicrobial swab, vigorously scrub the needleless connector or end cap on the extension tubing and allow to dry. Attach a passive disinfection cap.	
___	___	___	18. Label the dressing with the date, time of change, and initials. Resume fluid infusion, if indicated. Check that IV flow is accurate and system is patent. (Refer to Skill 15-3.)	
___	___	___	19. Apply an IV securement/stabilization device if not already in place as part of the dressing, as indicated, based on facility policy. Explain to the patient the purpose of the device and the importance of safeguarding the site when using the extremity.	
___	___	___	20. Remove equipment. Ensure the patient's comfort. Lower the bed, if not in the lowest position.	
___	___	___	21. Remove additional PPE, if used. Perform hand hygiene.	

Skill Checklists for Taylor's Clinical Nursing Skills. A Nursing Process Approach, 5th edition

Name ______________________ Date ______________________

Unit ______________________ Position ______________________

Instructor/Evaluator: ______________________ Position ______________________

SKILL 15-8

Accessing an Implanted Port

Excellent	Satisfactory	Needs Practice	**Goal:** The port is accessed with minimal to no discomfort to the patient; the patient experiences no trauma to the site or infection; and the patient verbalizes an understanding of care associated with the port.	**Comments**
___	___	___	1. Verify medical order and/or facility policy and procedure. Often, the procedure for accessing an implanted port and dressing changes will be a standing protocol. Gather equipment.	
___	___	___	2. Perform hand hygiene and put on PPE, if indicated.	
___	___	___	3. Identify the patient.	
___	___	___	4. Assemble equipment to the bedside stand or overbed table or other surface within reach.	
___	___	___	5. Close the curtains around the bed and close the door to the room, if possible. Explain what you are going to do, and why you are going to do it to the patient. Ask the patient about allergies to tape and skin antiseptics. If considering using a local anesthetic, inquire about allergies for these substances as well.	
___	___	___	6. If using a local anesthetic, explain the rationale and procedure to the patient. Apply the anesthetic as indicated to the port site. Allow sufficient time for the anesthetic to take effect.	
___	___	___	7. Place a waste receptacle or bag at a convenient location for use during the procedure.	
___	___	___	8. Adjust the bed to a comfortable working height, usually elbow height of the caregiver (VHACEOSH, 2016).	
___	___	___	9. Assist the patient to a comfortable position that provides easy access to the port site. Use the bath blanket to cover any exposed area other than the site.	
___	___	___	10. Apply a mask. Ask the patient to turn his/her head away from the access site. Alternately, have the patient put on a mask, depending on facility policy. Move the overbed table to a convenient location within easy reach. Set up a sterile field on the table. Open dressing supplies and add to the sterile field.	
___	___	___	11. Put on clean gloves. Palpate the location of the port. Assess site. Note the status of any surgical incisions that may be present. Remove gloves and discard.	

Excellent	Satisfactory	Needs Practice	SKILL 15-8 **Accessing an Implanted Port** *(Continued)*	Comments
___	___	___	12. Put on sterile gloves. Connect the needleless connector or end cap to the extension tubing on the noncoring needle. Using an antimicrobial swab, vigorously scrub the needleless connector or end cap on the extension tubing and allow to dry. Insert a syringe with 10-mL normal saline into the needleless connector or end cap. Fill the extension tubing with normal saline and apply clamp. Remove the syringe. Place on sterile field.	
___	___	___	13. Using the chlorhexidine swab, cleanse the port site, covering at least a 2- to 3-in area. ***Apply chlorhexidine using a gentle back and forth motion for at least 30 seconds*** (INS, 2016b). ***Do not wipe or blot. Allow to dry completely.***	
___	___	___	14. Using the nondominant hand, locate the port by palpating the edges through the skin. Hold the port stable, keeping the skin taut.	
___	___	___	15. Visualize the center of the port. Pick up the noncoring needle and extension tubing. Coil the extension tubing into the palm of your hand. Holding the needle at a 90-degree angle to the skin, insert ***through the skin into the port septum until the needle hits the back of the port.***	
___	___	___	16. Using an antimicrobial swab, vigorously scrub the needleless connector or end cap on the extension tubing and allow to dry. Insert the syringe with normal saline. ***Open the clamp on the extension tubing and flush with 3 to 5 mL of saline, while observing the site for fluid leak or infiltration. It should flush easily, without resistance.***	
___	___	___	***Alert: if an antimicrobial locking solution was used when the port was last locked, withdraw the solution from the port prior to flushing and discard*** (INS, 2016a, p. 182).	
___	___	___	17. Slowly pull back on the syringe plunger to aspirate for blood return. Do not allow blood to enter the syringe. If positive, instill the solution over 1 minute or by using a pulsatile flushing technique of 10 short boluses of 1 mL interrupted by brief pauses; flush the line according to facility policy. Remove the syringe. Insert the locking solution syringe and instill the volume of solution designated by facility policy over 1 minute or according to facility policy. Remove the syringe and reclamp the lumen. Alternately, if IV fluid infusion is to be initiated, do not flush with heparin.	

Excellent	Satisfactory	Needs Practice	SKILL 15-8 **Accessing an Implanted Port** *(Continued)*	Comments
___	___	___	18. If using a "Gripper" needle, remove the gripper portion from the needle by squeezing the sides together and lifting off the needle while holding the needle securely to the port with the other hand.	
___	___	___	19. Apply the skin protectant to the site, avoiding direct application to the needle insertion site. Allow to dry.	
___	___	___	20. Apply an antimicrobial dressing, a CVAD site dressing, and securement device, based on facility policy. Refer to Skill 15-7. Apply a passive disinfection cap to the needleless connector or end cap on the extension tubing.	
___	___	___	21. Remove equipment. Ensure the patient's comfort. Lower the bed, if not in the lowest position.	
___	___	___	22. Remove additional PPE, if used. Perform hand hygiene.	

Skill Checklists for Taylor's Clinical Nursing Skills.
A Nursing Process Approach, 5th edition

Name ______________________ Date ______________________

Unit ______________________ Position ______________________

Instructor/Evaluator: ______________________ Position ______________________

SKILL 15-9

Deaccessing an Implanted Port

Excellent	Satisfactory	Needs Practice	**Goal**: The port is flushed and locked without adverse effect and the needle is removed with minimal to no discomfort to the patient; the patient experiences no trauma or infection; and the patient verbalizes an understanding of port care.	**Comments**
___	___	___	1. Verify medical order and/or facility policy and procedure. Often, the procedure for deaccessing an implanted port will be a standing protocol. Gather equipment.	
___	___	___	2. Perform hand hygiene and put on PPE, if indicated.	
___	___	___	3. Identify the patient.	
___	___	___	4. Assemble equipment to the bedside stand or overbed table or other surface within reach.	
___	___	___	5. Close the curtains around the bed and close the door to the room, if possible. Explain what you are going to do and why you are going to do it to the patient.	
___	___	___	6. Adjust the bed to a comfortable working height, usually elbow height of the caregiver (VHACEOSH, 2016).	
___	___	___	7. Assist the patient to a comfortable position that provides easy access to the port site. Use the bath blanket to cover any exposed area other than the site.	
___	___	___	8. Put on gloves. Using an antimicrobial swab, vigorously scrub the needleless connector or end cap on the extension tubing and allow to dry. Insert the syringe with normal saline. Unclamp the extension tubing and check for a blood return as indicated in Skill 15-8. If positive, instill the solution over 1 minute or by using a pulsatile flushing technique of 10 short boluses of 1 mL interrupted by brief pauses; flush the line according to facility policy.	
___	___	___	9. Remove the syringe. Using an antimicrobial swab, vigorously scrub the needleless connector or end cap on the extension tubing and allow to dry. Insert the locking solution syringe and instill the volume of solution designated by facility policy over 1 minute or according to facility policy. Remove the syringe and clamp the lumen.	
___	___	___	10. Remove the dressing and/or stabilization device, noting any drainage and discard (Refer to Skill 15-7).	

Excellent	Satisfactory	Needs Practice	SKILL 15-9 **Deaccessing an Implanted Port** *(Continued)*	**Comments**
___	___	___	11. Stabilize the port on either side with the thumb and forefinger of your nondominant hand. Grasp the needle/wings with the fingers of the dominant hand. Firmly and smoothly, pull the needle straight up at a 90-degree angle from the skin to remove it from the port septum. Engage needle guard, if not automatic on removal.	
___	___	___	12. Apply gentle pressure with the gauze to the insertion site. Apply a small adhesive bandage over the port if any oozing occurs. Otherwise, a dressing is not necessary. Remove gloves.	
___	___	___	13. Ensure the patient's comfort. Lower the bed, if not in the lowest position. Put on one glove to handle the needle. Dispose of the needle with the extension tubing in the sharps container.	
___	___	___	14. Remove gloves and additional PPE, if used. Perform hand hygiene.	

Skill Checklists for Taylor's Clinical Nursing Skills. A Nursing Process Approach, 5th edition

Name ______________________ Date ______________________

Unit ______________________ Position ______________________

Instructor/Evaluator: ______________________ Position ______________________

SKILL 15-10

Removing a Peripherally Inserted Central Catheter (PICC)

Goal: The PICC is removed with minimal to no discomfort to the patient and the patient experiences no adverse effect or infection.

Excellent	Satisfactory	Needs Practice	Step	Comments
___	___	___	1. Verify medical order for PICC removal and facility policy and procedure. Gather equipment.	
___	___	___	2. Perform hand hygiene and put on PPE, if indicated.	
___	___	___	3. Identify the patient.	
___	___	___	4. Close the curtains around the bed and close the door to the room, if possible. Explain what you are going to do and why you are going to do it to the patient.	
___	___	___	5. Adjust the bed to a comfortable working height, usually elbow height of the caregiver (VHACEOSH, 2016).	
___	___	___	6. Assist the patient to a supine flat or Trendelenburg position with the arm straight and the catheter insertion site at or below heart level. Use the bath blanket to cover any exposed area other than the site.	
___	___	___	7. Put on gloves. Stabilize catheter hub with your nondominant hand. Remove the dressing and/or stabilization device, noting any drainage and discard (Refer to Skill 15-7).	
___	___	___	8. Instruct the patient to hold the breath, and perform a Valsalva maneuver as the last portion of the catheter is removed; if unable to do so, have the patient exhale (INS, 2016a).	
___	___	___	9. Using the dominant hand, remove the catheter slowly. Grasp the catheter close to the insertion site and slowly ease it out, keeping it parallel to the skin. Continue removing in small increments, using a smooth and constant motion.	
___	___	___	10. After removal, apply pressure to the site with sterile gauze until hemostasis is achieved (minimum 1 minute). Apply petroleum-based ointment and a sterile occlusive dressing.	
___	___	___	11. Measure the catheter and compare it with the length listed in the chart when it was inserted. Inspect the catheter for patency. Dispose of PICC according to facility policy.	
___	___	___	12. Remove gloves. Ensure the patient's comfort. Lower the bed, if not in the lowest position.	

Excellent	Satisfactory	Needs Practice	SKILL 15-10 **Removing a Peripherally Inserted Central Catheter (PICC)** *(Continued)*	Comments
____	____	____	13. Instruct the patient to remain in flat/supine position, if able, for 30 minutes postremoval.	
____	____	____	14. Remove additional PPE, if used. Perform hand hygiene.	
____	____	____	15. Leave the dressing in place for at least 24 hours (INS, 2016a). Change the dressing daily until the exit site has healed.	

Skill Checklists for Taylor's Clinical Nursing Skills. A Nursing Process Approach, 5th edition

Name ______________________ Date ______________________

Unit ______________________ Position ______________________

Instructor/Evaluator: ______________________ Position ______________________

SKILL 16-1

Performing Cardiopulmonary Resuscitation

Excellent	Satisfactory	Needs Practice	**Goal:** CPR is performed effectively without adverse effect to the patient.	Comments
___	___	___	1. Verify scene safety. Assess responsiveness. Look for no breathing or only gasping. Call for help, pull call bell, and call the facility emergency response number. Call for emergency equipment and the AED or defibrillator, if available.	
___	___	___	2. Put on gloves, if available. Position the patient supine on his or her back on a firm, flat surface, with arms alongside the body. If the patient is in bed, place a backboard or other rigid surface under the patient (often the footboard of the patient's bed). Position yourself at the patient's side.	
___	___	___	3. ***Provide defibrillation (if indicated) at the earliest possible moment, as soon as an AED becomes available.*** Refer to Skills 16-2 and Skill 16-3.	
___	___	___	4. Simultaneously look for no breathing or only gasping and check for a pulse, palpating the carotid pulse. This assessment should take at least 5 seconds and no more than 10 seconds. If you do not definitely feel a pulse within 10 seconds, begin CPR using the compression:ventilation ratio of 30 compressions to 2 breaths, starting with chest compressions (CAB sequence).	
___	___	___	Alternately, if there is no normal breathing but the patient has a pulse, see Step 14.	
___	___	___	5. Position the heel of one hand in the center of the chest between the nipples, directly over the lower half of the sternum. Place the heel of the other hand directly on top of the first hand. Extend or interlace fingers to keep fingers above the chest. Straighten arms and position shoulders directly over hands.	
___	___	___	6. Push hard and fast. Chest compressions should depress the sternum to a depth of at least 2 in (adult). Push straight down on the patient's sternum. Perform 30 chest compressions at a rate of 100/min, counting "1, 2, etc." up to 30, keeping elbows locked, arms straight, and shoulders directly over the hands. Allow full chest recoil (reexpand) after each compression. ***Do not lean on chest wall between compressions.*** Chest compression and chest recoil/relaxation times should be approximately equal.	
___	___	___	7. Ventilate using a barrier device (face mask or bag-valve-mask device, if available). Give 2 breaths (as described below) after	

Excellent	Satisfactory	Needs Practice	SKILL 16-1 **Performing Cardiopulmonary Resuscitation** *(Continued)*	Comments
			each set of 30 compressions. Cycles of 30 compressions and 2 ventilations are recommended (AHA, 2015a).	
___	___	___	8. Use the head tilt–chin lift maneuver to open the airway. Place one hand on the patient's forehead and apply firm, backward pressure with the palm to tilt the head back. Place the fingers of the other hand under the bony part of the lower jaw near the chin and lift the jaw upward to bring the chin forward and the teeth almost to occlusion.	
___	___	___	9. If trauma to the head or neck is present or suspected, use the jaw-thrust maneuver to open the airway. Place one hand on each side of the patient's head. Rest elbows on the flat surface under the patient, grasp the angle of the patient's lower jaw, and lift with both hands.	
___	___	___	10. Seal the patient's mouth and nose with the face shield, one-way valve mask, or Ambu bag (handheld resuscitation bag), if available. If not available, seal the patient's mouth with your mouth.	
___	___	___	11. Instill 2 breaths, each lasting 1 second, making the chest rise.	
___	___	___	12. If you are unable to ventilate or the chest does not rise during ventilation, reposition the patient's head and reattempt to ventilate. If still unable to ventilate, resume CPR. Each subsequent time the airway is opened to administer breaths, look for an object. If an object is visible in the mouth, remove it. If no object is visible, continue with CPR.	
___	___	___	13. After about 2 minutes (until prompted by AED or about 5 complete cycles of CPR), assess the patient's rhythm on the defibrillator. Defibrillate as indicated (see Skill 16-2 or Skill 16-3). If no pulse, continue CPR.	
___	___	___	14. Rescue breathing: If the patient has a pulse but remains without spontaneous breathing, continue with rescue breathing, without chest compressions. Administer rescue breathing at a rate of 1 breath every 5 to 6 seconds, for a rate of 10 to 12 breaths/min. If situation involves a possible opioid overdose, administer naloxone as per protocol. Check pulse about every 2 minutes. If no pulse, begin CPR (Step 5).	
___	___	___	15. If spontaneous breathing resumes, place the patient in the recovery position.	
___	___	___	16. Otherwise, continue CPR until advanced care providers take over, the patient starts to move, you are too exhausted to continue, or an advanced health care provider discontinues CPR.	
___	___	___	17. Remove gloves, if used. Perform hand hygiene.	

Skill Checklists for Taylor's Clinical Nursing Skills.
A Nursing Process Approach, 5th edition

Name ______________________ Date ______________________

Unit ______________________ Position ______________________

Instructor/Evaluator: ______________________ Position ______________________

Excellent	Satisfactory	Needs Practice	SKILL 16-2 **Performing Emergency Automated External Defibrillation** **Goal:** The defibrillation is performed correctly without adverse effect to the patient, and the patient regains signs of circulation, with organized electrical rhythm and pulse.	**Comments**
___	___	___	1. Verify scene safety. Assess responsiveness. Look for no breathing or only gasping. Call for help, pull call bell, and call the facility emergency response number. Call for emergency equipment and the AED or defibrillator, if available. Put on gloves, if available. Begin CPR (see Skill 16-1).	
___	___	___	2. ***Provide defibrillation at the earliest possible moment, as soon as AED becomes available.***	
___	___	___	3. Prepare the AED. Power on the AED. Push the power button. Some devices will turn on automatically when the lid or case is opened.	
___	___	___	4. Attach AED cables to the adhesive electrode pads (may be preconnected).	
___	___	___	5. Stop chest compressions. Peel away the covering from the electrode pads to expose the adhesive surface. Attach the electrode pads to the patient's chest. Place one pad on the upper right sternal border, directly below the clavicle. Place the second pad lateral to the left nipple, with the top margin of the pad a few inches below the axilla (anterolateral positioning). Alternately, if two or more rescuers are present, one rescuer should continue chest compressions while another rescuer attaches the AED pads. Attach the AED connecting cables to the AED box, if not preconnected.	
___	___	___	6. Once the pads are in place and the device is turned on, follow the prompts given by the device. Clear the patient and analyze the rhythm. Ensure no one is touching the patient. Loudly state a "Clear the patient" message. Press "Analyze" button to initiate analysis, if necessary. Some devices automatically begin analysis when the pads are attached. Avoid all movement affecting the patient during analysis.	
___	___	___	7. If a shockable rhythm is present, the device will announce that a shock is indicated and begin charging. Once the AED is charged, a message will be delivered to shock the patient.	

Excellent	Satisfactory	Needs Practice	SKILL 16-2 **Performing Emergency Automated External Defibrillation** *(Continued)*	Comments
___	___	___	8. ***Before pressing the "Shock" button, loudly state a "Clear the patient" message. Visually check that no one is in contact with the patient or the bed.*** Press the "Shock" button. If the AED is fully automatic, a shock will be delivered automatically.	
___	___	___	9. Immediately resume CPR, beginning with chest compressions. After about 2 minutes (until prompted by AED or about five complete cycles of CPR), allow the AED to analyze the heart rhythm. If a shock is not advised, resume CPR, beginning with chest compressions. Do not recheck to see if there is a pulse. Follow the AED voice prompts.	
___	___	___	10. Continue CPR until advanced care providers take over, the patient starts to move, you are too exhausted to continue, or an advanced health care provider discontinues CPR.	
___	___	___	11. Remove gloves, if used. Perform hand hygiene.	

Skill Checklists for Taylor's Clinical Nursing Skills. A Nursing Process Approach, 5th edition

Name ____________________ Date ____________________

Unit ____________________ Position ____________________

Instructor/Evaluator: ____________________ Position ____________________

SKILL 16-3

Performing Emergency Manual External Defibrillation (Asynchronous)

Excellent	Satisfactory	Needs Practice	**Goal:** The procedure is performed correctly without adverse effect to the patient; and the patient regains signs of circulation with organized electrical rhythm and pulse.	**Comments**
___	___	___	1. Verify scene safety. Look for no breathing or only gasping. Call for help, pull call bell, and call the facility emergency response number. Call for emergency equipment and the automated external defibrillator (AED) or defibrillator, if available. Put on gloves, if available. Begin CPR, as indicated (see Skill 16-1).	
___	___	___	2. ***Provide defibrillation at the earliest possible moment, as soon as AED becomes available.***	
___	___	___	3. Turn on the defibrillator.	
___	___	___	4. Expose the patient's chest, and apply electrode pads to the chest. Place one pad on the upper right sternal border, directly below the clavicle. Place the second pad lateral to the left nipple, with the top margin of the pad a few inches below the axilla (anterolateral positioning). Alternately, if two or more rescuers are present, one rescuer should continue chest compressions while another rescuer attaches the electrode pads. Assess the cardiac rhythm.	
___	___	___	5. Set the energy level for 360 J (joules) when using a monophasic defibrillator. Use clinically appropriate energy levels for biphasic defibrillators, beginning with 120 to 200 J, depending on device (Morton & Fontaine, 2018).	
___	___	___	6. If the patient remains in VF or pulseless VT, ***loudly state a "Clear the patient" message. Visually check that no one is in contact with the patient or the bed.*** Press the button to deliver the shock.	
___	___	___	7. After the shock, immediately resume CPR, beginning with chest compressions. After five cycles (about 2 minutes), reassess the cardiac rhythm. Continue until advanced care providers take over, the patient starts to move, you are too exhausted to continue, or an advanced health care provider discontinues CPR.	
___	___	___	8. If necessary, prepare to defibrillate subsequent shocks per ACLS protocol.	
___	___	___	9. Announce that you are preparing to defibrillate and follow the procedure described above.	

Excellent	Satisfactory	Needs Practice	SKILL 16-3 **Performing Emergency Manual External Defibrillation (Asynchronous)** *(Continued)*	Comments
___	___	___	10. If defibrillation restores a normal rhythm:	
___	___	___	a. Check for signs of circulation; check the central and peripheral pulses, and obtain a blood pressure reading, heart rate, and respiratory rate.	
___	___	___	b. If signs of circulation are present, check breathing. If breathing is inadequate, assist breathing. Administer rescue breathing at a rate of 1 breath every 5 to 6 seconds, for a rate of 10 to 12 breaths/min.	
___	___	___	c. If breathing is adequate, place the patient in the recovery position. Continue to assess the patient.	
___	___	___	d. Assess the patient's level of consciousness, cardiac rhythm, blood pressure, breath sounds, skin color, and temperature.	
___	___	___	e. Obtain baseline ABG levels (Skill 18-11) and a 12-lead ECG (Skill 16-4), if ordered.	
___	___	___	f. Provide supplemental oxygen, ventilation, and medications, as needed.	
___	___	___	g. Anticipate the possible use of targeted temperature management, including therapeutic hypothermia.	
___	___	___	11. Keep electrode pads on in case of recurrent VT or VF.	
___	___	___	12. Remove gloves, if used. Perform hand hygiene.	
___	___	___	13. Prepare the defibrillator for immediate reuse.	

Skill Checklists for Taylor's Clinical Nursing Skills. A Nursing Process Approach, 5th edition

Name ______________________ Date ______________________

Unit ______________________ Position ______________________

Instructor/Evaluator: ______________________ Position ______________________

SKILL 16-4

Obtaining an Electrocardiogram

Excellent	Satisfactory	Needs Practice	**Goal:** An ECG is obtained without any complications and the patient demonstrates an understanding of the need for and about the ECG.	**Comments**
___	___	___	1. Verify the order/prescription for an ECG in the patient's health record.	
___	___	___	2. Gather all equipment.	
___	___	___	3. Perform hand hygiene and put on PPE, if indicated.	
___	___	___	4. Identify the patient.	
___	___	___	5. Close curtains around the bed and close the door to the room, if possible. As you set up the machine to record a 12-lead ECG, explain the procedure to the patient. Tell the patient that the test records the heart's electrical activity, and it may be repeated at certain intervals. Emphasize that no electrical current will enter his or her body. Tell the patient the test typically takes about 5 minutes. Ask the patient about allergies to adhesive, as appropriate.	
___	___	___	6. Place the ECG machine close to the patient's bed, and plug the power cord into the wall outlet.	
___	___	___	7. If the bed is adjustable, raise it to a comfortable working height, usually elbow height of the caregiver (VHACEOSH, 2016).	
___	___	___	8. Ideally, position the patient supine in the center of the bed with the arms at the sides. Alternately, raise the head of the bed to a semi-Fowler's position, if necessary to promote comfort. Expose the patient's arms and legs, and drape appropriately. Encourage the patient to relax the arms and legs. Ensure the wrists do not touch the waist. Make sure the feet do not touch the bed's footboard.	
___	___	___	9. If necessary, prepare the skin for electrode placement. If an area is excessively hairy, clip the hair. ***Do not shave hair.*** Clean excess oil or other substances from the skin with skin cleanser and water. Use a gauze pad to vigorously rub and dry the skin.	

Excellent	Satisfactory	Needs Practice	SKILL 16-4 **Obtaining an Electrocardiogram** *(Continued)*	Comments
___	___	___	10. Apply the limb electrodes. Peel the contact paper off the self-sticking disposable electrode and apply directly to the prepared site, as recommended by the manufacturer. Connect the limb lead wires to the electrodes. The tip of each lead wire is lettered and color coded for easy identification. The white or RA lead goes to the right arm, just above the wrist bone; the green or RL lead to the right leg, just above the ankle bone; the red or LL lead to the left leg, just above the ankle bone; the black or LA lead to the left arm, just above the wrist bone.	
___	___	___	11. Expose the patient's chest. Apply the chest electrodes. Peel the contact paper off the self-sticking, disposable electrode and apply directly to the prepared site, as recommended by the manufacturer. Connect the chest lead wires to the electrodes. The tip of each lead wire is lettered and color coded for easy identification. The V_1 to V_6 leads are applied to the chest. Position chest electrodes as follows:	
___	___	___	• V_1: (Red) Fourth intercostal space at right sternal border	
___	___	___	• V_2: (Yellow) Fourth intercostal space at left sternal border	
___	___	___	• V_3: (Green) Exactly midway between V_2 and V_4	
___	___	___	• V_4: (Blue) Fifth intercostal space at the left midclavicular line	
___	___	___	• V_5: (Orange) Left anterior axillary line, same horizontal plane as V_4 and V_6	
___	___	___	• V_6: (Purple) Left midaxillary line, same horizontal plane as V_4 and V_5	
___	___	___	12. After the application of all the leads, ensure that the cables are not pulling on the electrodes or lying over each other. Make sure the paper-speed selector is set to the standard 25 mm/sec and that the machine is set to full voltage.	
___	___	___	13. Enter the appropriate patient identification data into the machine. Depending on facility policy, enter the patient's name, health record number, and age and sex.	
___	___	___	14. Ask the patient to relax and breathe normally. ***Instruct the patient to lie still and not to talk while the ECG is being recorded.***	

Excellent	Satisfactory	Needs Practice	SKILL 16-4 **Obtaining an Electrocardiogram** *(Continued)*	Comments
___	___	___	15. Press the AUTO button. Observe the tracing quality. The machine will record all 12 leads automatically, recording 3 consecutive leads simultaneously. Some machines have a display screen so you can preview waveforms before the machine records them on paper. Adjust waveform, if necessary. If any part of the waveform extends beyond the paper when you record the ECG, adjust the normal standardization to half-standardization and repeat. Note this adjustment on the ECG strip, because this will need to be considered in interpreting the results.	
___	___	___	16. When the machine finishes recording the 12-lead ECG, remove the electrodes and clean the patient's skin, if necessary, with adhesive remover for sticky residue.	
___	___	___	17. After disconnecting the lead wires from the electrodes, dispose of the electrodes. Return the patient to a comfortable position. Lower bed height and adjust the head of bed to a comfortable position.	
___	___	___	18. Clean the ECG machine per facility policy. If not done electronically from data entered into the machine, label the ECG with the patient's name, date of birth, location, date and time of recording, and other relevant information, such as symptoms that occurred during the recording. Note any deviations to the standard approach to the recording, such as alternative placement of leads.	
___	___	___	19. Remove additional PPE, if used. Perform hand hygiene.	

Skill Checklists for Taylor's Clinical Nursing Skills.
A Nursing Process Approach, 5th edition

Name ______________________ Date ______________________

Unit ______________________ Position ______________________

Instructor/Evaluator: ______________________ Position ______________________

SKILL 16-5

Applying a Cardiac Monitor

Excellent	Satisfactory	Needs Practice	**Goal:** A clear waveform, free from artifact, is displayed on the cardiac monitor.	**Comments**
___	___	___	1. Verify the order for cardiac monitoring in the patient's health record.	
___	___	___	2. Gather equipment.	
___	___	___	3. Perform hand hygiene and put on PPE, if indicated.	
___	___	___	4. Identify the patient.	
___	___	___	5. Close curtains around the bed and close the door to the room, if possible. Explain the procedure to the patient. Tell the patient that the monitoring records the heart's electrical activity. Emphasize that no electrical current will enter his or her body. Ask the patient about allergies to adhesive, as appropriate.	
___	___	___	6. For hardwire monitoring, plug the cardiac monitor into an electrical outlet and turn it on to warm up the unit while preparing the equipment and the patient. For telemetry monitoring, insert a new battery into the transmitter. Match the poles on the battery with the polar markings on the transmitter case. Press the button at the top of the unit, test the battery's charge, and test the unit to ensure that the battery is operational.	
___	___	___	7. Insert the cable into the appropriate socket in the monitor.	
___	___	___	8. Connect the lead wires to the cable. In some systems, the lead wires are permanently secured to the cable. For telemetry, if the lead wires are not permanently affixed to the telemetry unit, attach them securely. If they must be attached individually, connect each one to the correct outlet.	
___	___	___	9. Connect an electrode to each of the lead wires, carefully checking that each lead wire is in its correct outlet.	
___	___	___	10. If the bed is adjustable, raise it to a comfortable working height, usually elbow height of the caregiver (VHACEOSH, 2016).	

Excellent	Satisfactory	Needs Practice	SKILL 16-5 **Applying a Cardiac Monitor** *(Continued)*	**Comments**
____	____	____	11. Expose the patient's chest and determine electrode positions, based on which system and leads are being used. If necessary, clip the hair from an area about 10 cm in diameter around each electrode site. ***Do not shave hair.*** Clean excess oil or other substances from the skin with skin cleanser and water. Use a gauze pad to vigorously rub and dry the skin.	
____	____	____	12. Remove the backing from the pregelled electrode. Check the gel for moistness. If the gel is dry, discard it and replace it with a fresh electrode. ***Apply the electrode to the site and press firmly to ensure a tight seal.*** Repeat with the remaining electrodes to complete the three- or five-lead system.	
____	____	____	13. When all the electrodes are in place, connect the appropriate lead wire to each electrode. Check waveform for clarity, position, and size. ***To verify that the monitor is detecting each beat, compare the digital heart rate display with an auscultated count of the patient's heart rate.*** If necessary, use the gain control to adjust the size of the rhythm tracing, and use the position control to adjust the waveform position on the monitor.	
____	____	____	14. Set the upper and lower limits of the heart rate alarm, based on the patient's condition or unit policy.	
____	____	____	15. For telemetry, place the transmitter in the pouch in the patient gown. If no pouch is available in the gown, use a portable pouch. Tie the pouch strings around the patient's neck and waist, making sure that the pouch fits snugly without causing discomfort. If no pouch is available, place the transmitter in the patient's bathrobe pocket.	
____	____	____	16. Return the patient to a comfortable position. Lower the bed height and adjust the head of bed to a comfortable position.	
____	____	____	17. To obtain a rhythm strip, press the RECORD key, either at the bedside for monitoring or at the central station for telemetry. Analyze the strip, as appropriate. If the rhythm strip is a printed copy, label the strip with the patient's name and room number, date, time, and rhythm identification. Place the rhythm strip in the appropriate location in the patient's health record, based on facility policy.	
____	____	____	18. Remove additional PPE, if used. Perform hand hygiene.	

Skill Checklists for Taylor's Clinical Nursing Skills. A Nursing Process Approach, 5th edition

Name ______________________ Date ______________________

Unit ______________________ Position ______________________

Instructor/Evaluator: ______________________ Position ______________________

SKILL 16-6

Using a Transcutaneous (External) Pacemaker

Goal: The equipment is applied correctly without adverse effect to the patient.

Excellent	Satisfactory	Needs Practice		Comments
___	___	___	1. Verify the order for a transcutaneous pacemaker in the patient's health record.	
___	___	___	2. Gather all equipment.	
___	___	___	3. Perform hand hygiene and put on PPE, if indicated.	
___	___	___	4. Identify the patient.	
___	___	___	5. If the patient is responsive, explain the procedure to the patient. Explain that it involves some discomfort and that you will administer medication to keep him or her comfortable and help him or her to relax. ***Administer analgesia and sedation, as ordered, if not an emergency situation.***	
___	___	___	6. Close curtains around the bed and close the door to the room, if possible. Obtain vital signs.	
___	___	___	7. If necessary, clip the hair over the areas of electrode placement. ***Do not shave the area.*** Use a gauze pad to vigorously rub and dry the skin at the locations where the cardiac monitoring electrodes will be placed.	
___	___	___	8. Attach cardiac monitoring electrodes to the patient in the lead I, II, and III positions. Do this even if the patient is already on telemetry monitoring. If you select the lead II position, adjust the left leg (LL) electrode placement to accommodate the anterior pacing electrode and the patient's anatomy.	
___	___	___	9. Attach the patient monitoring electrodes to the ECG cable and into the ECG input connection on the front of the pacing generator. Set the selector switch to the "Monitor on" position.	
___	___	___	10. Note the ECG waveform on the monitor. Adjust the R-wave beeper volume to a suitable level and activate the alarm by pressing the "Alarm on" button. Set the alarm for 10 to 20 beats lower and 20 to 30 beats higher than the patient's target pacing rate.	
___	___	___	11. Press the "Start/Stop" button for a printout of the waveform.	

Excellent	Satisfactory	Needs Practice	SKILL 16-6 **Using a Transcutaneous (External) Pacemaker** *(Continued)*	Comments
___	___	___	12. Apply the two pacing electrodes. Make sure the patient's skin is clean and dry to ensure good skin contact. Pull the protective strip from the posterior electrode (marked "Back") and apply the electrode on the left side of the thoracic spinal column, just below the scapula.	
___	___	___	13. Apply the anterior pacing electrode (marked "Front"), which has two protective strips—one covering the gelled area and one covering the outer rim. Expose the gelled area and apply it to the skin in the anterior position, to the left of the precordium in the V_2 to the V_5 position. Move this electrode around to get the best waveform. Then expose the electrode's outer rim and firmly press it to the skin.	
___	___	___	14. Prepare to pace the heart. After making sure the energy output in milliamperes (mA) is on 0, connect the electrode cable to the monitor output cable.	
___	___	___	15. Check the waveform, looking for a tall QRS complex in lead II.	
___	___	___	16. Check the selector switch to "Pacer on." Select synchronous (demand) or asynchronous (fixed-rate or nondemand) mode, as prescribed. ***Tell the patient he or she may feel a thumping or twitching sensation. Reassure the patient you will provide analgesic medication if the discomfort is intolerable.***	
___	___	___	17. Set the pacing rate dial to a target pacing rate of 60 to 70 beats/min. Look for pacer artifact or spikes, which will appear as you increase the rate.	
___	___	___	18. Set the pacing current output (in mA), if not automatically done by the pacemaker. For patients with bradycardia, start with the minimal setting and ***slowly increase the amount of energy delivered to the heart by adjusting the "Output" mA dial. Do this until electrical capture is achieved: you will see a pacer spike followed by a widened QRS complex and a tall broad T wave that resembles a premature ventricular contraction.***	
___	___	___	19. Increase output by 2 mA or 10% to ensure capture. ***Do not go higher (unless prescribed or indicated) because of the increased risk of discomfort to the patient.*** Print a strip and place in the patient's health record.	

SKILL 16-6

Using a Transcutaneous (External) Pacemaker *(Continued)*

Excellent	Satisfactory	Needs Practice		Comments
___	___	___	20. Assess for effectiveness of pacing and mechanical capture: observe for pacemaker spike with subsequent capture; assess heart rate and rhythm (using right carotid, brachial, or femoral artery); assess blood pressure; assess for signs of improved cardiac output (increased blood pressure, improved level of consciousness, improved body temperature).	
___	___	___	21. Secure the pacing leads and cable to the patient's body.	
___	___	___	22. Remove PPE, if used. Perform hand hygiene.	
___	___	___	23. Continue to monitor the patient's heart rate and rhythm to assess ventricular response to pacing. Assess the patient's vital signs, skin color, level of consciousness, and peripheral pulses. Take blood pressure in both arms.	
___	___	___	24. Continue to assess the patient's pain and administer analgesia/sedation, as ordered, to ease the discomfort of chest wall muscle contractions (Morton & Fontaine, 2018).	
___	___	___	25. Perform a 12-lead ECG and additional ECG daily or with clinical changes.	
___	___	___	26. Continually monitor the ECG readings, noting capture, sensing, rate, intrinsic beats, and competition of paced and intrinsic rhythms. If the pacemaker is sensing correctly, the sense indicator on the pulse generator should flash with each beat.	

Skill Checklists for Taylor's Clinical Nursing Skills. A Nursing Process Approach, 5th edition

Name ______________________ Date ______________

Unit ______________________ Position ______________

Instructor/Evaluator: ______________________ Position ______________

SKILL 16-7

Obtaining an Arterial Blood Sample From an Arterial Catheter

Goal: A specimen is obtained without compromise to the patency of the arterial line.

Excellent	Satisfactory	Needs Practice		Comments
____	____	____	1. Verify the order for laboratory testing in the patient's health record.	
____	____	____	2. Gather all equipment.	
____	____	____	3. Perform hand hygiene and put on PPE, if indicated.	
____	____	____	4. Identify the patient.	
____	____	____	5. Close curtains around the bed and close the door to the room, if possible. Explain the procedure to the patient.	
____	____	____	6. Assemble equipment on overbed table or other surface within reach.	
____	____	____	7. Adjust the bed to a comfortable working height, usually elbow height of the caregiver (VHACEOSH, 2016).	
____	____	____	8. Compare specimen label with patient identification bracelet. Label should include patient's name and identification number, time specimen was collected, route of collection, identification of the person obtaining the sample, and any other information required by facility policy.	
____	____	____	9. Use blank labels to label the two blood sample collection tubes to be used for discard blood sample and discard flush.	
____	____	____	10. Assist the patient to a comfortable position that provides easy access to the sampling site. Use the bath blanket to cover any exposed area other than the sampling site. Place a waterproof pad under the site.	
____	____	____	11. Put on gloves and goggles or face shield.	
____	____	____	12. Temporarily silence the arterial pressure monitor alarms.	
____	____	____	13. Locate the stopcock nearest the arterial line insertion site. Remove the passive disinfection cap or nonvented cap from the stopcock. If a nonvented cap was removed, use an antimicrobial swab to vigorously scrub the sampling port on the stopcock. Allow to air dry.	

Excellent	Satisfactory	Needs Practice	SKILL 16-7 **Obtaining an Arterial Blood Sample From an Arterial Catheter** *(Continued)*	Comments
___	___	___	14. Attach the needleless Luer adapter to the Vacutainer. Connect the needleless adapter of the Vacutainer to the sampling port of the stopcock. Turn off the stopcock to the flush solution. Insert the labeled blood sample tube for the discard sample into the Vacutainer. Follow facility policy for the volume of discard blood to collect (usually 5 to 10 mL).	
___	___	___	15. Remove the discard syringe and dispose of appropriately, according to facility policy.	
___	___	___	16. Insert each blood sample collection tube into the Vacutainer, keeping the stopcock turned off to the flush solution. For each additional sample required, repeat this procedure. If coagulation tests are included in the required tests, obtain blood for this from the final sample. Apply the rubber cap to the ABG syringe hub, if necessary.	
___	___	___	17. After obtaining the final blood sample, turn off the stopcock to the Vacutainer. Activate the in-line flushing device.	
___	___	___	18. Turn off the stopcock to the patient. Attach a labeled discard blood sample tube to the Vacutainer. Activate the in-line flushing device.	
___	___	___	19. Turn off the stopcock to the sampling port. Remove the Vacutainer. Use an antimicrobial swab to vigorously scrub the sampling port on the stopcock. Allow to air dry. Place a new disinfection cap or sterile nonvented cap on the blood sampling port of the stopcock.	
___	___	___	20. Remove gloves. Reactivate the monitor alarms. Record date and time the samples were obtained on the labels, as well as the required information to identify the person obtaining the samples. If ABG was collected, record oxygen flow rate (or room air) on label. Apply labels to the specimens, according to facility policy. Place in biohazard bags; place ABG sample in bag with ice.	
___	___	___	21. Check the monitor for return of the arterial waveform and pressure reading.	
___	___	___	22. Return the patient to a comfortable position. Lower bed height, if necessary, and adjust head of bed to a comfortable position.	
___	___	___	23. Remove goggles and additional PPE, if used. Perform hand hygiene. Send specimens to the laboratory immediately.	

Skill Checklists for Taylor's Clinical Nursing Skills. A Nursing Process Approach, 5th edition

Name ______________________ Date ______________________

Unit ______________________ Position ______________________

Instructor/Evaluator: ______________________ Position ______________________

SKILL 16-8

Removing Peripheral Arterial Catheters

Goal: The line is removed intact and without injury to the patient.

Excellent	Satisfactory	Needs Practice		Comments
___	___	___	1. Verify the order for removal of the arterial catheter in the patient's health record.	
___	___	___	2. Gather all equipment.	
___	___	___	3. Perform hand hygiene and put on PPE, if indicated.	
___	___	___	4. Identify the patient.	
___	___	___	5. Close curtains around the bed and close the door to the room, if possible. Explain the procedure to the patient.	
___	___	___	6. Maintain an IV infusion of normal saline via another venous access during the procedure, as ordered or per facility guidelines.	
___	___	___	7. If the bed is adjustable, raise it to a comfortable working height, usually elbow height of the caregiver (VHACEOSH, 2016).	
___	___	___	8. Put on clean gloves, goggles, and gown.	
___	___	___	9. Turn off the monitor alarms and then turn off the flow clamp to the flush solution. Carefully remove the stabilization device and/or dressing over the insertion site. Remove any sutures using the suture removal kit; make sure all sutures have been removed.	
___	___	___	10. ***Withdraw the catheter using a gentle, steady motion. Keep the catheter parallel to the blood vessel during withdrawal. Watch for hematoma formation during catheter removal by gently palpating surrounding tissue. If hematoma starts to form, reposition your hands until optimal pressure is obtained to prevent further leakage of blood.***	
___	___	___	11. ***Immediately after withdrawing the catheter, apply pressure over and just above the cannula site with a sterile 4 × 4 gauze pad. Maintain pressure for at least 10 minutes, or per facility policy (longer if bleeding or oozing persists).*** Apply additional pressure to a femoral site or if the patient has a coagulation abnormality or is receiving anticoagulants (Infusion Nurses Society [INS], 2016).	

Excellent	Satisfactory	Needs Practice	SKILL 16-8 **Removing Peripheral Arterial Catheters** *(Continued)*	Comments
___	___	___	12. ***Assess distal pulses every 3 to 5 minutes while pressure is being applied.*** Note: Dorsalis pedis and posterior tibial pulses should be markedly weaker from baseline if sufficient pressure is applied to the femoral artery.	
___	___	___	13. Cover the site with an appropriate dressing and secure the dressing with tape. If stipulated by facility policy, make a pressure dressing for a femoral site by folding four sterile 4 × 4 gauze pads in half, and then applying the dressing.	
___	___	___	14. Cover the dressing with a tight adhesive bandage, per facility policy. Remove goggles and gloves. *If the catheter was in a femoral site*, use these additional interventions: Cover the bandage with a sandbag, depending on facility policy; maintain the patient on bed rest, with the head of the bed elevated less than 30 degrees, for 6 hours with the sandbag in place; instruct the patient not to lift his or her head while on bed rest; and use logrolling to assist the patient in using the bedpan, if needed.	
___	___	___	15. Lower the bed height. Remove additional PPE. Perform hand hygiene. Send specimens to the laboratory immediately.	
___	___	___	16. Observe the site for bleeding. Assess circulation in the extremity distal to the site by evaluating color, pulse, and sensation. Repeat this assessment every 15 minutes for the first 1 hour, every 30 minutes for the next 2 hours, hourly for the next 2 hours, then every 4 hours, or according to facility policy.	

Skill Checklists for Taylor's Clinical Nursing Skills.
A Nursing Process Approach, 5th edition

Name ______________________ Date ______________________

Unit ______________________ Position ______________________

Instructor/Evaluator: ______________________ Position ______________________

SKILL 17-1

Applying a Two-Piece Cervical Collar

Excellent	Satisfactory	Needs Practice	**Goal:** The patient's cervical spine is immobilized.	**Comments**
___	___	___	1. Review the medical record and nursing care plan to determine the need for placement of a cervical collar. Identify any movement limitations. Gather the necessary supplies.	
___	___	___	2. Perform hand hygiene and put on PPE, if indicated.	
___	___	___	3. Identify the patient.	
___	___	___	4. Assemble equipment to the bedside stand or overbed table or other surface within reach.	
___	___	___	5. Close curtains around the bed and close the door to the room, if possible. Explain what you are going to do and why you are going to do it to the patient.	
___	___	___	6. Assess the patient for any changes in neurologic status (see Fundamentals.	
___	___	___	7. Place the bed at an appropriate and comfortable working height, usually elbow height of the caregiver (VHACEOSH, 2016). Lower the side rails as necessary.	
___	___	___	8. Gently clean the patient's face and neck with a skin cleanser and water. If the patient has experienced trauma, inspect the area for broken glass or other material that could cut the patient or the nurse. Pat the area dry.	
___	___	___	9. If the patient has experienced trauma or injury, have a second caregiver in position to hold the patient's head firmly on either side above the ears. Measure from the bottom of the chin to the top of the sternum, and measure around the neck. Match these height and circumference measurements to the manufacturer's recommended size chart.	
___	___	___	10. Slide the flattened back portion of the collar under the patient's head. ***The center of the collar should line up with the center of the patient's neck. Do not allow the patient's head to move when passing the collar under the head.***	

SKILL 17-1

Applying a Two-Piece Cervical Collar *(Continued)*

Excellent	Satisfactory	Needs Practice		Comments
___	___	___	11. Place the front of the collar centered over the chin, while ensuring that the chin area fits snugly in the recess. Be sure that the front half of the collar overlaps the back half. Secure Velcro straps on both sides. Check to see that at least one finger can be inserted between collar and patient's neck.	
___	___	___	12. Raise the side rails. Place the bed in lowest position. Make sure the call bell is in reach.	
___	___	___	13. Reassess the patient's neurologic status and comfort level.	
___	___	___	14. Remove PPE, if used. Perform hand hygiene.	
___	___	___	15. ***Assess the skin under the cervical collar and at contact points on the chin, shoulder, and ear at least every 4 hours for any signs of skin breakdown. Remove the collar every 8 to 12 hours and inspect and cleanse the skin under the collar, drying well before replacement. When the collar is removed, if the patient has experienced trauma or injury, have a second person immobilize the cervical spine.***	

Skill Checklists for Taylor's Clinical Nursing Skills. A Nursing Process Approach, 5th edition

Name ____________________ Date ____________________

Unit ____________________ Position ____________________

Instructor/Evaluator: ____________________ Position ____________________

Excellent	Satisfactory	Needs Practice	SKILL 17-2 **Employing Seizure Precautions and Seizure Management** **Goal:** The patient remains free from injury and that the sequence of signs and symptoms is observed and recorded.	Comments
___	___	___	1. Review the health record and nursing care plan for conditions that would place the patient at risk for seizures. Review the medical orders and the nursing care plan for orders for seizure precautions.	
			Seizure Precautions	
___	___	___	2. Gather the necessary supplies.	
___	___	___	3. Perform hand hygiene and put on PPE, if indicated.	
___	___	___	4. Identify the patient.	
___	___	___	5. Assemble equipment to the bedside stand or overbed table or other surface within reach.	
___	___	___	6. Close curtains around the bed and close the door to the room, if possible. Explain what you are going to do and why you are going to do it to the patient.	
___	___	___	7. Place the bed in the lowest position with two to three side rails elevated. Apply padding to the side rails.	
___	___	___	8. Attach oxygen apparatus to oxygen access in the wall at the head of the bed. Place nasal cannula or mask equipment in a location where it can be easily reached, if needed.	
___	___	___	9. Attach suction apparatus to vacuum access in the wall at the head of the bed. Place suction catheter, oral airway, and resuscitation bag in a location where they are easily reached, if needed.	
___	___	___	10. Remove PPE, if used. Perform hand hygiene.	
			Seizure Management	
___	___	___	11. For patients with known seizures, be alert for the occurrence of an aura, if known. If the patient reports experiencing an aura, have the patient lie down.	
___	___	___	12. Once a seizure begins, close the curtains around the bed and close the door to the room, if possible.	
___	___	___	13. If the patient is seated, ease the patient to the floor.	

Excellent	Satisfactory	Needs Practice	SKILL 17-2 **Employing Seizure Precautions and Seizure Management** *(Continued)*	Comments
___	___	___	14. Remove patient's eyeglasses. Loosen any constricting clothing. Place something flat and soft, such as a folded blanket, under the head. Push aside furniture or other objects in area.	
___	___	___	15. If the patient is in bed, remove the pillow, place bed in lowest position, and raise side rails.	
___	___	___	16. Do not restrain patient. Guide movements, if necessary. Do not try to insert anything in the patient's mouth or open jaws.	
___	___	___	17. If possible, place patient on the side with the head flexed forward, head of bed elevated 30 degrees. Begin administration of oxygen, based on facility policy. Clear airway using suction, as appropriate.	
___	___	___	18. Provide supervision throughout the seizure and time the length of the seizure.	
___	___	___	19. Establish/maintain intravenous access, as necessary. Administer medications, as appropriate, based on medical order and facility policy.	
___	___	___	20. After the seizure, place the patient in a side-lying position. Clear airway using suction, as appropriate.	
___	___	___	21. Monitor vital signs, oxygen saturation, response to medications administered, and capillary glucose, as appropriate.	
___	___	___	22. Place the bed in the lowest position. Make sure the call bell is in reach.	
___	___	___	23. Reassess the patient's neurologic status and comfort level.	
___	___	___	24. Allow the patient to sleep after the seizure. On awakening, orient and reassure the patient. Reassess, as indicated.	
___	___	___	25. Remove PPE, if used. Perform hand hygiene.	

Skill Checklists for Taylor's Clinical Nursing Skills. A Nursing Process Approach, 5th edition

Name ________________ Date ________________

Unit ________________ Position ________________

Instructor/Evaluator: ________________ Position ________________

SKILL 17-3

Caring for a Patient in Halo Traction

Excellent	Satisfactory	Needs Practice	Goal: The patient maintains cervical alignment.	Comments
___	___	___	1. Review the health record and the nursing care plan to determine the type of device being used and prescribed care.	
___	___	___	2. Gather the necessary equipment.	
___	___	___	3. Perform hand hygiene and put on PPE, if indicated.	
___	___	___	4. Identify the patient.	
___	___	___	5. Assemble equipment to the bedside stand or overbed table or other surface within reach.	
___	___	___	6. Close curtains around the bed and close the door to the room, if possible. Explain what you are going to do and why you are going to do it to the patient.	
___	___	___	7. Assess the patient for possible need for nonpharmacologic, pain-reducing interventions or analgesic medication before beginning. Administer appropriate prescribed analgesic. Allow sufficient time for analgesic to achieve its effectiveness before beginning the procedure.	
___	___	___	8. Place a waste receptacle at a convenient location for use during the procedure.	
___	___	___	9. Adjust bed to comfortable working height, usually elbow height of the caregiver, if the patient will remain in bed (VHACEOSH, 2016). Alternatively, have the patient sit up, if appropriate.	
___	___	___	10. Assist the patient to a comfortable position that provides easy access to the head. Place a waterproof pad under the head if the patient is lying down.	
___	___	___	11. Monitor vital signs and perform a neurologic assessment, including level of consciousness, motor function, and sensation, per facility policy. This is usually at least every 2 hours for 24 hours, or possibly every hour for 48 hours.	
___	___	___	12. Examine the halo vest unit every 8 hours for stability, secure connections, and positioning. Make sure the patient's head is centered in the halo without neck flexion or extension. Check each bolt for loosening.	
___	___	___	13. Check the fit of the vest. With the patient in a supine position, you should be able to insert one or two fingers under the jacket at the shoulder and chest.	

Excellent	Satisfactory	Needs Practice	SKILL 17-3 **Caring for a Patient in Halo Traction** *(Continued)*	Comments
___	___	___	14. Put on nonsterile gloves, if appropriate. Remove patient's shirt or gown. Wash the patient's chest and back daily. Loosen the bottom Velcro straps. Protect the vest liner with a waterproof pad.	
___	___	___	15. Wring out a bath towel soaked in warm water (and skin cleanser, depending on facility policy). Pull the towel back and forth in a drying motion beneath the front.	
___	___	___	16. Thoroughly dry the skin in the same manner with a dry towel. Inspect the skin for tender, reddened areas or pressure spots. Do not use powder or lotion under the vest.	
___	___	___	17. Turn the patient on his or her side, less than 45 degrees if lying supine, and repeat the process on the back. Remove waterproof pad from the vest liner. Close the Velcro straps. Assist the patient with putting on a new shirt, if desired.	
___	___	___	18. Perform a respiratory assessment. Check for respiratory impairment, such as absence of breath sounds, the presence of adventitious sounds, reduced inspiratory effort, or shortness of breath.	
___	___	___	19. Assess the pin sites for redness, tenting of the skin; prolonged or purulent drainage; swelling; and bowing, bending, or loosening of the pins. Monitor body temperature.	
___	___	___	20. Perform pin-site care.	
___	___	___	21. Depending on medical order and facility policy, apply antimicrobial ointment to pin sites and a dressing.	
___	___	___	22. Remove gloves and dispose of them appropriately. Raise rails, as appropriate, and place the bed in the lowest position. Assist the patient to a comfortable position.	
___	___	___	23. Remove additional PPE, if used. Perform hand hygiene.	

Skill Checklists for Taylor's Clinical Nursing Skills. A Nursing Process Approach, 5th edition

Name ______________________ Date ______________________

Unit ______________________ Position ______________________

Instructor/Evaluator: ______________________ Position ______________________

SKILL 17-4

Caring for a Patient With an External Ventriculostomy (Intraventricular Catheter–Closed Fluid-Filled System)

Excellent	Satisfactory	Needs Practice	**Goal:** The patient maintains intracranial pressure at less than 15 mm Hg, and cerebral perfusion pressure at 50 to 70 mm Hg.	**Comments**
___	___	___	1. Review the medical orders and patient health record for specific information about ventriculostomy parameters.	
___	___	___	2. Gather the necessary supplies.	
___	___	___	3. Perform hand hygiene and put on PPE, if indicated.	
___	___	___	4. Identify the patient.	
___	___	___	5. Assemble equipment to the bedside stand or overbed table or other surface within reach.	
___	___	___	6. Close curtains around the bed and close the door to the room, if possible. Explain what you are going to do and why you are going to do it to the patient.	
___	___	___	7. Assess patient for any changes in neurologic status.	
___	___	___	8. Set the zero reference level. ***Assess the height of the ventriculostomy system to ensure that the stopcock is at the appropriate reference point: the tragus of the ear, the outer canthus of the patient's eye, or the patient's external auditory canal*** (American Association of Neuroscience Nurses [AANN], 2011) using carpenter level, bubble-line level, or laser level, according to facility policy. Adjust the height of the system, if needed.	
___	___	___	9. Set the pressure level based on prescribed pressure. Move the drip chamber to the ordered height. Assess the amount of CSF in the drip chamber if the ventriculostomy is draining.	
___	___	___	10. ***Zero the transducer.*** Turn the stopcock off to the patient. Remove the cap from the transducer, being careful not to touch the end of the cap. Press and hold the calibration button on the monitor until the monitor beeps. Return the cap to the transducer. ***Turn the stopcock off to the drip chamber to obtain an ICP reading and waveform tracing. After obtaining a reading, turn the stopcock off to the transducer.***	

Excellent	Satisfactory	Needs Practice	SKILL 17-4 **Caring for a Patient With an External Ventriculostomy (Intraventricular Catheter–Closed Fluid-Filled System)** *(Continued)*	Comments
___	___	___	11. ***Adjust the ventriculostomy height to prevent too much drainage, too little drainage, or inaccurate ICP readings.***	
___	___	___	12. Care for the insertion site according to the facility's policy. Maintain the system using strict sterile technique. Assess the site for any signs of infection, such as purulent drainage, redness, or warmth. Ensure the catheter is secured at site per facility policy. If the catheter is sutured to the scalp, assess integrity of the sutures.	
___	___	___	13. Calculate the CPP, if necessary. Calculate the difference between the systemic MAP and the ICP.	
___	___	___	14. Remove PPE, if used. Perform hand hygiene.	
___	___	___	15. Assess ICP, MAP, and CPP continuously or intermittently as prescribed (AACN, 2017). Note drainage amount, color, clarity. If there is an increase in the ICP, the value should be obtained more often, as often as every 15 minutes (AANN, 2011).	
___	___	___	16. Assess ICP drainage system at least every 4 hours, checking the insertion site, all drainage system tubing and parts, for cracks in the system, or leakage from insertion site or system. Label external ventriculostomy tubing and access ports clearly.	

Skill Checklists for Taylor's Clinical Nursing Skills.
A Nursing Process Approach, 5th edition

Name ______________________ Date ______________________

Unit ______________________ Position ______________________

Instructor/Evaluator: ______________________ Position ______________________

SKILL 17-5

Caring for a Patient With a Fiber Optic Intracranial Catheter

Goal: The patient maintains ICP less than 15 mm Hg, and CPP 50 to 70 mm Hg.

Excellent	Satisfactory	Needs Practice		Comments
___	___	___	1. Review the medical orders and health record for specific information about monitoring parameters.	
___	___	___	2. Perform hand hygiene and put on PPE, if indicated.	
___	___	___	3. Identify the patient.	
___	___	___	4. Close curtains around the bed and close the door to the room, if possible. Explain what you are going to do and why you are going to do it to the patient.	
___	___	___	5. Assess the patient for any changes in neurologic status.	
___	___	___	6. Assess ICP, MAP, and CPP continuously or intermittently as prescribed (AACN, 2017). Note ICP value and waveforms as shown on the monitor. If there is an increase in the ICP, the value should be obtained more often, as often as every 15 minutes (AANN, 2011).	
___	___	___	7. Care for the insertion site according to the facility's policy. Maintain the system using strict sterile technique. Assess the site for any signs of infection, such as drainage, redness, or warmth. Ensure the catheter is secured at site per facility policy.	
___	___	___	8. Calculate the CPP, if necessary. Calculate the difference between the systemic MAP and the ICP.	
___	___	___	9. Remove PPE, if used. Perform hand hygiene.	

Skill Checklists for Taylor's Clinical Nursing Skills. A Nursing Process Approach, 5th edition

Name ______________________ Date ______________________

Unit ______________________ Position ______________________

Instructor/Evaluator: ______________________ Position ______________________

SKILL 18-1

Obtaining a Nasal Swab

Goal: An uncontaminated specimen is obtained without injury to the patient and sent to the laboratory promptly.

Excellent	Satisfactory	Needs Practice		Comments
___	___	___	1. Verify the order for a nasal swab in the patient's health record. Gather equipment. Check the expiration date on the swab package.	
___	___	___	2. Perform hand hygiene and put on PPE, if indicated.	
___	___	___	3. Identify the patient.	
___	___	___	4. Explain the procedure to the patient. Discuss with the patient the need for a nasal swab. Explain to the patient the process by which the specimen will be collected.	
___	___	___	5. Check the specimen label with the patient identification bracelet. Label should include the patient's name and identification number, time specimen was collected, route of collection, identification of the person obtaining the sample, and any other information required by facility policy.	
___	___	___	6. Assemble equipment on overbed table or other surface within reach.	
___	___	___	7. Close curtains around the bed or close the door to the room, if possible.	
___	___	___	8. Put on goggles and face mask, or face shield and nonsterile gloves.	
___	___	___	9. Place the bed at an appropriate and comfortable working height, usually elbow height of the caregiver (VHACEOSH, 2016). Ask the patient to tip his or her head back slightly. Assist, as necessary.	
___	___	___	10. Peel open the swab kit packaging to expose the swab and collection tube. Remove the white plug from the collection tube and discard. Remove the swab from packaging by grasping the exposed end. Take care not to contaminate the swab by touching it to any other surface. Moisten with sterile water, depending on facility policy.	
___	___	___	11. Insert swab 2 cm into one naris and rotate against the anterior nasal mucosa for 3 seconds or five rotations, depending on facility policy, and then keep it in place for 15 seconds.	

Excellent	Satisfactory	Needs Practice	SKILL 18-1 **Obtaining a Nasal Swab** *(Continued)*	Comments
___	___	___	12. Remove the swab and repeat in the second naris, using the same swab.	
___	___	___	13. Insert the swab fully into the collection tube, taking care not to touch any other surface. The handle end of the swab should fit snugly into the collection tube and the end of swab should be in the culture medium at the distal end of the collection tube. Lightly squeeze the bottom of the collection tube as necessary, depending on type of tube in use in facility, to break the seal on the culture medium.	
___	___	___	14. Dispose of used equipment per facility policy. Remove gloves. Perform hand hygiene.	
___	___	___	15. Place label on the collection tube per facility policy. Place container in plastic, sealable biohazard bag.	
___	___	___	16. Remove face shield and other PPE, if used. Perform hand hygiene.	
___	___	___	17. Transport specimen to the laboratory immediately. If immediate transport is not possible, check with laboratory personnel or policy manual whether refrigeration is contraindicated.	

Skill Checklists for Taylor's Clinical Nursing Skills. A Nursing Process Approach, 5th edition

Name ______________________ Date ______________________

Unit ______________________ Position ______________________

Instructor/Evaluator: ______________________ Position ______________________

SKILL 18-2

Obtaining a Nasopharyngeal Swab

Excellent	Satisfactory	Needs Practice	**Goal:** An uncontaminated specimen is obtained without injury to the patient and sent to the laboratory promptly.	Comments
___	___	___	1. Verify the order for a nasopharyngeal swab in the patient's health record. Gather equipment. Check the expiration date on the swab package.	
___	___	___	2. Perform hand hygiene and put on PPE, if indicated.	
___	___	___	3. Identify the patient.	
___	___	___	4. Discuss with patient the need for a nasopharyngeal swab. Explain to patient the process by which the specimen will be collected. Inform the patient that he or she may experience slight discomfort and may gag.	
___	___	___	5. Check the specimen label with the patient's identification bracelet. Label should include the patient's name and identification number, time specimen was collected, route of collection, identification of person obtaining the sample, and any other information required by facility policy.	
___	___	___	6. Assemble equipment on overbed table or other surface within reach.	
___	___	___	7. Close curtains around the bed or close the door to the room, if possible.	
___	___	___	8. Put on goggles and face mask, or face shield and nonsterile gloves.	
___	___	___	9. Place the bed at an appropriate and comfortable working height, usually elbow height of the caregiver (VHACEOSH, 2016). Ask the patient to blow his or her nose into facial tissue. Ask the patient to cough into facial tissue, and then to tip back his or her head. Assist, as necessary.	
___	___	___	10. Peel open the swab packaging to expose the swab and collection tube. Remove the cap from the collection tube and discard. Remove the swab from packaging by grasping the exposed end. Take care not to contaminate the swab by touching it to any other surface.	
___	___	___	11. Ask the patient to open the mouth. Inspect the back of the patient's throat using the tongue depressor.	

Excellent	Satisfactory	Needs Practice	SKILL 18-2 **Obtaining a Nasopharyngeal Swab** *(Continued)*	Comments
____	____	____	12. Continue to observe the nasopharynx and gently insert the swab straight back into the nostril, aiming posteriorly along the floor of the nasal cavity. Insert approximately 6 in (adult) (approximately the distance from the nose to the ear) to the posterior wall of the nasopharynx. ***Do not insert the swab upward. Do not force the swab.*** Rotate the swab. Leave the swab in the nasopharynx for 15 to 30 seconds and remove. Take care not to touch the swab to the patient's tongue or sides of the nostrils.	
____	____	____	13. Insert the swab fully into the collection tube, taking care not to touch any other surface. The handle end of the swab should fit snugly into the collection tube and the end of swab should be in the culture medium at the distal end of the collection tube. Lightly squeeze the bottom of the collection tube as necessary, depending on type of tube in use in facility, to break the seal on the culture medium.	
____	____	____	14. Dispose of used equipment per facility policy. Remove gloves. Perform hand hygiene.	
____	____	____	15. Place label on the collection tube per facility policy. Place container in plastic, sealable biohazard bag.	
____	____	____	16. Remove other PPE, if used. Perform hand hygiene.	
____	____	____	17. Transport the specimen to the laboratory immediately. If immediate transport is not possible, check with laboratory personnel or policy manual whether refrigeration is contraindicated.	

Skill Checklists for Taylor's Clinical Nursing Skills.
A Nursing Process Approach, 5th edition

Name ____________________ Date ____________________

Unit ____________________ Position ____________________

Instructor/Evaluator: ____________________ Position ____________________

SKILL 18-3

Collecting a Sputum Specimen for Culture

Excellent	Satisfactory	Needs Practice	**Goal:** The patient produces an adequate sample from the lower respiratory tract.	Comments
___	___	___	1. Verify the order for a sputum specimen collection in the patient's health record. Gather equipment.	
___	___	___	2. Perform hand hygiene and put on PPE, if indicated.	
___	___	___	3. Identify the patient.	
___	___	___	4. Explain the procedure to the patient. Administer pain medication (if ordered) if the patient might have pain with coughing. If the patient can perform the task without assistance after instruction, leave the container at bedside with instructions to call the nurse as soon as a specimen is produced.	
___	___	___	5. Check specimen label with the patient's identification bracelet. Label should include the patient's name and identification number, time specimen was collected, route of collection, identification of the person obtaining the sample, and any other information required by facility policy.	
___	___	___	6. Assemble equipment on overbed table or other surface within reach.	
___	___	___	7. Close curtains around the bed and close the door to the room, if possible.	
___	___	___	8. Put on disposable gloves and goggles, safety glasses or face shield, as indicated.	
___	___	___	9. Place the bed at an appropriate and comfortable working height, usually elbow height of the caregiver (VHACEOSH, 2016). Lower side rail closest to you. Place patient in semi-Fowler's position. ***Have patient clear nose and throat and rinse mouth with water before beginning procedure.***	
___	___	___	10. Caution the patient to avoid spitting saliva secretion into the sterile container. Explain the importance of obtaining sputum from lower respiratory tract. ***Instruct the patient to inhale deeply two or three times and cough with exhalation.*** If the patient has had abdominal surgery, assist the patient to splint the abdomen.	

Excellent	Satisfactory	Needs Practice	SKILL 18-3 **Collecting a Sputum Specimen for Culture** *(Continued)*	Comments
___	___	___	11. If the patient produces sputum, open the lid to the container and have the patient expectorate the specimen into the container. Caution the patient to avoid touching the edge or the inside of the collection container.	
___	___	___	12. If patient believes he or she can produce more sputum for the specimen, have the patient repeat the procedure. Collect a volume of sputum based on facility policy.	
___	___	___	13. Close the container lid. Offer oral hygiene to the patient.	
___	___	___	14. Remove equipment and return the patient to a position of comfort. Raise side rails and lower bed.	
___	___	___	15. Remove gloves and goggles. Perform hand hygiene.	
___	___	___	16. Place label on the container per facility policy. Place container in plastic, sealable biohazard bag.	
___	___	___	17. Remove other PPE, if used. Perform hand hygiene.	
___	___	___	18. Transport the specimen to the laboratory immediately. If immediate transport is not possible, do not refrigerate specimens (Fischbach & Dunning, 2015).	

Skill Checklists for Taylor's Clinical Nursing Skills.
A Nursing Process Approach, 5th edition

Name ______________________________ Date ______________________

Unit ______________________________ Position ______________________

Instructor/Evaluator: ______________________ Position ______________________

SKILL 18-4

Collecting a Urine Specimen (Clean Catch, Midstream)

Goal: An adequate amount of urine is obtained from the patient without contamination.

Excellent	Satisfactory	Needs Practice	Step	Comments
____	____	____	1. Verify the order for a urine specimen collection in the patient's health record. Gather equipment.	
____	____	____	2. Perform hand hygiene and put on PPE, if indicated.	
____	____	____	3. Identify the patient.	
____	____	____	4. Explain the procedure to the patient. If the patient can perform the task without assistance after instruction, leave the container at bedside with instructions to call the nurse as soon as a specimen is produced.	
____	____	____	5. Check the specimen label with the patient's identification bracelet. Label should include the patient's name and identification number, time specimen was collected, route of collection, identification of the person obtaining the sample, and any other information required by facility policy.	
____	____	____	6. Assemble equipment on overbed table or other surface within reach.	
____	____	____	7. Have the patient perform hand hygiene, if performing self-collection.	
____	____	____	8. Close curtains around the bed and close the door to the room, if possible.	
____	____	____	9. Put on nonsterile gloves. Assist the patient to the bathroom, or onto the bedside commode or bedpan. Instruct the patient not to defecate or discard toilet paper into the urine.	
____	____	____	10. Instruct the female patient to separate the labia for cleaning of the area and during collection of urine. Female patients should use the towelettes or wet washcloth to clean each side of the urinary meatus, then the center over the meatus, from front to back, using a new wipe or a clean area of the washcloth for each stroke. Instruct the female patient to ***keep the labia separated after cleaning and during collection.*** Male patients should use a towelette to clean the area around the meatus of the penis, wiping in a circular motion away from the urethral meatus. Instruct the uncircumcised male patient to retract the foreskin before cleaning and during collection.	

Excellent	Satisfactory	Needs Practice	SKILL 18-4 **Collecting a Urine Specimen (Clean Catch, Midstream)** *(Continued)*	Comments
___	___	___	11. ***Do not let the container touch the perineal skin or hair during collection. Do not touch the inside of the container or the lid. Have patient void a small amount (approximately 25 to 30 mL/1 oz) of urine into the toilet, bedpan, or commode. The patient should then stop urinating briefly, and then continue voiding into the collection container.*** Collect the urine specimen (3 to 5 mL is sufficient), and then instruct the patient to finish voiding in the toilet, bedpan, or commode. Instruct the uncircumcised male patient to replace the foreskin after collection.	
___	___	___	12. Place lid on container. If necessary, transfer the specimen to appropriate containers/tubes for specific test ordered, according to facility policy.	
___	___	___	13. Assist the patient from the bathroom, off the commode, or off the bedpan. Provide perineal care, if necessary.	
___	___	___	14. Remove gloves and perform hand hygiene.	
___	___	___	15. Place label on the container per facility policy. Note specimen collection method, according to facility policy. Place container in plastic, sealable biohazard bag.	
___	___	___	16. Remove other PPE, if used. Perform hand hygiene.	
___	___	___	17. Transport the specimen to the laboratory as soon as possible. If unable to take the specimen to the laboratory immediately, refrigerate it (Fischbach & Dunning, 2015).	

Skill Checklists for Taylor's Clinical Nursing Skills. A Nursing Process Approach, 5th edition

Name ______________________ Date ______________________

Unit ______________________ Position ______________________

Instructor/Evaluator: ______________________ Position ______________________

SKILL 18-5

Obtaining a Urine Specimen From an Indwelling Urinary Catheter

Goal: An adequate amount of urine is obtained from the patient without contamination or adverse effect.

Excellent	Satisfactory	Needs Practice		Comments
___	___	___	1. Verify the order for a urine specimen collection in the patient's health record. Gather equipment.	
___	___	___	2. Perform hand hygiene and put on PPE, if indicated.	
___	___	___	3. Identify the patient.	
___	___	___	4. Explain the procedure to the patient.	
___	___	___	5. Check the specimen label with the patient's identification bracelet. Label should include the patient's name and identification number, time specimen was collected, route of collection, identification of person obtaining the sample, and any other information required by facility policy.	
___	___	___	6. Assemble equipment on overbed table or other surface within reach.	
___	___	___	7. Close curtains around the bed and close the door to the room, if possible.	
___	___	___	8. Put on nonsterile gloves.	
___	___	___	9. Clamp the catheter drainage tubing or bend it back on itself distal to the port. If an insufficient amount of urine is present in the tubing, allow the tubing to remain clamped up to 30 minutes, to collect a sufficient amount of urine, unless contraindicated. Remove lid from specimen container, keeping the inside of the container and lid free from contamination.	
___	___	___	10. ***Scrub aspiration port vigorously with alcohol or other disinfectant wipe and allow port to air dry.***	
___	___	___	11. Attach the syringe to the needleless port. Alternately, insert the blunt-tipped cannula into the port. Slowly aspirate enough urine for specimen (usually 3 to 5 mL is adequate; check facility requirements). Remove the syringe from the port. Engage the needle guard, if needle was used. ***Unclamp the drainage tubing.***	

Excellent	Satisfactory	Needs Practice	SKILL 18-5 **Obtaining a Urine Specimen From an Indwelling Urinary Catheter** *(Continued)*	Comments
____	____	____	12. If a needle or blunt-tipped cannula was used on the syringe, remove from the syringe before emptying the urine from the syringe into the specimen cup. Place the needle into a sharps collection container. ***Slowly inject urine into the specimen container. Take care to avoid touching the syringe tip to any surface. Do not touch the edge or inside of the collection container.***	
____	____	____	13. Replace lid on container. If necessary, transfer the specimen to appropriate containers/tubes for specific test ordered, according to facility policy. Dispose of syringe in a sharps collection container.	
____	____	____	14. Remove gloves and perform hand hygiene.	
____	____	____	15. Place label on the container per facility policy. Note specimen collection method, according to facility policy. Place container in plastic sealable biohazard bag.	
____	____	____	16. Remove other PPE, if used. Perform hand hygiene.	
____	____	____	17. Transport the specimen to the laboratory as soon as possible. If unable to take the specimen to the laboratory immediately, refrigerate it (Fischbach & Dunning, 2015).	

Skill Checklists for Taylor's Clinical Nursing Skills.
A Nursing Process Approach, 5th edition

Name ______________________ Date ______________________

Unit ______________________ Position ______________________

Instructor/Evaluator: ______________________ Position ______________________

SKILL 18-6

Testing Stool for Occult Blood

Excellent	Satisfactory	Needs Practice	**Goal:** An uncontaminated stool sample is obtained, following collection guidelines, and then transported to the laboratory within the recommended time frame.	**Comments**
___	___	___	1. Verify the order for a stool specimen collection in the patient's health record. Gather equipment.	
___	___	___	2. Perform hand hygiene and put on PPE, if indicated.	
___	___	___	3. Identify the patient.	
___	___	___	4. Discuss with the patient the need for a stool sample. Explain to the patient the process by which the stool will be collected, either from a bedpan, commode, or plastic receptacle in the toilet.	
___	___	___	5. If sending the specimen to the laboratory, check specimen label with patient identification bracelet. Label should include the patient's name and identification number, time specimen was collected, route of collection, identification of the person obtaining the sample, and any other information required by facility policy.	
___	___	___	6. Assemble equipment on overbed table or other surface within reach.	
___	___	___	7. Close curtains around the bed or close the door to the room, if possible.	
___	___	___	8. Place the plastic collection receptacle in the toilet, if applicable. Assist the patient to the bathroom or onto the bedside commode, or onto the bedpan. Instruct the patient not to urinate or discard toilet paper with the stool.	
___	___	___	9. After the patient defecates, assist the patient out of the bathroom, off the commode, or remove the bedpan. Perform hand hygiene and put on disposable gloves.	
			If using gFOBT:	
___	___	___	10. Open flap on sample side of card. With wooden applicator, apply a small amount of stool from the center of the bowel movement onto one window of the testing card. With the opposite end of the wooden applicator, obtain another sample of stool from another area and apply a small amount of stool onto second window of testing card.	
___	___	___	11. Close flap over stool samples.	

SKILL 18-6

Testing Stool for Occult Blood *(Continued)*

Excellent	Satisfactory	Needs Practice		Comments
___	___	___	12. If sending stool to the laboratory, label the specimen card per facility policy. Place in a sealable plastic biohazard bag and send to the laboratory immediately.	
___	___	___	13. If testing at the point of care, wait 3 to 5 minutes before developing. Open flap on opposite side of card and place two drops of developer over each window and ***wait the time stated in the manufacturer's instructions.***	
___	___	___	14. Observe card for any blue areas.	
			If using FIT:	
___	___	___	15. Open flap on sample side of card. With applicator, brush, or sampling probe, apply a small amount of stool from the center of the bowel movement onto the top half of window of the testing card. With the opposite end of the device, obtain another sample of stool from another area and apply a small amount of stool onto the bottom half of window of testing card.	
___	___	___	16. Use the applicator to mix the samples and spread samples over entire window. Close flap over sample. Allow card to dry.	
___	___	___	17. If sending to the laboratory, label the specimen card per facility policy. Place in a sealable plastic biohazard bag and send to the laboratory immediately.	
___	___	___	18. If testing at the point of care, open collection card according to manufacturer's instructions. Add three drops of developer to center of sample on Sample Pad. Developer should flow through the test (T) line and through the control (C) line. Snap Test Device closed.	
___	___	___	19. Wait 5 minutes, or time specified by manufacturer. Observe card for pink color on the test (T) line. The control (C) line must also turn pink within 5 minutes. If the control (C) line turns pink, read and report the result.	
___	___	___	20. After reading results, discard testing slide appropriately, according to facility policy. Remove gloves and any other PPE, if used. Perform hand hygiene.	

Skill Checklists for Taylor's Clinical Nursing Skills. A Nursing Process Approach, 5th edition

Name ____________________ Date ____________________

Unit ____________________ Position ____________________

Instructor/Evaluator: ____________________ Position ____________________

SKILL 18-7
Collecting a Stool Specimen

Goal: An uncontaminated specimen is obtained and sent to the laboratory promptly.

Excellent	Satisfactory	Needs Practice		Comments
____	____	____	1. Verify the order for a stool specimen collection in the patient's health record. Gather equipment.	
____	____	____	2. Perform hand hygiene and put on PPE, if indicated.	
____	____	____	3. Identify the patient.	
____	____	____	4. Discuss with the patient the need for a stool sample. Explain to the patient the process by which the stool will be collected, either from a bedpan, commode, or plastic receptacle in the toilet to catch stool without urine. Instruct the patient to void first and not to discard toilet paper with stool. Tell the patient to call you as soon as a bowel movement is completed.	
____	____	____	5. Check specimen label with the patient's identification bracelet. Label should include the patient's name and identification number, time specimen was collected, route of collection, identification of the person obtaining the sample, and any other information required by facility policy.	
____	____	____	6. Assemble equipment on overbed table or other surface within reach.	
____	____	____	7. After the patient has passed a stool, put on gloves. Use the tongue blades to obtain a sample, free of blood or urine, and place it in the designated clean specimen container.	
____	____	____	8. Collect as much of the stool as possible to send to the laboratory.	
____	____	____	9. Place lid on container. Dispose of used equipment per facility policy. Remove gloves and perform hand hygiene.	
____	____	____	10. Place label on the container per facility policy. Place container in plastic, sealable biohazard bag.	
____	____	____	11. Remove other PPE, if used. Perform hand hygiene.	
____	____	____	12. Transport the specimen to the laboratory while stool is still warm. If immediate transport is impossible, check with laboratory personnel or policy manual whether refrigeration is contraindicated.	

Skill Checklists for Taylor's Clinical Nursing Skills.
A Nursing Process Approach, 5th edition

Name ______________________ Date ______________________

Unit ______________________ Position ______________________

Instructor/Evaluator: ______________________ Position ______________________

SKILL 18-8

Obtaining a Capillary Blood Sample for Glucose Testing

Goal: The blood glucose level is measured accurately without adverse effect.

Excellent	Satisfactory	Needs Practice		Comments
___	___	___	1. Check the patient's health record or nursing care plan for monitoring schedule. You may decide that additional testing is indicated based on nursing judgment and the patient's condition.	
___	___	___	2. Gather equipment. Check expiration date on blood test strips.	
___	___	___	3. Perform hand hygiene and put on PPE, if indicated.	
___	___	___	4. Identify the patient. Explain the procedure to the patient and instruct the patient about the need for monitoring blood glucose.	
___	___	___	5. Close curtains around the bed and close the door to the room, if possible.	
___	___	___	6. Turn on the monitor.	
___	___	___	7. Enter the patient's identification number or scan his or her identification bracelet, if required, according to facility policy.	
___	___	___	8. Put on nonsterile gloves.	
___	___	___	9. Prepare lancet using aseptic technique.	
___	___	___	10. Remove test strip from the vial. ***Recap container immediately.*** Test strips also come individually wrapped. ***Check that the code number for the strip matches the code number on the monitor screen.***	
___	___	___	11. Insert the strip into the meter according to directions for that specific device. Alternately, strip may be placed in meter after collection of sample on test strip, depending on meter in use.	
___	___	___	12. ***Have the patient wash hands with skin cleanser and warm water and dry thoroughly. Alternately, cleanse the skin with an alcohol swab. Allow skin to dry completely.***	
___	___	___	13. Choose a skin site that is intact, warm, and free of calluses and edema (Van Leeuwen & Bladh, 2017).	
___	___	___	14. Hold lancet perpendicular to skin and pierce skin with lancet.	

Excellent	Satisfactory	Needs Practice	SKILL 18-8 **Obtaining a Capillary Blood Sample for Glucose Testing** *(Continued)*	Comments
___	___	___	15. Encourage bleeding by lowering the hand, making use of gravity. Lightly stroke the finger, if necessary, until a sufficient amount of blood has formed to cover the sample area on the strip, based on monitor requirements (check instructions for monitor). Take care not to squeeze the finger, not to squeeze at puncture site, or not to touch puncture site or blood.	
___	___	___	16. Gently touch a drop of blood to the test strip without smearing it. Depending on meter in use, insert strip into meter after collection of sample on test strip.	
___	___	___	17. Apply pressure to puncture site with a cotton ball or dry gauze. ***Do not use alcohol wipe.***	
___	___	___	18. Read blood glucose results and document the results in EHR or other designated location, based on facility policy. Inform patient of test result.	
___	___	___	19. Turn off meter, remove test strip, and dispose of supplies appropriately. Place lancet in sharps container.	
___	___	___	20. Remove gloves and any other PPE, if used. Perform hand hygiene.	

Skill Checklists for Taylor's Clinical Nursing Skills. A Nursing Process Approach, 5th edition

Name ______________________ Date ______________

Unit ______________________ Position ______________

Instructor/Evaluator: ______________________ Position ______________

Excellent	Satisfactory	Needs Practice	SKILL 18-9 **Using Venipuncture to Collect a Venous Blood Sample** **Goal:** An uncontaminated specimen is obtained without injury to the patient and sent to the laboratory promptly.	**Comments**
____	____	____	1. Gather the necessary supplies. Check product expiration dates. Identify ordered tests and select the appropriate blood collection tubes.	
____	____	____	2. Perform hand hygiene and put on PPE, if indicated.	
____	____	____	3. Identify the patient.	
____	____	____	4. Explain the procedure to the patient. Allow the patient time to ask questions and verbalize concerns about the venipuncture procedure.	
____	____	____	5. Check the specimen label with the patient's identification bracelet. Label should include the patient's name and identification number, time specimen was collected, route of collection, identification of the person obtaining the sample, and any other information required by facility policy.	
____	____	____	6. Assemble equipment on overbed table or other surface within reach.	
____	____	____	7. Close curtains around the bed and close the door to the room, if possible.	
____	____	____	8. Provide for good light. Artificial light is recommended. Place a trash receptacle within easy reach.	
____	____	____	9. Assist the patient to a comfortable position, either sitting or lying. If the patient is lying in bed, raise the bed to a comfortable working height, usually elbow height of the caregiver (VHACEOSH, 2016).	
____	____	____	10. Determine the patient's preferred site for the procedure based on his or her previous experience. Expose the arm, supporting it in an extended position on a firm surface, such as a tabletop. Position self on the same side of the patient as the site selected. Apply a tourniquet to the upper arm on the chosen side approximately 3 to 4 in above the potential puncture site. Apply sufficient pressure to impede venous circulation but not arterial blood flow.	
____	____	____	11. Put on gloves. Assess the veins using inspection and palpation to determine the best puncture site.	

Excellent	Satisfactory	Needs Practice	SKILL 18-9 **Using Venipuncture to Collect a Venous Blood Sample** *(Continued)*	Comments
___	___	___	12. ***Release the tourniquet. Check that the vein has decompressed.***	
___	___	___	13. Attach the needle to the Vacutainer device. Place first blood collection tube into the Vacutainer, but not engaged in the puncture device in the Vacutainer.	
___	___	___	14. ***Clean the patient's skin at the selected puncture site with the antimicrobial swab. If using chlorhexidine, use a gentle back and forth motion for at least 30 seconds or use the procedure recommended by the manufacturer*** (INS, 2016a). ***If using alcohol, wipe in a circular motion spiraling outward. Allow the skin to dry before performing the venipuncture. Do not wipe or blot. Allow to dry completely.***	
___	___	___	15. Reapply the tourniquet approximately 3 to 4 in above the identified puncture site. Apply sufficient pressure to impede venous circulation but not arterial blood flow. ***After disinfection, do not palpate the venipuncture site unless sterile gloves are worn.***	
___	___	___	16. Hold the patient's arm in a downward position with your nondominant hand. Align the needle and Vacutainer device with the chosen vein, holding the Vacutainer and needle in your dominant hand. Use the thumb or first finger of your nondominant hand to apply pressure and traction to the skin about 1 to 2 in below the identified puncture site (Van Leeuwen & Bladh, 2017).	
___	___	___	17. ***Inform the patient that he or she is going to feel a pinch.*** With the bevel of the needle up, insert the needle into the vein at a 15 to 30 degree angle to the skin (Van Leeuwen & Bladh, 2017).	
___	___	___	18. Grasp the Vacutainer securely to stabilize it in the vein with your nondominant hand, and push the first collection tube into the puncture device in the Vacutainer, until the rubber stopper on the collection tube is punctured. You will feel the tube push into place on the puncture device. Blood will flow into the tube automatically.	
___	___	___	19. ***Remove the tourniquet as soon as blood flows adequately into the tube.***	
___	___	___	20. Continue to hold the Vacutainer in place in the vein and continue to fill the required tubes, removing one and inserting another. Gently rotate each tube as you remove it.	

Excellent	Satisfactory	Needs Practice	SKILL 18-9 **Using Venipuncture to Collect a Venous Blood Sample** *(Continued)*	Comments
___	___	___	21. After you have drawn all required blood samples, remove the last collection tube from the Vacutainer. ***Place a gauze pad over the puncture site and slowly and gently remove the needle from the vein. Engage needle guard. Do not apply pressure to the site until the needle has been fully removed.***	
___	___	___	22. Apply gentle pressure to the puncture site for 2 to 3 minutes or until bleeding stops.	
___	___	___	23. After bleeding stops, apply an adhesive bandage.	
___	___	___	24. Remove equipment and return the patient to a position of comfort. Raise side rail and lower bed.	
___	___	___	25. Discard Vacutainer and needle in sharps container.	
___	___	___	26. Remove gloves and perform hand hygiene.	
___	___	___	27. Place label on the container per facility policy. Place container in plastic, sealable biohazard bag.	
___	___	___	28. Check the venipuncture site to see if a hematoma has developed.	
___	___	___	29. Remove other PPE, if used. Perform hand hygiene.	
___	___	___	30. Transport the specimen to the laboratory immediately. If immediate transport is not possible, check with laboratory personnel or policy manual whether refrigeration is contraindicated.	

Skill Checklists for Taylor's Clinical Nursing Skills. A Nursing Process Approach, 5th edition

Name ______________________ Date ______________________

Unit ______________________ Position ______________________

Instructor/Evaluator: ______________________ Position ______________________

SKILL 18-10

Obtaining a Venous Blood Specimen for Culture and Sensitivity

Excellent	Satisfactory	Needs Practice	**Goal:** An uncontaminated specimen is obtained without injury to the patient and sent to the laboratory promptly.	Comments
___	___	___	1. Gather the necessary supplies. Check product expiration dates. Identify ordered number of blood culture sets and select the appropriate blood collection bottles (at least one anaerobic and one aerobic bottle). ***If tests are ordered in addition to the blood cultures, collect the blood culture specimens before other specimens.***	
___	___	___	2. Perform hand hygiene and put on PPE, if indicated.	
___	___	___	3. Identify the patient.	
___	___	___	4. Explain the procedure. Allow the patient time to ask questions and verbalize concerns about the venipuncture procedure.	
___	___	___	5. Check specimen label with the patient's identification bracelet. Label should include the patient's name and identification number, time specimen was collected, route of collection, identification of person obtaining the sample, and any other information required by facility policy.	
___	___	___	6. Assemble equipment on overbed table or other surface within reach.	
___	___	___	7. Close curtains around the bed and close the door to the room, if possible.	
___	___	___	8. Provide for good light. Artificial light is recommended. Place a trash receptacle within easy reach.	
___	___	___	9. Assist the patient to a comfortable position, either sitting or lying. If the patient is lying in bed, raise the bed to a comfortable working height, usually elbow height of the caregiver (VHACEOSH, 2016).	
___	___	___	10. Determine the patient's preferred site for the procedure based on his or her previous experience. Expose the arm, supporting it in an extended position on a firm surface, such as a tabletop. Position self on the same side of the patient as the site selected. Apply a tourniquet to the upper arm on the chosen side approximately 3 to 4 in above the potential puncture site. Apply sufficient pressure to impede venous circulation, but not arterial blood flow.	

Excellent	Satisfactory	Needs Practice	SKILL 18-10 **Obtaining a Venous Blood Specimen for Culture and Sensitivity** *(Continued)*	Comments
___	___	___	11. Put on nonsterile gloves. Assess the veins using inspection and palpation to determine the best puncture site.	
___	___	___	12. ***Release the tourniquet. Check that the vein has decompressed.***	
___	___	___	13. Attach the butterfly needle extension tubing to the Vacutainer device.	
___	___	___	14. Move collection bottles to a location close to the arm.	
___	___	___	15. ***Clean the patient's skin at the selected puncture site with the antimicrobial swab, according to facility policy. If using chlorhexidine, use a gentle back and forth motion for at least 30 seconds or use the procedure recommended by the manufacturer (INS, 2016a). Allow the skin to dry before performing the venipuncture. Do not wipe or blot. Allow to dry completely.***	
___	___	___	16. Using a new antimicrobial swab, clean the stoppers of the culture bottles with the appropriate antimicrobial, per facility policy. Cover bottle top with sterile gauze square, based on facility policy.	
___	___	___	17. Reapply the tourniquet approximately 3 to 4 in above the identified puncture site. Apply sufficient pressure to impede venous circulation, but not arterial blood flow. ***After disinfection, do not palpate the venipuncture site unless sterile gloves are worn.***	
___	___	___	18. Hold the patient's arm in a downward position with your nondominant hand. Align the butterfly needle with the chosen vein, holding the needle in your dominant hand. Use the thumb or first finger of your nondominant hand to apply pressure and traction to the skin about 1 to 2 in below the identified puncture site (Van Leeuwen & Bladh, 2017). ***Do not touch the insertion site.***	
___	___	___	19. ***Inform the patient that he or she is going to feel a pinch.*** With the bevel of the needle up, insert the needle into the vein at a 15 to 30 degree angle to the skin (Malarkey & McMorrow, 2012; Van Leeuwen & Bladh, 2017). You should see a flash of blood in the extension tubing close to the needle when the vein is entered.	

SKILL 18-10

Obtaining a Venous Blood Specimen for Culture and Sensitivity *(Continued)*

Excellent	Satisfactory	Needs Practice		Comments
___	___	___	20. ***Keeping the specimen bottle upright,*** fill the aerobic bottle first (Fischbach & Dunning, 2015; Laboratory Alliance of Central New York, LLC, 2017; Van Leeuwen & Bladh, 2017). Grasp the butterfly needle securely to stabilize it in the vein with your nondominant hand, and push the Vacutainer onto the first collection bottle (aerobic bottle), until the rubber stopper on the collection bottle is punctured. You will feel the bottle push into place on the puncture device. Blood will flow into the bottle automatically. Fill to the level indicated on the bottle; do not overfill (Fischbach & Dunning, 2015).	
___	___	___	21. ***Remove the tourniquet as soon as blood flows adequately into the bottle.***	
___	___	___	22. Continue to hold the butterfly needle in place in the vein. Once the first bottle is filled, remove it from the Vacutainer and insert the second bottle. After the blood culture specimens are obtained, continue to fill any additional required tubes, removing one and inserting another. Gently rotate each bottle and tube as you remove it.	
___	___	___	23. After you have drawn all required blood samples, remove the last collection tube from the Vacutainer. ***Place a gauze pad over the puncture site and slowly and gently remove the needle from the vein. Engage needle guard. Do not apply pressure to the site until the needle has been fully removed.***	
___	___	___	24. Apply gentle pressure to the puncture site for 2 to 3 minutes or until bleeding stops.	
___	___	___	25. After bleeding stops, apply an adhesive bandage.	
___	___	___	26. Remove equipment and return patient to a position of comfort. Raise side rails and lower bed.	
___	___	___	27. Discard Vacutainer and butterfly needle in sharps container.	
___	___	___	28. Remove gloves and perform hand hygiene.	
___	___	___	29. Place label on the container, per facility policy. Place containers in plastic, sealable biohazard bag. Refer to facility policy regarding the need for separate biohazard bags for blood culture specimens and other blood specimens.	
___	___	___	30. Check the venipuncture sites to see if a hematoma has developed.	
___	___	___	31. Remove other PPE, if used. Perform hand hygiene.	
___	___	___	32. Transport the specimen to the laboratory immediately. If immediate transport is not possible, check with laboratory personnel or policy manual as to appropriate handling.	

Skill Checklists for Taylor's Clinical Nursing Skills. A Nursing Process Approach, 5th edition

Name ______________________ Date ______________________

Unit ______________________ Position ______________________

Instructor/Evaluator: ______________________ Position ______________________

SKILL 18-11

Obtaining an Arterial Blood Specimen for Blood Gas Analysis

Goal: An uncontaminated specimen is obtained without injury to the patient or damage to the artery and sent to the laboratory promptly.

Excellent	Satisfactory	Needs Practice		Comments
___	___	___	1. Gather the necessary supplies. Check product expiration dates. Identify ordered arterial blood gas analysis. Check the chart to make sure the patient has not been suctioned within the past 20 to 30 minutes. Check facility policy and/or procedure for guidelines on administering local anesthesia for arterial punctures. Administer anesthetic and allow sufficient time for full effect before beginning procedure.	
___	___	___	2. Perform hand hygiene and put on PPE, if indicated.	
___	___	___	3. Identify the patient.	
___	___	___	4. Explain the procedure to the patient. Tell the patient you need to collect an arterial blood sample and the needlestick will cause some discomfort but that he or she must remain still during the procedure.	
___	___	___	5. Check specimen label with the patient's identification bracelet. Label should include patient's name and identification number, time specimen was collected, route of collection, identification of person obtaining the sample, amount of oxygen the patient is receiving, type of oxygen administration device, patient's body temperature, and any other information required by facility policy.	
___	___	___	6. Assemble equipment on overbed table or other surface within reach.	
___	___	___	7. Close curtains around the bed and close the door to the room, if possible.	
___	___	___	8. Provide for good light. Artificial light is recommended. Place a trash receptacle within easy reach.	
___	___	___	9. If the patient is on bed rest, ask him or her to lie in a supine position, with the head slightly elevated and the arms at the sides. Ask an ambulatory patient to sit in a chair and support the arm securely on an armrest or a table. Place a waterproof pad under the site and a rolled towel under the wrist.	

Excellent	Satisfactory	Needs Practice	SKILL 18-11 **Obtaining an Arterial Blood Specimen for Blood Gas Analysis** *(Continued)*	Comments
___	___	___	10. ***Perform Allen's test before obtaining a specimen from the radial artery.***	
___	___	___	a. Have the patient clench the fist to minimize blood flow into the hand.	
___	___	___	b. Using your index and middle fingers, press on the radial and ulnar arteries. Hold this position for a few seconds.	
___	___	___	c. Without removing your fingers from the arteries, ask the patient to unclench the fist and hold the hand in a relaxed position. The palm will be blanched because pressure from your fingers has impaired the normal blood flow.	
___	___	___	d. Release pressure on the ulnar artery. If the hand becomes flushed, which indicates that blood is filling the vessels, it is safe to proceed with the radial artery puncture. This is considered a positive test. If the hand does not flush, perform the test on the other arm.	
___	___	___	11. Put on nonsterile gloves. Locate the radial artery and lightly palpate it for a strong pulse.	
___	___	___	12. ***Clean the patient's skin at the puncture site with the antimicrobial swab, according to facility policy. If using chlorhexidine, use a gentle back and forth motion for at least 30 seconds or use the procedure recommended by the manufacturer*** (INS, 2016a). ***Do not wipe or blot. Allow to dry completely. After disinfection, do not palpate the site unless sterile gloves are worn.***	
___	___	___	13. Stabilize the hand with the wrist extended over the rolled towel, palm up. Palpate the artery above the puncture site with the index and middle fingers of your nondominant hand while holding the syringe over the puncture site with your dominant hand. ***Do not directly touch the area to be punctured.***	
___	___	___	14. Hold the needle bevel up at a 45- to 60-degree angle at the site of maximal pulse impulse, with the shaft parallel to the path of the artery.	
___	___	___	15. ***Inform the patient that he or she is going to feel a pinch.*** Puncture the skin and arterial wall in one motion. Watch for blood backflow in the syringe. Pulsating blood will flow into the syringe. Do not pull back on the plunger. Collect 2 to 3 mL (Hess et al., 2016).	

Excellent	Satisfactory	Needs Practice	SKILL 18-11 **Obtaining an Arterial Blood Specimen for Blood Gas Analysis** *(Continued)*	Comments
___	___	___	16. After collecting the sample, withdraw the syringe while your nondominant hand is beginning to place pressure proximal to the insertion site with the 2 × 2 gauze. ***Press a gauze pad firmly over the puncture site until the bleeding stops—at least 5 minutes. If the patient is receiving anticoagulant therapy or has a blood dyscrasia, apply pressure for 10 to 15 minutes; if necessary, ask a coworker to hold the gauze pad in place while you prepare the sample for transport to the laboratory, but do not ask the patient to hold the pad.***	
___	___	___	17. When the bleeding stops and the appropriate time has lapsed, apply a small adhesive bandage or small pressure dressing (fold a 2 × 2 gauze into fourths and firmly apply tape, stretching the skin tight).	
___	___	___	18. Once the sample is obtained, check the syringe for air bubbles. If any appear, remove them by holding the syringe upright and slowly ejecting some of the blood onto a 2 × 2 gauze pad.	
___	___	___	19. Engage the needle guard and remove the needle. Place the airtight cap on the syringe. Gently rotate the syringe. Do not shake.	
___	___	___	20. Place label on the syringe per facility policy. Place syringe in plastic, sealable biohazard bag. Insert the syringe into a cup or bag of ice water.	
___	___	___	21. Remove equipment and return the patient to a position of comfort. Raise side rail and lower bed.	
___	___	___	22. Discard the needle in sharps container. Remove gloves and perform hand hygiene.	
___	___	___	23. Check the puncture site for bleeding and to see if a hematoma has developed.	
___	___	___	24. Remove other PPE, if used. Perform hand hygiene.	
___	___	___	25. Transport the specimen to the laboratory immediately.	